Inflammatory Bowel Disease: A Clinical Case Approach to Pathophysiology, Diagnosis, and Treatment

FALK SYMPOSIUM 122

Inflammatory Bowel Disease: A Clinical Case Approach to Pathophysiology, Diagnosis, and Treatment

Edited by

M. Campieri
Dipartimento di Medicina Interna
e Gastroenterologia
Policlinico S. Orsola
Bologna, Italy

C. Fiocchi
Case Western Reserve University
School of Medicine (BRB)
Gastroenterology Division
Cleveland, OH, USA

S.B. Hanauer
University of Chicago
Pritzker School of Medicine
Gastroenterology Section
Chicago, IL, USA

D.P. Jewell
Gastroenterology Unit
The Radcliffe Infirmary
University of Oxford
Oxford, UK

D. Rachmilewitz
Division of Medicine
Shaare Zedek Medical Center
Jerusalem, Israel

J. Schölmerich
Klinik und Poliklinik für Innere
Medizin I
Klinikum der Universität
Regensburg
Regensburg, Germany

Proceedings of Falk Symposium 122 held in Bologna, Italy, June 22–23, 2001

KLUWER ACADEMIC PUBLISHERS
DORDRECHT / BOSTON / LONDON

Library of Congress Cataloging-in-Publication Data is available.

ISBN 0–7923–8772–4

Published by Kluwer Academic Publishers, BV
P.O. Box 17, 3300 AA Dordrecht, The Netherlands.

Sold and distributed in North, Central and South America
by Kluwer Academic Publishers,
101 Philip Drive, Norwell, MA 02061, USA.

In all other countries, sold and distributed
by Kluwer Academic Publishers, Distribution Center,
P.O. Box 322, 3300 AH Dordrecht, The Netherlands.

Printed on acid-free paper

Printed and bound in Great Britain by MPG Books, Bodmin, Cornwall.

Contents

SECTION VII: MISCELLANEOUS TOPICS

SECTION VIII: COMPLICATIONS OF ILEAL-POUCH ANASTOMOSIS

List of principal authors

V Annese
Division of Gastroenterology and Endoscopy "C.S.S.-IRCCS" Hospital
I-71013 San Giovanni Rotondo (FG)
Italy

HA Büller
Sophia Children's Hospital
Department of Pediatrics
Dr. Molewaterplein 60
NL-3015 GJ Rotterdam
The Netherlands

M Campieri
Dipartimento di Medicina Interna
e Gastroenterologia
Policlinico S. Orsola
Via Massarenti 9
I-40138 Bologna
Italy

R Caprilli
Dipartimento di Scienze Cliniche
Cattedra di Gastroenterologia I
Università "La Sapienza" di Roma
Policlinico Umberto I
Viale del Policlinico
I-00161 Roma
Italy

SM Collins
McMaster University Medical Centre
Division of Gastroenterology, R-4W8
1200 Main Street West
Hamilton
Ontario L8N 3Z5
Canada

J-F Colombel
Clinique des Maladies de l'Appareil Digestif et de la Nutrition
Hôpital Huriez
CHRU Lille
F-59037 Lille
France

S Cucchiara
Department of Pediatric Gastroenterology
University of Rome "La Sapienza"
Viale Regina Elena 324
I-00161 Rome
Italy

G D'Haens
Imelda Ziekenhuis
Radiologie
Imeldalaan 9
B-2820 Bonheiden
Belgium

MC Dubinsky
Cedars-Sinai IBD Center
8631 West Third Street
Suite 245E
Los Angeles, CA 90048
USA

A Ekbom
Department of Medical Epidemiology
Karolinska Institutet
PO Box 281
S-17177 Stockholm
Sweden

VW Fazio
Department of Colorectal Surgery
Cleveland Clinic Foundation
9500 Euclid Avenue
Cleveland, OH 44195-5044
USA

RN Fedorak
University of Alberta
Division of Gastroenterology
519 Robert Newton Research Building
Edmonton
Alberta T5G 2C2
Canada

C Fiocchi
Case Western Reserve University
School of Medicine (BRB)
Gastroenterology Division
10900 Euclid Avenue
Cleveland, OH 44106-4952
USA

MA Gassull
Department of Gastroenterology
Hospital Universitari Germans Trias i Pujol
Carretera del Canyet s/u
E-08916 Badalona
Catalunya
Spain

K Geboes
Laboratory for Histo- & Cytochemie
University Hospital St. Rafael
Minderbroedersstraat 12
B-3000 Leuven
Belgium

P Gionchetti
Dipartimento di Medicina Interna
Università di Bologna
Policlinico S. Orsola
Via Massarenti, 9
I-40138 Bologna
Italy

SB Hanauer
University of Chicago
Department of Medicine
Gastroenterology Section
5758 S. Maryland Avenue
Chicago, IL 60637-1463
USA

H Herfarth
Klinik und Poliklinik für Innere Medizin I
Klinikum der Universität Regensburg
D-93042 Regensburg
Germany

DP Jewell
Gastroenterology Unit
University of Oxford, Nuffield Department of Medicine
Gibson Laboratories, 2nd Floor
Radcliffe Infirmary, Block 21
Woodstock Rd
Oxford, OX2 6HE, UK

MA Kamm
St Mark's Hospital
Northwick Park
Watford Road
Harrow
Middlesex HA1 3UJ
UK

JA Katz
Case Western Reserve University School of Medicine
Division of Gastroenterology
11100 Euclid Avenue
Cleveland, OH 44106-5066
USA

JF Markowitz
North Shore University Hospital
Division of Pediatric GI/Nutrition
300 Community Drive
Manhasset, NY 11030-3801
USA

RS McLeod
Mount Sinai Hospital
University of Toronto
600 University Ave., Rm 449
Toronto, Ontario M5G 1X5
Canada

SGM Meuwissen
Department of Gastroenterology
Free University Hospital
de Boelelaan 1117
P.O. Box 7057
NL-1007 MB Amsterdam
The Netherlands

M Parkes
Gastroenterology Unit
The Radcliffe Infirmary
Woodstock Road
Oxford OX2 6HE
UK

A Pera
Unità Operativa Autonoma di Gastroenterologia
Ospedale Mauriziano Umberto I
Largo Turati, 62
I-10128 Torino
Italy

DK Podolsky
Gastrointestinal Unit
Center for the Study of Inflammatory Bowel Diseases
Harvard School
Massachusetts General Hospital
55 Fruit Street, GRJ 719
Boston, MA 02114-2696
USA

G Poggioli
Department of Clinical Surgery
University of Bologna
Policlinico S. Orsola
Via Massarenti, 9
I-40138 Bologna
Italy

C Prantera
Divisione di Gastroenterologia
Azienda Ospedaliera S. Camillo Forlanini
Via Portuense, 292
I-00149 Roma
Italy

DH Present
Mount Sinai Medical Center
12 East 86th Street
New York, NY 10028
USA

D Rachmilewitz
Division of Medicine
Shaare Zedek Medical Center
P.O. Box 3235
91031 Jerusalem
Israel

JM Rhodes
Department of Medicine
University of Liverpool
Liverpool
L69 3GA
UK

G Riegler
Seconda Università di Napoli
Dipartimento "F. Magrassi"
Via Vincenzo Mosca, 39
I-80129 Napoli
Italy

G Rogler
Cellular and Molecular Medicine
University of California at San Diego UCSD
9500 Gilman Drive
La Jolla, CA 92093-0651
USA

DB Sachar
Division of Gastroenterology
The Mount Sinai Medical Center
Box 1069
One Gustave L. Levy Place
New York, NY 10029-6574
USA

WJ Sandborn
E19B
Division of Gastroenterology and Hepatology
Mayo Clinic
200 First Street SW
Rochester, MN 55905
USA

J Schölmerich
Klinik und Poliklinik für Innere Medizin I
Klinikum der Universität Regensburg
D-93042 Regensburg
Germany

EF Stange
Zentrum für Innere Medizin I
Robert Bosch Krankenhaus
Auerbachstr. 110
D-70276 Stuttgart
Germany

GC Sturniolo
Dipartimento di Scienze Chirurgiche e Gastroenterologiche
Policlinico Universitario
Via Giustiniani, 2
I-35127 Padova
Italy

LR Sutherland
Department of Community Health Sciences
The University of Calgary
3330 Hospital Drive N.W.
Calgary, Alberta T2N 4N1
Canada

SJH van Deventer
Department of Gastroenterology
Academic Medical Center
University of Amsterdam
Meibergdreef 9
NL-1105 AZ Amsterdam
The Netherlands

M Vecchi
Department of Internal Medicine
IRCCS Ospedale Policlinico
University of Milan
Via della Pace, 9
I-20122 Milan
Italy

M Zeitz
Department of Medicine I
Benjamin Franklin Medical School
Free University Berlin
Hindenburgdamm 30
D-12200 Berlin
Germany

G Zoli
Ospedale SS. Annunziata
Via Vicini 2
I-44042 Cento (FE)
Italy

Section I
Genetics of IBD

1
Genetics of IBD – case presentation

V. ANNESE and A. ANDRIULLI

Interest in the genetic predisposition to inflammatory bowel disease (IBD) has increased progressively since its familial occurrence was brought to our attention by Kirsner *et al.*[1]. Between 6% and 32% of patients with IBD have an affected first- or second-degree relative[2]. The prevalence of a family history is highest in Jewish patients and in patients with early onset of disease. This finding might suggest a greater contribution of genetic predisposition in patients with early onset of disease. This hypothesis has been recently supported by the demonstration of stronger linkage on chromosomes 1, 3, 12 and 16 in families with at least one member with early onset of IBD (less than 20 years)[3,4]. The familial component of the disease, which documents its heritability, provides the opportunity to use genetic technology in the search for causative factors to dissect the possible molecular causes.

Along the effort for a genome-wide search, 186 families with two or more affected members have been identified in 20 different General and University Hospitals in Italy. The main characteristics of these families are summarized in Table 1.

The majority of families identified are sib pairs with two affected members with the same proportion of CD and UC families; however, in 20% of families, both CD and UC were reported in different members (mixed families).

Here we describe two families with peculiar clinical characteristics.

Table 1 Characteristics of IBD families collected in a multicentre Italian study

	Crohn's disease	*Ulcerative colitis*	*Mixed*	*Total*
Sib pairs	18	52	41	111
Affected members	13	27	35	75
2 affected	27	72	64	163
3 affected	4	6	8	18
4 affected	—	1	1	2

CASE REPORT 1

G.M. at the age of 22 years in 1984 started to complain of abdominal pain, intermittent diarrhoea, and weight loss. She was the oldest of a large family with 14 children (Figure 1). The main laboratory values were: ESR 45, CRP × 3, Hb 11.9 and albumin 3.1g/L. A colonoscopy was performed with demonstration of aftoid erosions of the right colon and caecum, and ulcers of the caecal valve. The histology showed a patchy chronic inflammation extending into the submucosa. No granulomas or crypt abscess were found. A small bowel follow-through showed mucosal nodularity and areas of cobblestoning of the distal ileum in the last 20–30 cm. A diagnosis of Crohn's ileocolitis was established and the total CDAI was calculated as 210. The symptoms were successfully controlled by sulphasalazine therapy. She was married and had a 2-year-old daughter. All sibs and relatives were in good health and so also were the grandfathers and grandmothers, with the exception of the paternal grandmother who had died at the age of 78 years from breast cancer. At that time, no other intestinal complaints were recorded in the family. The father was a farmer but all the family members lived in an urban community in a large house. The economic situation was rather low but the domestic hygiene very accurate.

Subsequently, in 1992, 1993 and 1995, three other sibs had a diagnosis of Crohn's disease established. All four members of this family had ileocolonic localization; three of them also had perianal fistulas, and two articolar manifestations. In two subjects, perianal fistulas were resistant to azathioprine and metronidazole; therapy with Remicade was started with healing of fistulas, but with relapse 2–3 months later. In the last 2 years, three additional members of the family have been referred with abdominal pain and occasional rectal bleeding, but so far, have refused any investigations. The family was evaluated in more detail (Figure 2). The family includes 1 proband, 3 affected sibs, and 3 sibs with gastrointestinal symptoms which might be due to IBD. All IBD has occurred in the same generation. There are, however, 7 sibs, 19 nephews, 10 spouses, 2 relatives, 4 grandparents, 5 uncles, and 37 cousins with no symptoms of IBD.

We also looked at some subclinical markers in this particular family, namely the presence of ANCA (antineutrophil cytoplasmic antibodies) and ASCA (anti-*Saccharomyces cerevisiae* antibodies) (Figure 3). ANCA were absent in all members and ASCA were found in the father of proband and the majority of

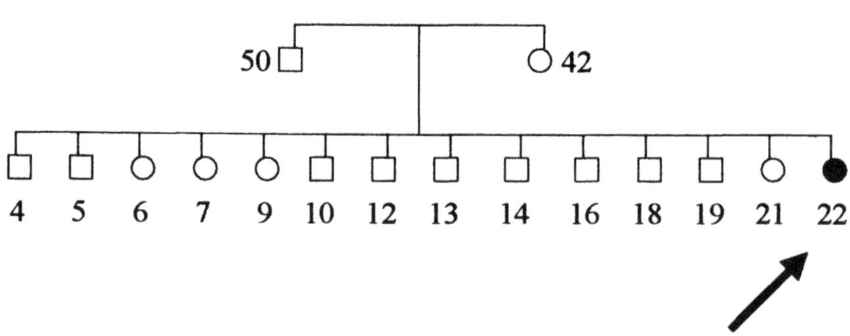

Figure 1 Pedigree of the proband (arrow) of Case report 1 in 1984

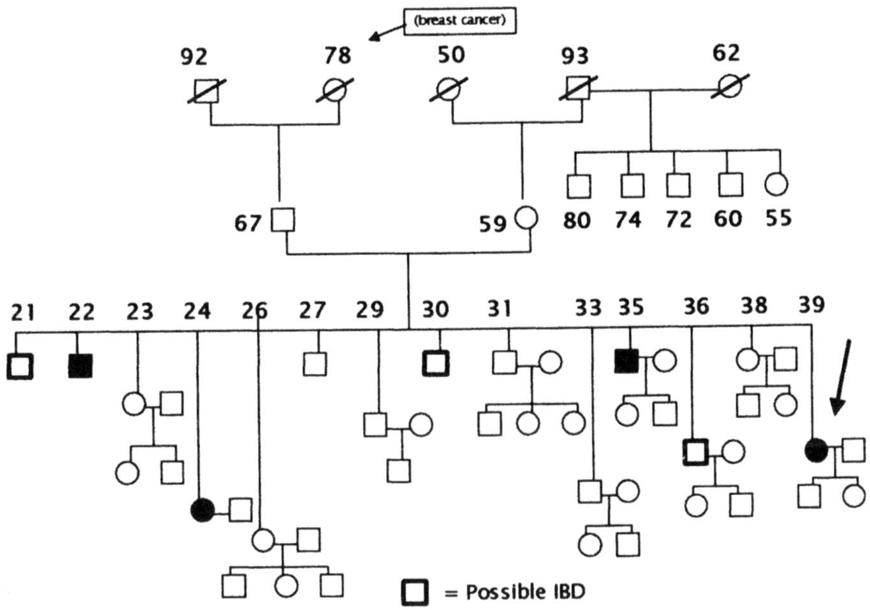

Figure 2 Pedigree of proband of Case report 1 in 2001

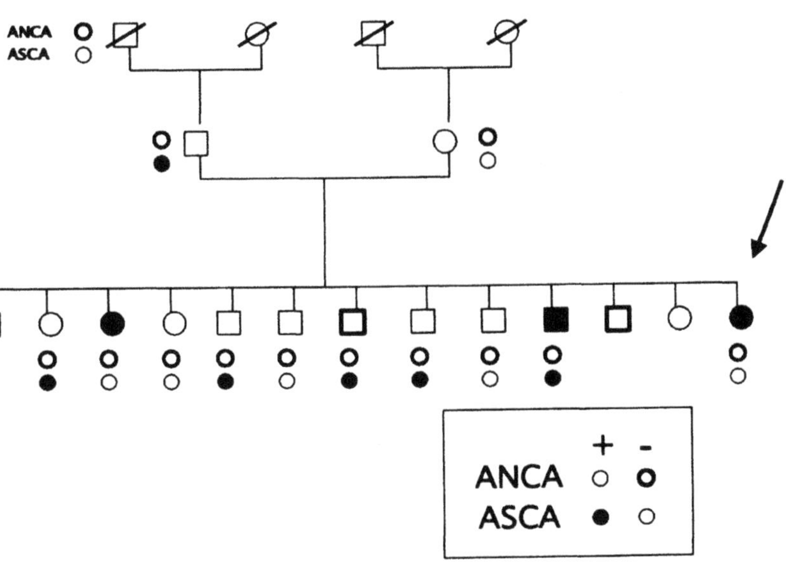

Figure 3 Presence of ANCA and ASCA within the pedigree of Case report 1

offspring. Interestingly, ASCA were found in two of the four affected members and all those members with suspected IBD. It will be interesting to investigate in the future whether the members unaffected by the presence of ASCA carry a greater risk of developing the disease.

CASE REPORT 2

P.R. and P.A. are monozygotic twins. Their family history was negative, except for type I diabetes in the grandmother. The past history was not relevant: they were both housewives with healthy children. They both had had a measles infection in childhood and had used estroprogestins. No symptoms were reported up to the age of 30 years.

P.R., in May 1990 at the age of 30 years, complained of an episode of severe abdominal pain, vomiting and abdominal distension. Subsequently, since January of 1992 she has had recurring episodes of crampy abdominal pain. In May 1992, a double-contrast barium enema showed a deformation and stiffness of the caecum, a granular surface of the transverse colon, and narrowing of the terminal ileum. A further small bowel follow-through confirmed a 10-cm narrowing of the terminal ileum with a 5-mm-wide lumen. At ultrasonography, a 7-mm thickness of terminal ileum wall and 5-mm thickness of the right colon wall was found. The upper GI endoscopy was negative. A diagnosis of Crohn's disease was established.

P.A. started to complain of nausea, vomiting, and sideropenic anaemia in February 1992. In January 1993, she had a small-bowel enema, which showed a 3-cm-long narrowing of the terminal ileum with a dilated loop and stiffness of the caecum. Ultrasonography showed an 8-mm thickness of terminal ileum wall. At colonoscopy, mucosal lesions were found throughout the colon with rectal sparing. The histology confirmed the features of Crohn's disease.

The clinical history of these two twins was remarkably similar. They were both poorly compliant to medical management and therapy and reported recurring episodes of subocclusions. Curiously, they were operated on in November 1994 on the same day by the same surgeon with a similar resection of terminal ileum and right colon. So far, they have not reported any clinical relapse; however, an anastomotic relapse has been found at endoscopy and ultrasonography.

References

1. Kirsner J, Spencer J. Familial occurrences of ulcerative colitis, regional enteritis and ileocolitis. Ann Intern Med. 1963;59:133–4.
2. Ahmad T, Satsangi J, McGovern D, Bunce M, Jewell DP. Review article: the genetics of inflammatory bowel disease. Aliment Ther Pharmacol. 2001;15:731–48.
3. Brant S, LaBuda M, Lee S *et al.* Younger age at diagnosis identifies families with greater linkage evidence for IBD1 loci on chromosome 1p, 3q, and 16. Gastroenterology 1999;166: A673 (abstract).
4. Van Heel D, Satsangi J, Carey A, Jewell D. Chromosome 12 linkage for IBD is greater in families identified by early age at diagnosis. Gut 2000; 46(Suppl 11): A6 (abstract).

2
Intestinal permeability in Crohn's disease: genetic, environmental, or inflammatory?

J. A. KATZ

INTRODUCTION

Intestinal permeability refers to the barrier function of the intestine that prevents potentially harmful substances from penetrating the mucosa and reaching the internal environment of the body[1]. The physiology and pathophysiology of the intestinal permeability barrier remains incompletely understood, but includes the mucous layer, the brush border cell membrane, paracellular tight junctions, immune defences, mesenteric lymph nodes, and the reticuloendothelial system in the liver and spleen[2]. Crohn's disease (CD) is associated with increased intestinal permeability[3,4], a phenomenon that may play a role in the pathophysiology of the disease[5]. One hypothesis is that increased permeability allows increased antigen trafficking across the mucosa, with subsequent increased stimulation of the gut immune system, leading eventually to tissue damage and the symptoms of CD. However, it remains unclear whether increased intestinal permeability is a primary inherited defect, and therefore critical in the induction of inflammation, or is a secondary acquired abnormality, caused by pre-existing but subclinical inflammation[2,5].

Despite nearly two decades of research, it remains uncertain whether changes in intestinal permeability are inherited primary or acquired secondary phenomena. Studies in mice with a genetically engineered abnormal intestinal barrier function have documented inflammatory changes by 6 weeks of age[6]. This provides direct support for the idea that abnormal intestinal permeability can be genetically predetermined and an early event in the development of inflammatory bowel disease (IBD) in animal models. On the other hand, some animal models show that abnormal barrier function is a result of inflammation and improves with treatment[7].

The identification 15 years ago of increased intestinal permeability in a subset of first-degree relatives of patients with CD first suggested a genetic link between abnormal permeability and human IBD[4]. This finding has been supported by a number of subsequent studies[4,8–12], although not all studies have confirmed abnormal permeability in relatives of CD patients[13–16]. Importantly, none of the studies of first-degree relatives of CD patients has included a careful systematic search for occult intestinal inflammation. This paper will review the data on intestinal permeability and its role in CD and also present new data on permeability and subclinical gut inflammation.

INTESTINAL PERMEABILITY IN CROHN'S DISEASE PATIENTS

Early permeability studies in IBD have shown abnormally high intestinal permeability in some, but not all, patients with CD[9,17]. This fact alone makes it significantly less likely that genetically predetermined abnormalities in intestinal barrier function are a primary aetiological factor in all patients with CD. Rather, most data in CD patients show a close correlation between intestinal permeability and inflammation. Abnormal permeability improves after treatment of active CD with an elemental diet or corticosteroids[18,19]. Changes in permeability occurr in parallel with an improvement in measures of clinical disease activity. In over half of these CD patients, intestinal permeability fell to the normal range[19]. More recently, probiotic therapy has restored normal barrier function in an animal model of IBD[7], and therapy with infliximab, a chimeric monoclonal antibody to tumour necrosis factor α (TNF-α) restored normal gut permeability[20].

In prospective follow-up studies of CD patients in clinical remission, increases in intestinal permeability have been closely correlated with risk of clinical relapse[21,22]. Among 72 patients with quiescent CD (defined as a CDAI < 150) for at least 6 months, 26/37 patients with raised baseline permeability relapsed within 1 year compared with 6/35 patients with normal permeability at baseline ($p < 0.001$)[22]. Logistic regression analysis showed a significant correlation between the lactulose–mannitol ratio and the probability of relapse. There was no association between permeability, the location of CD, and relapse. A 2-year study of 130 CD patients in remission for a mean of 13 months also reported a significant correlation between elevated permeability at baseline and risk of relapse in the following 4 months. The relative risk of relapse in CD patients with elevated permeability was 4.4 (95% CI 1.55–12.51; $p < 0.05$)[21]. Similar results have been found using permeability studies to predict clinical relapse after surgical induction of remission[23]. None of these studies evaluated the endoscopic or histological integrity of the bowel at the time of permeability testing. However, faecal calprotectin, a stable calcium-binding protein found in granulocytes and used as an objective and quantitative marker of inflammation, has been correlated with permeability abnormalities and disease relapse in CD[24]. These data suggest that permeability abnormalities in CD are secondary to gut inflammation.

Although elevated permeability in CD patients may be a surrogate marker for mucosal inflammation below the threshold of clinical symptoms, it still remains possible that in CD a defect in gut barrier function is a primary genetically predetermined defect. Abnormal intestinal permeability has been reported in radiographically normal small bowel in CD patients, suggesting that the permeability defect could exist independently of intestinal inflammation[25]. This clinical finding is supported by *in-vitro* data, documenting increased epithelial permeability to ovalbumin in macroscopically and microscopically non-inflamed ileal mucosa from patients with CD[26]. Although long-term longitudinal follow-up studies of serial permeability measurements in persons at risk for CD do not exist, a recent case report highlights the potential significance of permeability abnormalities predating the later development of CD. In this report, a young woman with a strong family history of CD was documented to have abnormal intestinal permeability 8 years prior to a subsequent diagnosis of CD[27]. Extensive evaluation performed immediately after identification of the permeability abnormality, including radiographic and endoscopic studies, failed to show any evidence of gut inflammation. Although an isolated case, this report supports the concept of a permeability defect playing an early role in the pathogenesis of CD.

INTESTINAL PERMEABILITY IN FIRST-DEGREE RELATIVES AND SPOUSES OF CROHN'S DISEASE PATIENTS

Relatives of CD patients have a greater risk of developing CD. However, there exists, at present, no means of identifying precisely which healthy relatives are likely to develop symptomatic CD. In 1986, Hollander and colleagues demonstrated an increased intestinal permeability to PEG 400 in asymptomatic relatives of CD patients[4]. These investigators suggested that increased intestinal permeability might be an inherited pathophysiologically important subclinical marker of CD. The number of subjects studied by Hollander *et al.* was small and the techniques for measuring urinary PEG 400 concentrations complex, raising questions about the broad applicability of their findings. When further studies examining larger groups of relatives and using several different permeability probes were performed, no statistically significant differences in permeability between the relatives of CD patients and healthy control subjects could be found[14,15,28] (Table 1).

Recently, however, May *et al.* have critically re-evaluated the issue of increased intestinal permeability in healthy relatives of CD patients[11]. These investigators argued that, if approximately 10% of these relatives are statistically likely to

Table 1 Permeability studies in relatives and spouses of patients with Crohn's disease

Elevated in relatives	*Normal in relatives*	*Elevated in spouses*
Hollander *et al.*[4]	Teahon *et al.*[14]	Peeters *et al.*[13]
Katz *et al.*[16]	Ruttenberg *et al.*[28]	Breslin *et al.*[30]
Valpiani *et al.*[51]	Munkholm *et al.*[15]	Söderholm *et al.*[31]*
Pironi *et al.*[29]		
Ainsworth *et al.*[52]		
May *et al.*[11]		
Hilsden *et al.*[10]*		
Peeters *et al.*[13]		
Söderholm *et al.*[31]*		

*Permeability measured in response to acetylsalicylic acid challenge.

develop symptomatic CD, then the group of relatives analysed as a whole would be unlikely to show altered permeability. Instead, about 10% of relatives should be expected to have a permeability defect. Indeed, these investigators found that approximately 10% of asymptomatic first-degree relatives of CD patients had abnormally high permeability when tested using the lactulose–mannitol ratio[11]. Importantly, these investigators then used the same logic to reanalyse the raw data from a previous study by Katz and colleagues[16], and again found that approximately 10% of first-degree relatives of CD patients had abnormally high permeability. In addition to abnormal baseline permeability, a proportion of first-degree relatives of CD patients have an exaggerated increase in intestinal permeability in response to acetylsalicylic acid (ASA) compared with controls[10,29].

The identification of abnormal intestinal permeability in first-degree relatives suggests, but does not prove, a genetic basis for this trait. Indeed, several studies have reported that some spouses of CD patients also have elevated permeability[13,30], and pedigree analysis of families with CD has failed to show any specific genetic pattern to account for the presence of CD and abnormal permeability[13]. These data argue that elevated permeability in relatives and spouses results from some shared environmental factor or, alternatively, from subclinical disease.

These conflicting results can be partly reconciled by a recent study, which evaluated permeability with and without ASA challenge in CD patients, first-degree relatives, spouses and controls[31]. Baseline permeability was higher in patients and spouses than in controls and relatives. However, after ingestion of ASA, although permeability increased in all groups, patients and relatives had similar increases, while spouses were similar to controls. These findings suggest that baseline permeability is determined by environmental factors, while ASA stimulated permeability changes are a function of the genetically controlled integrity of the mucosal barrier[31]. In other words, both environmental and genetic factors may be at work!

ARE PERMEABILITY ABNORMALITIES SECONDARY TO INTESTINAL INFLAMMATION?

In addition to genetic or environmental causes, it remains possible that elevated intestinal permeability in relatives and spouses represents subclinical or 'silent' CD[5]. Although clinical studies have yet to adequately address this hypothesis, ample evidence from animal studies and data from other chronic inflammatory conditions supports a close relationship between permeability and intestinal inflammation. In the rat model of trinitrobenzene sulphonic acid-induced colitis, a rapid increase in intestinal permeability is detectable immediately before increases in tissue proinflammatory cytokines tumour necrosis factor α (TNF-α), interleukin-1β (IL-1β), and interleukin-6 (IL-6)[32]. Non-steroidal anti-inflammatory drugs (NSAIDs) increase intestinal permeability within 12 h[33], and, in patients taking NSAIDs for more than 6 months, approximately 50% will have scintigraphic abnormalities on ^{111}indium (^{111}In)-labelled white blood cell scans, irrefutable evidence of small intestinal inflammation[34]. In patients with untreated coeliac disease, the mean sucrose excretion and lactulose–mannitol ratio are significantly increased compared with healthy controls, and both decline significantly after initiation of a gluten-free diet[35]. Using ^{51}Cr-EDTA, Mielants *et al.* found a significant increase in permeability in patients with spondyloarthropathy not taking NSAIDs compared with controls[36]. Interestingly, when ileocolonoscopy was performed in these rheumatological patients, a subset had chronic intestinal inflammation histologically consistent with CD, as well as abnormal permeability in the absence of any gastrointestinal symptoms[36].

Clinical studies in patients with CD have also produced evidence linking abnormal permeability to gut inflammation. In 34 patients with active CD, Teahon and colleagues measured ^{51}Cr-EDTA permeability and faecal excretion of ^{111}In-labelled white blood cells, both of which were abnormal[19]. After induction of remission using an elemental diet in 27/34 patients, there was a significant decrease in both the urine excretion of ^{51}Cr-EDTA and the faecal excretion of ^{111}In-labelled white blood cells[19]. Relatives of CD patients with increased permeability have a significant increase in the CD45RO isoform, a marker of increased antigen exposure, on circulating $CD19^{+}$ B lymphocytes[37]. Importantly, in this study, relatives with normal permeability failed to display an increased number of CD45RO-expressing cells. Despite the accumulation of findings from both clinical and basic investigations supporting a link between intestinal permeability and intestinal inflammation, this relationship has yet to be directly confirmed. No study to date has specifically examined intestinal permeability together with objective endoscopic and histological findings in CD patients or their relatives.

CAN SUBCLINICAL INFLAMMATION EXIST IN CROHN'S DISEASE?

It is well established that endoscopic inflammation correlates poorly with clinical symptoms in CD and is commonly present in the absence of clinical symptoms[38,39]. Asymptomatic intestinal inflammation can be found in other chronic inflammatory disorders as well. Subclinical gut inflammation has been detected in more than half of patients with spondyloarthropathy[40,41]. Over time, 7% of these patients have been diagnosed with IBD[42]. Coeliac disease exists as a latent form in approximately 10% of family members of symptomatic patients; many of these healthy family members display histological evidence for increased intraepithelial lymphocytes and/or partial villous atrophy[43]. Such relatives, not surprisingly, often have abnormal intestinal permeability as well[44]. Thus, low-grade intestinal inflammation without clinical intestinal symptoms clearly is common in patients with chronic immunological conditions and is even present in some of their asymptomatic relatives.

Histological inflammation can also exist without detectable endoscopic inflammation. Both lymphocytic and microscopic colitis are characterized by the presence of endoscopically normal colonic mucosa and chronic histological inflammation[45]. D'Haens *et al.* have recently shown that, in early recurrent CD, both histological and immunological mucosal abnormalities can exist in the absence of endoscopic disease[46]. Notably, even morphologically normal intestinal mucosa from patients with CD spontaneously produces increased amounts of TNF-α, interleukin 1β (IL-1β) and interleukin 6 (IL-6)[47]. It is clear, therefore, that immunological abnormalities can exist without endoscopic or histological abnormalities.

DO RELATIVES WITH ELEVATED INTESTINAL PERMEABILITY HAVE SILENT CROHN'S DISEASE?

Recently, we have begun to investigate whether abnormal intestinal permeability in healthy first-degree relatives of CD patients is due to subclinical intestinal inflammation. Specifically, we have been attempting to correlate intestinal permeability with objective evidence of intestinal inflammation as determined by endoscopic appearance, histological assessment, and measurement of mucosal cytokine levels[48]. Twenty-eight symptom-free first-degree relatives and 12 control subjects (healthy subjects undergoing colon cancer screening) have been studied to date. Intestinal permeability was measured by the lactulose–mannitol ratio and complete ileocolonoscopy was performed with mucosal biopsies obtained from the terminal ileum (TI), ascending and descending colon, and rectum for histological and cytokine determination. IL-6, interleukin 8 (IL-8), interleukin 12 (IL-12), and TNF-α were measured in the undernatant of mucosal organ cultures using ELISA. Among the relatives, 7% had elevated permeability, 7% had endoscopic ileitis, and 11% had histological ileitis and/or colitis; none of the controls showed endoscopic or histological ileitis. Compared with controls, the mucosal biopsies from relatives generated significantly higher levels of IL-8 (25.4 ± 54.5 pg/μg vs. 5.3 ± 2.6 pg/μg; $p = 0.005$) (Figure 1) and IL-6 (0.25 ± 0.3 vs. 0.08 ± 0.05 pg/μg; $p = 0.02$) (Figure 2). IL-12 was detected in 32% of relatives but only 17% of controls; these differences were not statistically significant ($p = 0.08$). TNF-α was undetectable in all samples. The three relatives with histological inflammation had levels of IL-8 significantly greater ($p = 0.04$) than those of inflammation-free relatives. Two relatives with endoscopic ileitis had significantly greater IL-6 levels ($p = 0.04$) than the other relatives without endoscopic inflammation. In this small sample, no direct correlation was observed between permeability and the presence or absence of inflammation or specific cytokine levels.

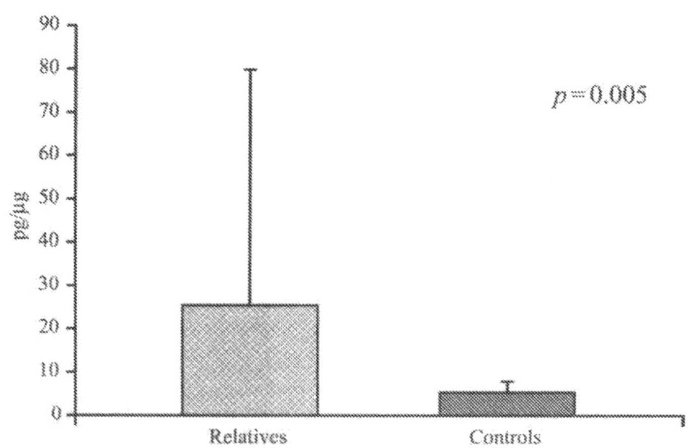

Figure 1 IL-8 concentration measured by ELISA from organ cultures of intestinal biopsies. Relatives $n = 28$ and controls $n = 12$. (From Katz *et al.*[48])

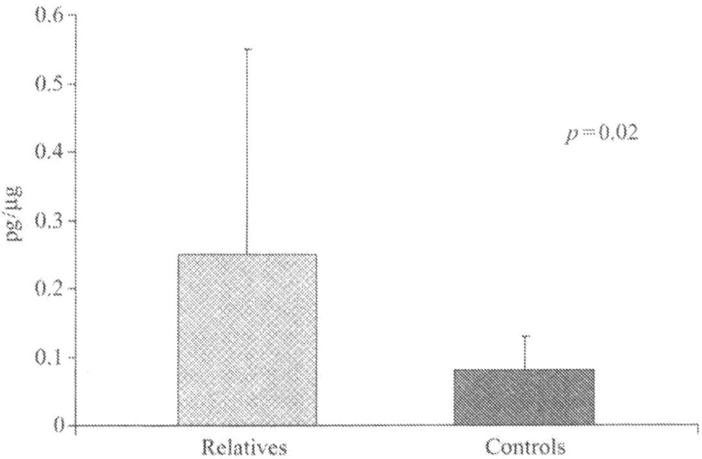

Figure 2 IL-6 concentration measured by ELISA from organ cultures of mucosal biopsies. Relatives $n=28$ and controls $n=12$. (From Katz *et al.*[48])

Our preliminary results do not yet allow us to determine the precise significance of abnormal permeability among relatives of CD patients. However, it appears that some healthy first-degree relatives of CD patients produce abnormally high levels of mucosal inflammatory cytokines compared with normal controls, and some of them also display active intestinal inflammation. The apparent lack of correlation between abnormal permeability, inflammation or elevated cytokine production may be due to small sample size. This preliminary report demonstrates, for the first time, the objective evidence of intestinal inflammation and immune abnormalities in healthy relatives of CD patients and suggests that subclinical CD may be more common than previously suspected.

CONCLUSION

The significance of abnormal intestinal permeability in the pathogenesis of Crohn's disease remains uncertain. The preponderance of evidence from studies in patients with Crohn's disease argues that permeability closely parallels inflammation, and is thus a secondary phenomenon. However, permeability studies in relatives of patients with Crohn's disease suggest that alterations in gut barrier function may predate any inflammation, and therefore may be important aetiological factors. Whether this finding in relatives is genetically predetermined, environmentally acquired or a combination of both influences is unknown. Preliminary study of family members of CD patients has documented the presence of asymptomatic inflammation at the endoscopic, histological and immune function levels, suggesting that subclinical CD may exist in relatives of affected patients, but these results have yet to be correlated with elevated intestinal permeability. The recent association of a mutation in the NOD2 gene with CD will hopefully lead to a more fundamental understanding of the pathophysiology of this illness[49,50]. Investigation of intestinal permeability and its relationship with NOD2, and other as-yet-undiscovered genes, may ultimately lead to a better understanding of the mechanisms controlling gut barrier function and their significance in the development of Crohn's disease.

Acknowledgements

This work was supported by a research grant from the Crohn's and Colitis Foundation of America.

References

1. Hollander D. Intestinal permeability in health and disease. In: Kirsner JB, ed, Inflammatory Bowel Disease. 5th edn. Philadelphia: W.B. Saunders Company; 2000:45–54.
2. Bjarnason I, MacPherson A, Hollander D. Intestinal permeability: an overview. Gastroenterology. 1995;108:1566–81.
3. Olaison G, Sjödahl R, Tagesson C. Abnormal intestinal permeability in Crohn's disease. A possible pathogenic factor. Scand J Gastroenterol. 1990;25:321–8.
4. Hollander D, Vadheim C, Brettholz E *et al.* Increased intestinal permeability in patients with Crohn's disease and their relatives. Ann Intern Med. 1986;105:883–5.
5. Hollander D. Permeability in Crohn's disease: altered barrier function in healthy relatives? Gastroenterology. 1993;104:1848–73.
6. Hermiston M, Gordon J. Inflammatory bowel disease and adenomas in mice expressing a dominant negative N-cadherin. Science. 1995;270:1203–7.
7. Soper PR, Cornish A, McKaigney C *et al.* Oral administration of VSL #3 is effective in restoring epithelial ion transport and barrier function in IL-10−/− mice. Gastroenterology. 2001;120(suppl 1):A673.
8. Adenis A, Colombel J-F, Lecouffe P *et al.* Increased pulmonary and intestinal permeability in Crohn's disease. Gut. 1992;33:678–82.
9. Bjarnason I, O'Morain C, Levi AJ, Peters TJ. Absorption of 51-chromium-labelled ethylenediaminetetracetate in inflammatory bowel disease. Gastroenterology. 1983;85:318–22.
10. Hilsden RJ, Meddings JB, Sutherland LR. Intestinal permeability changes in response to acetylsalicylic acid in relatives of patients with Crohn's disease. Gastroenterology. 1996;110: 1395–403.
11. May G, Sutherland L, Meddings J. Is small intestinal permeability really increased in relatives of patients with Crohn's disease? Gastroenterology. 1993;104:1627–32.
12. Pironi L, Miglioli M, Ruggeri E *et al.* Relationship between intestinal permeability to [51Cr]EDTA and inflammatory activity in asymptomatic patients with Crohn's disease. Dig Dis Sci. 1990;35(5):582–8.
13. Peeters M, Geypens B, Claus D *et al.* Clustering of increased small intestinal permeability in families with Crohn's disease. Gastroenterology. 1997;113:802–7.
14. Teahon K, Smethurst P, Levi A *et al.* Intestinal permeability in patients with Crohn's disease and their first degree relatives. Gut. 1992;33:320–3.
15. Munkholm P, Langholz E, Hollander D *et al.* Intestinal permeability in patients with Crohn's disease and ulcerative colitis and their first degree relatives. Gut. 1994;35:68–72.
16. Katz K, Hollander D, Vadheim C *et al.* Intestinal permeability in patients with Crohn's disease and their healthy relatives. Gastroenterology. 1989;97:927–31.
17. Pearson AD, Eastman EJ, Laker MF *et al.* Intestinal permeability in children with Crohn's disease and coeliac disease. Br Med J. 1982;285:20–1.
18. Wyatt J, Vogelsang H, Lochs H. Effect of corticosteroids on intestinal permeability in patients with active Crohn's disease. Gastroenterology. 1992;102:A947.
19. Teahon K, Smethurst P, Pearson M *et al.* The effect of elemental diet on intestinal permeability and inflammation in Crohn's disease. Gastroenterology. 1991;101:84–9.
20. Suenaert P, Bulteel V, Lemmens L *et al.* Anti-TNF treatment restores gut barrier function in Crohn's disease. Gastroenterology. 2001;120(suppl 1):A518.

21. D'Inca R, Leo VD, Corrao G *et al.* Intestinal permeability test as a predictor of clinical course in Crohn's disease. Am J Gastroenterol. 1999;94:2956–60.
22. Wyatt J, Vogelsang H, Hubl W *et al.* Intestinal permeability and the prediction of relapse in Crohn's disease. Lancet. 1993;341:1437–9.
23. Pironi L, Miglioli M, Ruggeri E *et al.* Intestinal permeability (IP) to 51Cr-EDTA and postoperative recurrence of Crohn's disease (CD): A follow-up study. Gastroenterology. 1991;100:A239.
24. Tibble JA, Sigthorsson G, Bridger S *et al.* Surrogate markers of intestinal inflammation are predictive of relapse in patients with inflammatory bowel disease. Gastroenterology. 2000;119: 15–22.
25. Peeters M, Ghoos Y, Maes B *et al.* Increased permeability of macroscopically normal small bowel in Crohn's disease. Dig Dis Sci. 1994;39:2170–6.
26. Söderholm JD, Peterson KH, Olaison G *et al.* Epithelial permeability to proteins in the noninflamed ileum of Crohn's disease. Gastroenterology. 1999;117:65–72.
27. Irvine EJ, Marshall JK. Increased intestinal permeability precedes the onset of Crohn's disease in a subject with familial risk. Gastroenterology. 2000;119:1740–4.
28. Ruttenberg D, Young GO, Wright JP, Isaacs S. PEG-400 excretion in patients with Crohn's disease, their first-degree relatives, and healthy volunteers. Dig Dis Sci. 1992;37(5):705–8.
29. Pironi L, Miglioli M, Ruggeri E *et al.* Effect of non-steroidal anti-inflammatory drugs (NSAID) on intestinal permeability of first degree relatives of patients with Crohn's disease. Gastroenterology. 1992;102:A679.
30. Breslin NP, Price LM, Hershfield NB *et al.* Intestinal permeability is altered in the spouses of patients with Crohn's disease (abstract). Gastroenterology. 1998;114:A942.
31. Söderholm JD, Olaison G, Lindberg E *et al.* Different intestinal permeability patterns in relatives and spouses of patients with Crohn's disease: an inherited defect in mucosal defense? Gut. 1999;44:96–100.
32. Tateishi H, Mitsuyama K, Toyonaga A *et al.* Role of cytokines in experimental colitis: relation to intestinal permeability. Digestion. 1997;58:271–81.
33. Bjarnason I, Hayllar J, MacPherson AJ, Russell AS. Side effects of nonsteroidal anti-inflammatory drugs on the small and large intestine in humans. Gastroenterology. 1993;104:1832–47.
34. Bjarnson I, Zanelli G, Smith T *et al.* Nonsteroidal antiinflammatory drug induced inflammation in humans. Gastroenterology. 1987;93:480–9.
35. Smecuol E, Bai JC, Vazquez H *et al.* Gastrointestinal permeability in celiac disease. Gastroenterology. 1997;112:1129–36.
36. Mielants H, Vos MD, Goemaere S *et al.* Intestinal permeability in inflammatory rheumatic diseases. II. Role of disease. J Rheumatol. 1991;18:394–400.
37. Yacyshyn BR, Meddings JB. CD45RO expression on circulating CD19+ B cells in Crohn's disease correlates with intestinal permeability. Gastroenterology. 1995;108:132–7.
38. Cellier C, Sahmoud T, Froguel E *et al.* Correlations between clinical activity, endoscopic severity, and biological parameters in colonic and ileocolonic Crohn's disease. A multicenter prospective study of 121 cases. Gut. 1994;35:231–5.
39. Modigliani R, Mary J-Y, Simon J-F *et al.* Clinical, biological, and endoscopic picture of attacks of Crohn's disease. Evolution on prednisolone. Gastroenterology. 1990;98:811–18.
40. Mielants H, Veys EM, Cuvelier C *et al.* HLA-B27 related arthritis and bowel inflammation. Part 2: Ileocolonoscopy and bowel histology in patients with HLA-B27 related arthritis. J Rheumatol. 198;12:294–8.
41. DeVos M, Cuveliae C, Mielants H *et al.* Ileocolonoscopy in seronegative spondyloarthropathy. Gastroenterology. 1989;96:339–44.
42. DeVos M, Mielants H, Cuvelier C *et al.* Long-term evolution of gut inflammation in patients with spondyloarthropathy. Gastroenterology. 1996;110:1696–703.
43. Auricchio S, Mazzacca G, Tosi R *et al.* Coeliac disease as a familial condition: identification of asymptomatic coeliac patients within family groups. Gastroenterol Int. 1988;1:25–31.
44. Elberg RMv, Uil JJ, Mulder CJJ, Heymans HSA. Intestinal permeability in patients with coeliac disease and relatives of patients with celiac disease. Gut. 1993;34:354–7.
45. Saul SH. The watery diarrhea–colitis syndrome. A review of collagenous and microscopic/lymphocytic colitis. Int J Surg Pathol. 1993;1:65–82.
46. D'Haens GR, Geboes K, Peeters M *et al.* Early lesions of recurrent Crohn's disease caused by infusion of intestinal contents in excluded ileum. Gastroenterology. 1998;114:262–7.

47. Reimund JM, Wittersheim C, Dumont S *et al.* Increased production of tumor necrosis factor-alpha, interleukin-1 beta, and interleukin-6 by morphologically normal intestinal biopsies from patients with Crohn's disease. Gut. 1996;39:684–9.
48. Katz JA, Willis JE, Cooper GS *et al.* Subclinical intestinal inflammation and immune abnormalities in healthy relatives of Crohn's disease (CD) patients. Gastroenterology. 2001;120(suppl 1): A140.
49. Ogura Y, Bonen DK, Inohara N *et al.* A frameshift mutation in NOD2 associated with susceptibility to Crohn's disease. Nature. 2001;411:603–6.
50. Hugot JP, Chamaillard M, Zouali H *et al.* Associations of NOD2 leucine-rich repeat variants with susceptibility to Crohn's disease. Nature. 2001;411:599–603.
51. Valpiani D, Ornigotti L, Ricca-Rosellini S *et al.* Intestinal permeability in patients with Crohn's disease and in first grade relatives. Gastroenterology. 1992;102:A708.
52. Ainsworth M, Eriksen J, Rasmussen JW. Intestinal permeability of 51Cr-labelled ethylenediaminetetraacetic acid in patients with Crohn's disease and their healthy relatives. Scand J Gastroenterol. 1989;24:993–8.

3
Screening for IBD susceptibility: subclinical markers

J.-F. COLOMBEL, S. JOOSSENS, P. VANDEWALLE, S. VERMEIRE, B. SENDID, V. ANNESE, P. RUTGEERTS and D. POULAIN

The strongest risk factor for IBD is having a relative with the disease. Familial clustering can be measured by the ratio of the risk to siblings compared with the general population risk (λs), estimated to be 15–35 for Crohn's disease (CD) and 7–12 for ulcerative colitis (UC)[1,2]. In recent years, there has been a great interest in searching for subclinical markers of IBD in families. Their presence in 'unaffected' members may either indicate the genetic and/or environmental factor predisposing to a disease, or identify those in whom an earlier phase of the disease process is occurring. Data concerning intestinal permeability are reviewed in depth in this book by J. Katz and we will concentrate, among proposed serological markers (Table 1), on the two most studied, i.e. antineutrophil cytoplasmic autoantibodies (ANCA) and anti-*Saccharomyces cerevisiae* mannan antibodies (ASCA).

Intestinal permeability is increased in patients with CD and a proportion of their healthy relatives. Hollander *et al.*[3] first reported an increased permeability in 78% of healthy relatives from patients with CD. Additional results were controversial,

Table 1 Potential serological subclinical markers in IBD

Antibodies	*Increased frequency in healthy relatives*	*IBD*	*Reference*
ANCA	+ but not consistent	UC	10–16
ASCA	+	CD	22–24, 27
Antigoblet cells	+	CD/UC	30
Antipancreas	−	CD	15, 31
Lymphocytotoxic	+	CD	32
Antitropomyosin	−	UC	33

ASCA: anti-*Saccharomyces cerevisiae* mannan antibodies; ANCA: antineutrophil cytoplasmic antibodies; CD: Crohn's disease; UC: ulcerative colitis.

mainly due to a lack of standardization in methodology[4,5]. More recent studies detected an increased permeability index in 10–25% of healthy relatives[6,7]. Reports of an increased sensitivity of healthy first-degree relatives to NSAID challenge were interesting. A significantly higher proportion of relatives showed an increased permeability compared with controls[8]. One can speculate on a genetically determined hypersensitivity of the bowel mucosa to environmental factors. This hypothesis, however, conflicts with the finding that permeability is also increased in 30% of spouses of CD patients[7,9]. Soderhölm *et al.* suggested that baseline permeability (increased in both subsets of spouses and relatives) may be determined by environmental factors while permeability provoked by acetylsalicylic acid (only increased in relatives) may be a function of the genetically determined state of the mucosal barrier[9].

ANCA were first described in sera from patients with systemic vasculitides such as Wegener's granulomatosis. They were subsequently found in many inflammatory disorders. UC-associated ANCA is characterized by perinuclear highlighting on indirect immunofluorescence microscopy and has been described commonly as pANCA. In 1992, Shanahan *et al.* found an increased frequency of pANCA in healthy relatives (16%) of UC patients compared with controls (3%) with a higher rate of positivity in relatives from ANCA-positive patients[10]. Another family study reported ANCA positivity in 30% of the first-degree relatives of UC patients[11]. These results were, however, not confirmed[12–16]. Moreover, the frequency of pANCA was not significantly increased in healthy monozygotic twins with UC compared with healthy controls[17]. These studies overall did not support the hypothesis that pANCA is a subclinical marker for susceptibility to UC.

ASCA, an antibody against oligomannosidic epitopes of the yeast *Saccharomyces cerevisiae,* has been associated with CD but not with UC. Reported prevalence is 60–70% in patients with CD, 10–15% in patients with UC, and 0–5% in control subjects[18–21]. In a first set of CD families, ASCA were detected in 35/51 (69%) patients with CD and in 13/66 (20%) of healthy relatives versus 1/163 controls ($p<0.001$)[22]. The presence of ASCA in healthy relatives was observed in 12 of 20 families and was not restricted to a few particular multiplex families. The prevalence of ASCA in relatives did not depend on the ASCA status of affected members. In 15 families, children with CD were born of healthy parents and in eight of these 15 families, at least one of the parents was ASCA-positive. This led us to suppose that ASCA in parents is at least as potent a risk factor for children to develop CD as parental CD. Conversely, Sutton *et al.* did not find a significantly increased frequency of ASCA in unaffected relatives (9.3%) of CD patients in comparison with healthy controls (4%). However, they demonstrated a high concordance of seropositivity rates in affected family members with seronegative or seropositive probands and intra-class correlation of quantitative ASCA levels in both affected and unaffected family members[23]. Familial aspects of ASCA were further investigated in a large series of Belgian families having one, two or more than two affected members[24]. Overall, ASCA prevalence was the same in both sporadic (63.4%) and familial (62.1%) CD. Within pure CD families, ASCA were present in 54.2% of CD patients with two members affected versus 74.7% in CD patients with three or more members affected ($p=0.002$) (Figure 1). More recently, through collaborative efforts, higher ASCA titres have been found in families with three or more members affected than in families with two members affected ($p=0.01$)[25]. Further, the Belgian study indicated that CD patients from mixed families show a serological response different from sporadic cases and pure familial CD with a significantly lower (33.3%) ASCA prevalence (Figure 1). Conversely, ASCA prevalence in UC patients from mixed families was higher than in sporadic cases (32.4% vs. 8%) ($p<0.001$)[24]. This suggests that mixed families may represent a different entity from pure CD families as far as immunological response is concerned.

ASCA were present in 28/135 (20.7%) unaffected relatives of CD patients which was higher than in the control group ($p<0.001$)[24]. The prevalence of ASCA in relatives did not depend on the ASCA status of affected members, thus disproving the claim that ASCA might be a marker of disease heterogeneity[23]. Until now, no data were available to assume that familial and sporadic CD are different entities. However, ASCA were present in 21.3% of healthy relatives of familial CD versus 8.7% of healthy relatives of sporadic CD ($p=0.006$)[25]. These data give additional arguments for the hypothesis that ASCA is an expression of the familial load of the disease. The lack of concordance for the marker in marital couples[24] may further indicate that its presence in families is due in part to a genetic factor or childhood environmental exposure. We recently showed that familiality of ASCA might occur in control families independently from CD with evidence for vertical transmission of the marker from mother to child[26]. However, the claim that ASCA may represent a specific marker of susceptibility for CD was challenged by Annese *et al.* who found that the frequency of ASCA in healthy relatives of UC and mixed families did not differ from that of CD families[27].

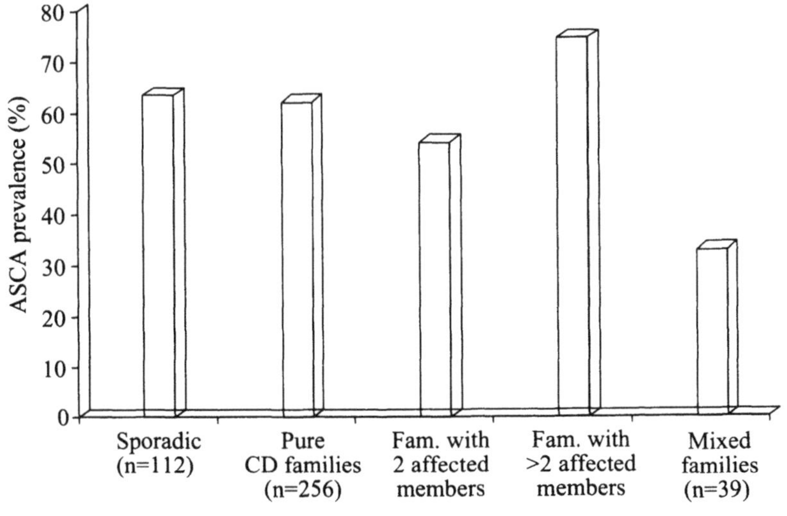

Figure 1 Prevalence of ASCA in sporadic CD, pure CD families and mixed families. From Reference 24

Studies in families suggest that unravelling the origin of ASCA may offer new clues to the pathophysiology of CD. ASCA are not an epiphenomenon related to disease activity and titres are relatively constant over time[24]. In the same study, no relationship between ASCA presence and titres and intestinal permeability was found in CD patients and their healthy relatives[24]. Different hypotheses concerning the origin of ASCA in IBD can be proposed[28]. One must take into account the widespread distribution of oligomannosides shared by many molecules present in a wide variety of organisms. The role of dietary yeasts has been explored without definitive conclusions and no data are available about endogenous yeasts. A second hypothesis is that yeast mannan oligomannosides could correspond to epitopes shared by other micro-organisms. Finally, the ubiquitous character of mannose residue sequences raises a third hypothesis: some *S. cerevisiae* oligomannosides could share structural homologies with oligomannosides expressed on human glycoconjugates acting as autoantigens or neoautoantigens.

The presence of subclinical markers in families does not have clinical implications yet. Very interestingly, Irvine and Marshall recently described a 24-year-old woman with a positive family history of CD who had no evidence of CD but had an elevated gut permeability to ^{51}Cr-EDTA at age 13. Repeated investigation after the onset of symptoms at age 21 revealed ileocolonic CD. In this case, a permeability defect was clearly identified to precede the onset of CD in a subject at increased risk[29]. More studies are needed, however, to assess the relevance of screening unaffected relatives.

References

1. Orholm M, Munkholm P, Langholz E, Nielsen OH, Sorensen TIA, Binder V. Familial occurrence of inflammatory bowel disease. N Engl J Med. 1991;324:84–8.
2. Peeters M, Nevens H, Baert F. Familial aggregation in Crohn's disease: increased age-adjusted risk and concordance in clinical characteristics. Gastroenterology. 1996;111:597–603.
3. Hollander D, Vadheim CM, Brettholz E, Petersen GM, Delahunty T, Rotter JI. Increased intestinal permeability in patients with Crohn's disease and their relatives – a possible aetiological factor. Ann Intern Med. 1986;105:883–5.
4. Teahon K, Smethurst P, Levi AJ, Menzies IS, Bjarnason I. Intestinal permeability in patients with Crohn's disease and their first degree relatives. Gut. 1992;33:320–3.
5. Ainsworth M, Eriksen J, Rasmussen JW, Schaffalitzky De Muckadell OB. Intestinal permeability of Cr-labelled ethylenediaminetetraacetic acid in patients with Crohn's disease and their first degree relatives. Scand J Gastroenterol. 1989;24:993–8.
6. May G, Sutherland L, Meddings J. Is small intestinal permeability really increased in relatives of patients with Crohn's disease? Gastroenterology. 1993;104:1627–32.
7. Peeters M, Geypens B, Claus D *et al.* Clustering of increased small intestinal permeability in families with Crohn's disease. Gastroenterology. 1997;113:802–7.
8. Hilsden RJ, Meddings JB, Sutherland LR. Intestinal permeability changes in response to acetylsalicylic acid in relatives of patients with Crohn's disease. Gastroenterology. 1996;110:1395–403.
9. Söderholm JD, Olaison G, Lindberg E *et al.* Different intestinal permeability patterns in relatives and spouses of patients with Crohn's disease: an inherited defect in mucosal defence? Gut. 1999;44:96–100.
10. Shanahan F, Duerr RH, Rotter JI *et al.* Neutrophil autoantibodies in ulcerative colitis: familial aggregation and genetic heterogeneity. Gastroenterology. 1992;103:456–61.
11. Seibold F, Slametschka D, Gregor M, Weber P. Neutrophil autoantibodies: a genetic marker in primary sclerosing cholangitis and ulcerative colitis. Gastroenterology. 1994;107:532–6.
12. Reumaux D, Colombel JF, Delecourt L, Noel LH, Cortot A, Duthilleul P. Anti-neutrophil cytoplasmic auto-antibodies (ANCA) in patients with ulcerative colitis (UC): influence of disease activity and familial study. Adv Exp Med Biol. 1993;336:515–18.

13. Lee JC, Lennard-Jones JE, Cambridge G. Antineutrophil antibodies in familial inflammatory bowel disease. Gastroenterology. 1995;108:428–33.
14. Bansi DS, Lo S, Chapman RW, Fleming KA. Absence of antineutrophil cytoplasmic antibodies in relatives of UK patients with primary sclerosing cholangitis and ulcerative colitis. Eur J Gastroenterol Hepatol. 1996;8:111–16.
15. Papo M, Quer JC, Pastor RM *et al.* Antineutrophil cytoplasmic antibodies in relatives of patients with inflammatory bowel disease. Am J Gastroenterol. 1996;91:1512–15.
16. Folwaczny C, Noehl N, Endres SP, Loeschke K, Fricke H. Antineutrophil and pancreatic autoantibodies in first-degree relatives of patients with inflammatory bowel disease. Scand J Gastroenterol. 1998;33:523–8.
17. Yang P, Jarnerot G, Danielsson D, Tysk C, Lindberg E. pANCA in monozygotic twins with inflammatory bowel disease. Gut. 1995;36:887–90.
18. McKenzie H, Main J, Pennington CR, Parratt D. Antibody to selected strains of Saccharomyces cerevisiae (baker's and brewer's yeast) and Candida albicans in Crohn's disease. Gut. 1990;31:536–8.
19. Quinton JF, Sendid B, Reumaux D *et al.* Anti-*Saccharomyces cerevisiae* mannan antibodies combined with antineutrophil cytoplasmic antibodies in inflammatory bowel disease: prevalence and diagnostic role. Gut. 1998;42:788–91.
20. Ruemmele FM, Targan SR, Levy G, Dubinsky M, Braun J, Seidman EG. Diagnostic accuracy of serological assays in pediatric inflammatory bowel disease . Gastroenterology. 1998;115:822–9.
21. Peeters M, Joossens S, Vermeire S, Vlietinck R, Bossuyt X, Rutgeerts P. Diagnostic value of anti-*Saccharomyces cerevisiae* and antineutrophil cytoplasmic autoantibodies in inflammatory bowel disease. Am J Gastroenterol. 2001;96:730–4.
22. Sendid B, Quinton JF, Charrier G. Anti-*Saccharomyces cerevisiae* mannan antibodies in familial Crohn's disease. Am J Gastroenterol. 1998;93:1306–10.
23. Sutton CL, Yang H, Li Z, Rotter JL, Targan SR, Braun J. Familial expression of anti-*Saccharomyces cerevisiae* mannan antibodies in affected and unaffected relatives of patients with Crohn's disease. Gut. 2000;45:58–63.
24. Vermeire S, Peeters M, Vlietinck R *et al.* Anti-*Saccharomyces cerevisiae* antibodies (ASCA), phenotypes of IBD, and intestinal permeability: a study in IBD families. Inflamm Bowel Dis. 2001;7:8–15.
25. Joossens S, Vermeire S, Vandewalle P *et al.* ASCA (Anti-Saccharomyces cerevisiae antibodies) in healthy relatives of sporadic and familial Crohn's disease patients. Gastroenterology. 2001; abstract.
26. Poulain D, Sendid B, Fajardy I, Danze PM, Colombel JF. Mother to child transmission of anti-*S. cerevisiae* mannan antibodies (ASCA) in non IBD families (letter). Gut. 2000;47:780.
27. Annese V, Andreoli A, Andriulli A *et al.* Familial expression of anti-Saccharomyces cerevisiae mannan antibodies in Crohn's disease and ulcerative colitis. Am J Gastroenterol. 2001;96:2407–12.
28. Sendid B, Colombel JF, Jacquinot PM *et al.* Specific antibody response to oligomannosidic epitopes in Crohn's disease. Clin Diagn Lab Immunol. 1996;3:219–26.
29. Irvine EJ, Marshall JK. Increased intestinal permeability precedes the onset of Crohn's disease in a subject with familial risk. Gastroenterology. 2000;119:1740–4.
30. Folwaczny C, Noehl N, Tschop K *et al.* Goblet cell autoantibodies in patients with inflammatory bowel disease and their first-degree relatives. Gastroenterology. 1997;113:101–6.
31. Seibold F, Mork H, Tanza S *et al.* Pancreatic autoantibodies in Crohn's disease: a family study. Gut. 1997;40:481–4.
32. Korsmeyer SJ, Williams RC Jr., Wilson ID, Strickland RG. Lymphocytotoxic antibody in inflammatory bowel disease. A family study. N Engl J Med. 1975;293:1117–20.
33. Biancone L, Monteleone G, Marasco R, Pallone F. Autoimmunity to tropomyosin isoforms in ulcerative colitis patients and unaffected relatives. Clin Exp Immunol. 1998;113:198–205.

4
Genetics of IBD: chromosomal studies

M. PARKES and D. P. JEWELL

INTRODUCTION

Investigating the genetic basis of inflammatory bowel disease (IBD) has been an area of intense scientific interest over the last five years and, with recent exciting advances, promises to provide profound insights into the pathogenesis of Crohn's disease and ulcerative colitis. A number of strong and replicated regions of linkage have been identified in different parts of the genome, and the various techniques of fine mapping are being applied to characterize these further. The goal in each case is to define the disease-predisposing genetic variant, as has been achieved recently for the *IBD1* locus on chromosome 16[1–3].

THE RATIONALE FOR LINKAGE STUDIES: EPIDEMIOLOGY

Early evidence for the importance of genetic susceptibility came from epidemiological studies. Particularly striking were those demonstrating substantially higher concordance in monozygotic compared with dizygotic twins: for Crohn's disease 35% vs. 7% respectively, and for ulcerative colitis 11% vs. 3%[4–6].

Family studies also showed that the siblings of patients with IBD were at substantially greater risk of developing disease than were members of the general population – formalized as the λs ratio. For Crohn's disease, this ratio is 20–35 and, for ulcerative colitis, it is 8–15[7,8]. Although the high λs ratio undoubtedly reflects some contribution from the shared family environment, the consistent message from epidemiological studies has been that the genetic contribution to the pathogenesis of Crohn's disease is greater than that for ulcerative colitis and, indeed, greater than most other common diseases, such as type 1 diabetes ($\lambda s = 10$–15), hypertension ($\lambda s = 2$–3) or schizophrenia ($\lambda s = 5$–10).

DEFINING A MODEL

While genetic susceptibility is important, it is clear from studies of multiply affected families that inheritance does not follow a monogenic pattern, at least in most cases. Instead, the complex pattern of inheritance is thought to reflect the action of several susceptibility genes, as well as an important role for environmental triggers, both of which facts substantially magnify the complexity of the task of identifying susceptibility genes.

A number of other factors also contribute to the complexity of the picture and may hinder gene identification. These include:

- The probable presence of significant heterogeneity within each phenotypically defined disease category, the terms 'ulcerative colitis' and 'Crohn's disease' encompassing a number of conditions that are non-overlapping or only partially overlapping in their genetic predisposition.
- The fact that the phenotype of Crohn's disease or ulcerative colitis does not 'breed true', and up to 30% of multiplex families will contain cases of both[7,9].
- The likely finding for any given genotype of both variable penetrance (the probability that a person with a given genotype will manifest the trait) and variable expression (differing manifestations of the same phenotype for a given genotype), both depending on the genetic and environmental context of the particular susceptibility allele.

Thus, the terms Crohn's disease and ulcerative colitis probably represent groups of closely related polygenic disorders. Within each disease category, there is likely to be considerable overlap in the nature of the susceptibility genes; and, between each category, there may be some overlap, perhaps determined by genes that confer overall susceptibility to the IBD phenotype, but also some major differences, representing those genes that confer the disease-specific phenotypes.

LOCATING POLYGENES: AN OVERVIEW

There are broadly two strategies that can be used to identify complex disease susceptibility genes.

(1) Candidate gene studies focus on genes implicated for one of a number of reasons, such as work in animal models of IBD, the known function of the gene or its pattern of expression. Most are in the form of an association study, comparing the frequency of a particular allele in a panel of IBD patients to its frequency in a matched control population[10]. For a rigorous assessment, all polymorphisms present in the gene must be detected and studied, and possible linkage disequilibrium with neighbouring polymorphisms must be taken into account. Positive association may arise if the polymorphism is functionally significant and causing disease (i.e. it lies in an exon or regulatory sequence) or if it is in linkage disequilibrium with such a variant by virtue of proximity and a number of other factors, such as the presence of a discernible founder effect, the population history, the position on the chromosome and so on.

(2) Genome scanning and fine mapping is undertaken using the hypothesis-free methods of positional cloning. These are based on no prior assumptions

regarding disease pathogenesis. Instead, they rely on a systematic screen of polymorphic markers distributed across the human genome in large panels of multiply affected families, looking for regions which show linkage to disease susceptibility[11]. The linkage analysis typically used is the affected sibling or relative pair method which, being non-parametric, does not require specification of a model of inheritance. Regions of linkage are those where the affected sibling or relative pairs show significantly greater allele sharing than expected by chance alone and where this finding can be replicated in an independent panel of families[12]. Such regions tend to be very large in genetic terms, and require refinement using techniques such as linkage disequilibrium mapping[13].

Both approaches have their problems. Before too much credence can be attached to the results of any candidate gene study it is necessary to see evidence of replicability in independent datasets, and preferably also evidence of linkage in addition to association. Poorly designed candidate gene studies have all too frequently resulted in positive but unreplicable findings. Genome scans have been helpful in defining large regions in which susceptibility genes are likely to lie, but linkage disequilibrium mapping has yet to achieve successful widespread application in polygenic diseases, and methodologies for resolving the large regions remain clouded in uncertainty.

In many respects, the strengths and weaknesses of the two broad strategies described above are mutually exclusive, and thus the optimal strategy at present is probably to combine the two. Linkages identified in the course of genome scans that are both *strong* and *replicable* define intervals of the genome within which all genes are potential positional candidates. They can then be further prioritized on the basis of function, either known or predicted from database homology searches, expression patterns as defined by microarray studies etc. This whole process should be greatly facilitated by the increasing volume of data being made available regarding genomic sequence[14], the position of single nucleotide polymorphisms (SNPs)[15] and identification and mapping of transcripts.

GENOME SCANS IN IBD PROVIDE REPLICATED LINKAGE RESULTS

To date, seven genome scans have been published in IBD, focusing on Crohn's disease alone or combining Crohn's disease and ulcerative colitis[16–22]. These studies have used panels of multiply affected families and hypothesis-free non-parametric methods of linkage analysis as outlined above.

Compared with genome scans in other complex diseases, where results have proven frustratingly discrepant[23,24], such studies in IBD have proven highly successful. Seven regions have been identified where the linkage data are both strong enough to at least satisfy the criteria for 'suggestive linkage' as proposed by Kruglyak and Lander ('suggestive' linkage Lod ≥ 2.2, 'significant' linkage Lod ≥ 3.6)[12], and replicable in at least one independent dataset.

These candidate intervals are found on chromosomes 1p, 3p, 5q, 6p, 12q, 14q and 16 ('p' denotes the short arm and 'q' the long arm of the chromosome).

The exciting progress with regard to the chromosome 16 linkage is described elsewhere by Judy Cho. A brief overview of the remaining regions is given below in chromosome numerical order.

There are, of course, many other regions of the genome of potential interest, and which have shown strong evidence for linkage in individual datasets or weaker evidence in more than one panel. However, given that genome scanning is based on multiple tests, and thus very susceptible to type-1 error, it is rational to focus attention on regions where the evidence is both strong and replicable.

Chromosome 1p

In a genome scan from Chicago and Johns Hopkins, Baltimore, Cho *et al.*[18] studied a panel of 297 affected relative pairs (Crohn's disease 175, ulcerative colitis 26, mixed 96) and identified peak linkage at the telomeric end of chromosome 1p, with a Lod score of 2.6. They also reported the interesting observation of an epistatic (gene–gene) interaction between this locus and the chromosome 16 locus. Currently, the power of available linkage programs to detect such multiplicative interactions and conditional gene effects is rather low. It will, however, expand and bring with it the potential to reveal novel linkages and a better understanding of gene–gene and gene–environment interactions.

Replication and fine mapping of the 1p linkage has been undertaken by studying a population isolate – the Chaldeans who migrated to North America from Iraq in the 16th century[25]. Strong linkage was also seen in this independent panel. Furthermore, it was possible to identify a consensus haplotype of SNPs and microsatellite alleles that appears to co-segregate with disease susceptibility, and refine the 1p locus to a region of approximately 1 cM. Although linkage to this region has not been strong in other panels, this fine mapping is clearly exciting. With a region so refined, and given the availability of ever more sequence data, SNPs and methods for gene identification, there must be genuine optimism that an IBD susceptibility gene will be identified from this candidate region in the near future.

Chromosome 3p

The locus on chromosome 3p21 was first implicated in the Oxford IBD genome scan of 186 sib pairs with IBD (Crohn's disease 81, ulcerative colitis 64, mixed 41)[17]. A Lod score of 2.48 was observed for IBD – evidence which is suggestive of linkage but not significant according to accepted criteria[12]. Supportive evidence for this locus has, however, been seen in three additional datasets, with Lod scores of 2.4[22], 1.4[26] and 1.7 for IBD[27].

Fine mapping in the Oxford panel indicates that the region may be more strongly linked to Crohn's disease (Lod = 4.2) than ulcerative colitis (Lod = 0.75), although the difference between the results just fails to achieve statistical significance in formal tests for heterogeneity[28]. This study also identified a positive transmission disequilibrium test (TDT) result in the Crohn's disease panel at marker D3S1611 ($p = 0.005$). Although this marker was not studied in the fine mapping paper of Hampe *et al.*[26], a number of other putative associations were reported. These may provide tentative clues as to the high-resolution localization of a susceptibility gene in this transcript-rich region, although some caution is required in interpreting these data as correction for multiple tests and for the study of multiply affected families is required.

There are many tempting positional candidate genes in this region including the chemokine-receptor gene cluster and integrin β9, both of which are involved in leukocyte trafficking and immunoregulation; the TGF-β receptor 1 gene, which plays an important role in epithelial restitution; hMLH1, a DNA mismatch repair gene which causes hereditary non-polyposis colon cancer when mutated; and GNAI2, a G-protein gene which, when knocked out in mice, leads to the development of an IBD-like illness and adenocarcinoma of the colon[29]. The CCR5 gene deletion which protects from HIV has been studied in IBD in more than one dataset, but results have been negative[27], as they have for GNAI2[30]. There are some association data for hMLH1[31] but these have yet to be replicated elsewhere and so must be regarded as preliminary.

Chromosome 5q

Peak linkage in the Canadian genome scan of 158 sib pairs was observed at a locus on chromosome 5q31. In the subgroup of families with young onset of Crohn's disease, the Lod score was 3.9. There is good evidence that genetic susceptibility is more important in young-onset cases and similar heterogeneity was observed on chromosome 16[32].

Linkage to this region was also seen in a genome scan from Los Angeles, in Jewish families containing multiple cases of Crohn's disease[20]. In this subgroup, a Lod score of 2.2 was observed.

This region is of potential interest for two other reasons. It is syntenic with two loci implicated in a genome scan using a mouse model of IBD[33], which may facilitate fine mapping, for example using congenic strains. Furthermore, it also encodes a cluster of immunoactive cytokine genes which are clearly attractive candidate genes. Further evaluation of these is awaited.

Chromosome 6p and the HLA complex

The region of the human leukocyte antigen (HLA) complex on the short arm of chromosome 6 was one of the first to which the techniques of allelic association study were applied. Early studies from Japan using serological genotyping of HLA Class II alleles detected a positive association with HLA-DR2: this allele was present in 70% of ulcerative colitis patients compared with 30% of controls[34]. This finding was replicated in two further Japanese datasets using molecular genotyping, both of which implicated the DRB1*1502 allele of DR2[35,36]. In non-Japanese populations, the role of HLA DRB1*1502 is less clear. There is some evidence that it is associated with an increased risk of ulcerative colitis in Jewish populations[37] but, in non-Jewish European populations, DRB1*1502 is rare and not associated with IBD. HLA-DR2 may also be associated particularly with extensive disease[34,38].

In a UK-based study, Satsangi and colleagues used techniques of linkage analysis and association study to investigate the role of the HLA Class II region in non-Jewish Caucasians with IBD[39]. Linkage to the HLA-DRB1 and -DQB1 loci was detected using the affected sibling pair method in ulcerative colitis

($p = 0.017$) but not Crohn's disease ($p = 0.3$). Furthermore, the results of an association study using 348 IBD patients and 472 ethnically matched controls suggested that HLA Class II alleles might determine disease behaviour in ulcerative colitis.

A number of different allelic associations have been reported in Crohn's disease from different groups around the world. Association with DR4 has been reported particularly from Japan[40,41], and studies from California suggest an association of the DR1-DQ5 haplotype with Crohn's disease susceptibility[37]. However, these results have proven difficult to replicate in independent datasets – a requirement to protect against the type-1 error to which genetic studies are particularly prone, and without which the validity of any reported associations must be questioned.

Interest in the contribution of genes in this region to the pathogenesis of Crohn's disease has been rekindled by the results of recent linkage studies. In a panel of 49 families with more than one case of Crohn's disease, Yang *et al.* identified evidence for linkage with $p = 0.001$, and haplotype sharing by disease concordant pairs of 0.6 ($p = 0.002$)[42]. The genome scan of Hampe *et al.* and Rioux *et al.* demonstrated Lod scores of 2.1 and 2.3 respectively for this region for all IBD[19,22], although the latter was predominantly a Crohn's disease panel, and in an expanded Oxford panel of 284 affected sib pairs, a Lod score of 3.0 was observed for all IBD.

Fine mapping of this region is confounded by the strong and extensive linkage disequilibrium that is observed here. Before a causative role can be ascribed to any gene on the basis of demonstrable association, the fact that it may be secondary to linkage disequilibrium must be considered. Nonetheless, strong and replicable associations with subphenotypes of ulcerative colitis have been observed, as is discussed in Chapter 4, and there is increasing evidence to implicate the TNF-α gene which lies in the middle of the HLA complex.

A number of SNPs have been detected within the promoter region of the TNF-α gene, with data suggesting that some of these determine levels of TNF production. Such a role has been attributed to the relatively recently described −1031 polymorphism, where the substitution of thymidine for cytosine results in increased production of this pro-inflammatory cytokine. Association between this SNP and Crohn's disease was first observed in a Japanese population[43] where the frequency of the C allele in 107 Crohn's disease patients was 24% and in healthy controls 16%. This finding has subsequently been replicated in association studies on two independent panels of UK Caucasian Crohn's disease patients[44,45]. In a case-control study, the allele frequency in 121 patients with Crohn's disease was 27.6% compared to 18.4% in controls ($p = 0.005$), and, in a panel which included a number of multiply affected families, a significant distortion of alleleic transmission was observed in a TDT ($p = 0.01$)[45].

A number of factors testify to the validity of this result. The association is with a functionally significant polymorphism within a gene known to encode a molecule of great significance to the pathogenesis of Crohn's disease. Association is seen not only in more than one dataset, but also in panels of different ethnicity – increasing the likelihood that the result is true, and reducing the chance that it is due to linkage disequilibrium. And finally the association is found at a locus at which strong and replicated linkage has been observed – both in sib pair linkage studies and using the TDT, which has properties of both linkage and association. Functional studies are awaited with interest.

Chromosome 12

The strongest linkage in the Oxford IBD genome scan of 186 sib pairs (Crohn's disease 81, ulcerative colitis 64, mixed 41) was found on the long arm of chromosomes 12 (two point Lod = 5.47)[17]. This finding has subsequently been replicated in a number of additional independent datasets[19,20,46–48]. However, it has not been found in all family panels, and the evidence for linkage observed in the recent mega-analysis of worldwide genotyping data from the International IBD Genetics Consortium was relatively modest, with a Lod score of 1.8[49]. Furthermore, one study claimed to exclude this region for a locus-specific $\lambda s > 2$[50].

There are many precedents for failure to replicate linkages in complex diseases and many possible explanations, particularly relating to heterogeneity and power[51,52]. A recent study of 581 affected relative pairs (Crohn's disease 252, ulcerative colitis 138, mixed 191) indicates that heterogeneity may indeed be an issue with regard to the chromosome 12 locus. A multipoint Lod score of 3.91 was seen for ulcerative colitis-only families, compared with 1.66 for Crohn's disease-only families. This difference was statistically significant in two tests for heterogeneity, suggesting that this locus is likely to make a substantially stronger contribution to ulcerative colitis than Crohn's disease.

Success in fine mapping the chromosome 12 locus has been limited to date. In the linkage studies published to date, peak linkage is observed in different positions across a 40-cM segment[17,19,20,46–48]. This probably reflects the poor resolution of allele methods of linkage analysis[53] but might also point to the presence of more than one susceptibility gene in this region. A precedent for the latter comes from fine mapping in mouse models of type 1 diabetes[54].

Preliminary data from Oxford have demonstrated positive evidence for association (particularly with ulcerative colitis) at three adjacent microsatellite markers within a 150 kb segment[55]. The alleles implicated also show strong linkage disequilibrium, suggesting that the distortion observed is likely to be true. Duerr and colleagues also observed a positive TDT result at one of these microsatellite markers (D12S83) but with distortion at a different allele[46]. TDT analysis in the combined Oxford/Pittsburgh panel did not corroborate the earlier findings from the independent datasets (M. Parkes and R. Duerr, unpublished data) and so additional work typing SNPs in the region is required to ascertain whether there is evidence for association at this locus or not.

Two positional candidate gene studies – of interferon γ (IFN-γ) and integrin β_7 – have been negative[56,57], although the study of IFN-γ focused on a single (dinucleotide repeat) polymorphism and thus cannot completely exclude a role for this gene. Preliminary association with the gene for the vitamin D receptor has been reported but awaits replication[58].

Chromosome 14

Both Ma *et al.*[20] and Duerr *et al.*[21] found significant evidence for linkage to chromosome 14q11 (Lod = 2.8 and 3.6, respectively) in Crohn's disease-dominated panels, thereby together satisfying the criteria for a 'confirmed' locus.

It has subsequently been replicated in a Belgian panel again predominantly containing multiplex Crohn's disease families[59]. This is clearly a region of interest.

SUMMARY

Genome searches in IBD have been almost uniquely successful among polygenic diseases in providing strong and replicated regions of linkage. The identification of the NOD2 mutations that underlie the evidence for linkage so widely observed on chromosome 16 provides grounds for optimism that other IBD genes will be cloned[1–3]. Indeed, the identification of NOD2 should itself facilitate this process by allowing stratification of multiplex families into those which do and those which do not carry NOD2 mutations. Technological advances will also undoubtedly play a role[60], as will progress in the fields of bioinformatics and statistics[61]. Identifying the genetic basis of IBD will provide the key to understanding the pathogenesis of Crohn's disease and ulcerative colitis, with far-reaching implications for the way IBD is managed in the future.

References

1. Hugot JP, Chamaillard M, Zouali H *et al.* Association of NOD2 leucine-rich repeat variants with susceptibility to Crohn's disease. Nature. 2001;411(6837):599–603.
2. Ogura Y, Bonen DK, Inohara N *et al.* A frameshift mutation in NOD2 associated with susceptibility to Crohn's disease. Nature. 2001;411(6837):603–6.
3. Hampe J, Cuthbert A, Croucher PJ *et al.* Association between insertion mutation in NOD2 gene and Crohn's disease in German and British populations. Lancet. 2001;357(9272):1925–8.
4. Tysk C, Lindberg E, Järnerot G *et al.* Ulcerative colitis and Crohn's disease in an unselected population of monozygotic and dizygotic twins. A study of heritability and the influence of smoking. Gut. 1988;29:990–6.
5. Orholm M, Binder V, Sorenson T *et al.* Inflammatory bowel disease in a Danish twin register. Gut. 1996;39(Suppl 3):A187.
6. Subhani J, Montgomery S, Pounder R *et al.* Concordance rates of twins and siblings in IBD. Gastroenterology. 1998:A3113.
7. Satsangi J, Rosenberg WMC, Jewell DP. The prevalence of inflammatory bowel disease in relatives of patients with Crohn's disease. Euro J Gastroenterol Hepatol. 1994;6:413–16.
8. Probert CSJ, Jayanthi V, Hughes AO *et al.* Prevalence and family risk of ulcerative colitis and Crohn's disease: an epidemiological study among Europeans and South Asians in Leicestershire. Gut. 1993;34:1547–51.
9. Kirsner JB. Genetic aspects of inflammatory bowel disease. Clin Gastroenterol. 1973;2:557.
10. Cardon LR, Bell JI. Association study designs for complex diseases. Nat Rev Genet. 2001;2(2):91–9.
11. Lander ES, Schork NJ. Genetic dissection of complex traits. Science. 1994;265:2037–48.
12. Kruglyak L, Lander E. Genetic dissection of complex traits: guidelines for interpreting and reporting linkage results. Nature Genet. 1995;11:241–7.
13. Strachan T, Read A. Human Molecular Genetics. Oxford, UK: BIOS Scientific Publishers Limited, 1996.
14. McPherson JD, Marra M, Hillier L *et al.* A physical map of the human genome. Nature. 2001;409(6822):934–41.
15. Sachidanandam R, Weissman D, Schmidt SC *et al.* A map of human genome sequence variation containing 1.42 million single nucleotide polymorphisms. Nature. 2001;409(6822):928–33.
16. Hugot JP, Laurent-Puig P, Gower-Rousseau C *et al.* Mapping of a susceptibility locus for Crohn's disease on chromosome 16. Nature. 1996;379:821–3.
17. Satsangi J, Parkes M, Louis E *et al.* Two-stage genome-wide search in inflammatory bowel disease: evidence for susceptibility loci on chromosomes 3, 7 and 12. Nature Genet. 1996; 14(2):199–202.

18. Cho JH, Nicolae DL, Gold LH *et al.* Identification of novel susceptibility loci for inflammatory bowel disease on chromosomes 1p, 3q and 4q: evidence for epistasis between 1p and IBD1. Proc Natl Acad Sci USA. 1998;95:7502–7.
19. Hampe J, Schreiber S, Shaw SH *et al.* A genomewide analysis provides evidence for novel linkages in inflammatory bowel disease in a large European cohort. Am J Hum Genet. 1999;64(3): 808–16.
20. Ma Y, Ohmen JD, Li Z *et al.* A genome-wide search identifies potential new susceptibility loci for Crohn's disease. Inflamm Bowel Dis. 1999;5(4):271–8.
21. Duerr RH, Barmada MM, Zhang L *et al.* High-density genome scan in Crohn disease shows confirmed linkage to chromosome 14q11–12. Am J Hum Genet. 2000;66(6):1857–62.
22. Rioux JD, Silverberg MS, Daly MJ *et al.* Genomewide search in Canadian families with inflammatory bowel disease reveals two novel susceptibility loci. Am J Hum Genet. 2000;66(6): 1863–70.
23. Lernmark A, Ott J. Sometimes it's hot, sometimes it's not. Nature Genet. 1998;19(3):213.
24. Bell JI, Lathrop GM. Multiple loci for multiple sclerosis. Nature Genet. 1996;13:377–8.
25. Cho JH, Nicolae DL, Ramos R *et al.* Linkage and linkage disequilibrium in chromosome band 1p36 in American Chaldeans with inflammatory bowel disease. Hum Mol Genet. 2000;9(9): 1425–32.
26. Hampe J, Lynch NJ, Daniels S *et al.* Fine mapping of the chromosome 3p susceptibility locus in inflammatory bowel disease. Gut. 2001;48(2):191–7.
27. Paavola P, Helio T, Kiuru M *et al.* Genetic analysis in Finnish families with inflammatory bowel disease supports linkage to chromosome 3p21. Eur J Hum Genet. 2001;9(5):328–34.
28. Parkes M, Satsangi J, Jewell DP. Fine mapping the IBD linkage on chromosome 3. Gastroenterology. 1999;116:A792.
29. Rudolph U, Finegold MJ, Rich SS *et al.* Ulcerative colitis and adenocarcinoma of the colon in Gαi2-deficient mice. Nature Genet. 1995;10:143–9.
30. Zhang WJ, Koltun WA, Tilberg AF *et al.* Absence of GNAI2 codon 179 oncogene mutations in inflammatory bowel disease. Inflamm Bowel Dis. 2000;6(2):103–6.
31. Pokomy RM, Hofmeister A, Galanduk S *et al.* Crohn's disease and ulcerative colitis are associated with the DNA repair gene MLH1. Ann Surg. 1997;225:437.
32. Brant SR, Panhuysen CI, Bailey-Wilson JE *et al.* Linkage heterogeneity for the IBD1 locus in Crohn's disease pedigrees by disease onset and severity [In Process Citation]. Gastroenterology. 2000;119(6):1483–90.
33. Mahler M, Bristol IJ, Sundberg JP *et al.* Genetic analysis of susceptibility to dextran sulfate sodium-induced colitis in mice. Genomics. 1999;55(2):147–56.
34. Asakura H, Tsuchiya M, Aiso S *et al.* Association of the human leukocyte DR2 antigen with Japanese ulcerative colitis. Gastroenterology. 1982;82:413–18.
35. Sigimura K, Asakura H, Mizuki W *et al.* Analysis of genes within the HLA region affecting susceptibility to ulcerative colitis. Hum Immunol. 1993;36:112.
36. Kobayashi K *et al.* HLA-DR, DQ and T cell antigen receptor constant beta genes in Japanese patients with ulcerative colitis. Clin Exp Immunol. 1990;80:400.
37. Toyoda H, Wang S-J, Yang H *et al.* Distinct association of HLA Class II genes with inflammatory bowel disease. Gastroenterology. 1993;104:741–8.
38. McConnell R. Ulcerative colitis – genetics feature. Scand J Gastroenterol. 1983;18:14.1.
39. Satsangi J, Welsh KI, Bunce M *et al.* Contribution of genes of the major histocompatibility complex to susceptibility and disease phenotype in inflammatory bowel disease. Lancet. 1996;347:1212–17.
40. Fujita K, Naito S, Okabe N *et al.* Immunological studies in Crohn's disease. 1. Association with the HLA system in Japanese. J Clin Lab Immunol. 1984;14:99.
41. Kobayashi K. Crohn's disease in the Japanese is associated with the HLA-DRw53. Clin Exp Immunogenet. 1990;7:101.
42. Yang H, Plevy SE, Taylor K *et al.* Linkage of Crohn's disease to the major histocompatibility complex region is detected by multiple non-parametric analyses. Gut. 1999;44(4):519–26.
43. Negoro K, Kinouchi Y, Hiwatashi N *et al.* Crohn's disease is associated with novel polymorphisms in the 5′-flanking region of the tumor necrosis factor gene. Gastroenterology. 1999; 117(5):1062–8.
44. Kinouchi Y, van Heel D, Cardon L *et al.* Transmission disequilibrium testing confirms the association of the TNF 1031 C allele with Crohn's disease. Gastroenterology. 2000;118:A2321.

45. van Heel DA, Kinouchi Y, Cardon LR *et al.* Transmission disequilibrium testing confirms the association of the TNF a -1031C allele with Crohn's disease. Gut. 2001;48(Supplement 1): A319.
46. Duerr RH, Barmada MM, Zhang L *et al.* Linkage and association between inflammatory bowel disease and a locus on chromosome 12. Am J Hum Genet. 1998;63(1):95–100.
47. Curran ME, Lau KF, Hampe J *et al.* Genetic analysis of inflammatory bowel disease in a large European cohort supports linkage to chromosomes 12 and 16. Gastroenterology. 1998;115(5): 1066–71.
48. Akolkar P, Gulwani B, Lin X *et al.* Fine mapping of regions linked to Crohn's disease on chromosomes 12 and 16. Am J Hum Genet. 1998;63(4):A279 (abst. A).
49. International IBD Genetics Consortium. International collaboration provides convincing linkage replication in complex disease through analysis of a large pooled data set: Crohn disease and chromosome 16. Am J Hum Genet. 2001;68(5):1165–71.
50. Rioux JD, Daly MJ, Green T *et al.* Absence of linkage between inflammatory bowel disease and selected loci on chromosomes 3, 7, 12 and 16. Gastroenterology. 1998;115(5):1062–5.
51. Suarez B, Hampe C, Eerdewegh PV. Problems of replicating linkage claims in psychiatry. In: Gershon E, Cloniger C, editors, Genetic Approaches to Mental Disorders. Washington DC: Am. Psychiatric Press, 1994:23–46.
52. Mandal DM, Sorant AJ, Pugh EW *et al.* Environmental covariates: effects on the power of sib-pair linkage methods. Genet Epidemiol. 1999;17(Suppl 1):S643–8.
53. Kruglyak L, Lander ES. Limits on fine mapping of complex traits [letter]. Am J Hum Genet. 1996;58(5):1092–3.
54. Podolin PL, Denny P, Armitage N *et al.* Localization of two insulin-dependent diabetes (Idd) genes to the Idd 10 region on mouse chromosome 3. Mamm Genome. 1998;9(4):283–6.
55. Parkes M, Satsangi J, Merriman A *et al.* Precision mapping of chromosome 12 linkage in IBD: evidence of a haplotype association. Gastroenterology. 1998;114(4):A1058.
56. Hampe J, Hermann B, Bridger S *et al.* The interferon-gamma gene as a positional and functional candidate gene for inflammatory bowel disease. Int J Colorectal Dis. 1998;13(5–6):260–3.
57. Heel DV, Carey A, Jewell D. Novel polymorphism in the Beta 7 integrin gene: family based association studies in IBD. Gut. 2001;43:3 (abstract).
58. Simmons JD, Mullighan C, Welsh KI *et al.* Vitamin D receptor gene polymorphism: association with Crohn's disease susceptibility. Gut. 2000;47(2):211–14.
59. Vermeire S, Vlietinck R, Peeters M *et al.* Replication of linkage on 14q11 in IBD. Gastroenterology. 2000;118:A338.
60. Weaver T. High-throughput SNP discovery and typing for genome-wide genetic analysis. Trends Genet. 2000;Suppl 1:36–42.
61. Chakravarti A. To a future of genetic medicine. Nature. 2001;409(6822):822–3.

5 Defining clinical activity in Crohn's disease

D. B. SACHAR

An ancient tradition calls for answering a question with a question. For example, when the late F. T. de Dombal addressed the question of how to measure how bad a particular case of Crohn's disease was, he responded with the question: 'What do we mean by "bad"?'[1]. Similarly, faced with the question, 'What is the best measure of disease activity in Crohn's disease?', my first response is, 'Who wants to know?' This response is the key to formulating a useful answer to the persistent question of how best to measure disease activity, since the choice will depend upon whether the questioner is a basic laboratory scientist, a clinical laboratory investigator, a clinical trialist, a pathologist, a radiologist, a surgeon, an endoscopist, a health policy administrator, a patient, or a treating physician. Let us consider each of these scenarios individually.

BASIC LABORATORY SCIENTISTS

The basic scientist will seek an objective biochemical or cellular marker of inflammatory activity in blood or tissue. For both theoretical and logistical simplicity, blood *cytokine* markers have proved popular for this purpose[2], with circulating interleukin-1 receptor antagonist[3,4] and interleukin-6[5,6] both having shown positive correlation with other biological and clinical indicators of Crohn's disease activity. Other circulating biochemical markers of inflammation that have been applied to earlier studies of Crohn's disease include *collagen* degradation products like serum C-terminal telopeptide of type I collagen, S-ICTP[7]; *coagulation proteins* like factor VIII[8] and factor XIIIA subunit[9]; and measures of *cellular adhesion* like circulating soluble intercellular adhesion molecule-1, sICAM-1[10], or direct microscopic assessment of leukocyte adhesiveness/aggregation[11].

More recently, however, attention has been turning away from peripheral blood and focusing increasingly on cytokine expression at the gut tissue level itself[12–14], on TNF synthesis by gut mucosal mononuclear cells[15], and even on subcellular migration of key mediators like NF-kappa B[16]. What all these basic laboratory studies have in common, of course, are a quest for objectivity and reproducibility and an exploration of the underlying pathophysiology of the inflammatory bowel diseases, often regardless of the dichotomy between laboratory indicators of 'inflammatory activity' and clinical measures of 'disease severity'[17].

CLINICAL LABORATORY INVESTIGATORS

The methods and goals of basic and clinical laboratory investigators overlap to a large and healthy extent. What sometimes distinguishes their efforts, though, is a relatively greater interest by the latter group in establishing direct correlations between physiological markers of inflammation and clinical assessments of disease course. Moreover, most clinical laboratory scientists try to employ techniques that are at least potentially, even if not routinely, accessible to clinicians.

The avenues explored by clinical laboratory investigators of Crohn's disease tend to fall into three principal groups: intestinal permeability markers that 'leak' *out* of the gut, inflammatory and permeability markers that 'leak' *into* the gut, and inflammatory indicators excreted in the urine. The first group comprises measurements of macromolecular absorption from the gut, either sugars as with lactulose/L-rhamnose ratios[18,19] or ^{51}chromium-labelled ethylene diamine tetraacetate, EDTA[20–22]. Happily for the patients, investigators, and technicians, these measurements are made from simple urine collections.

The second category of markers, however, requires stool collections of various thoroughness and duration. Relatively complex tests include measurement of immunoglubulin G in gut lavage fluid[23], assays of leukotriene-B4 in rectal dialysis fluid[24], and radioactive counts of ^{111}indium-labelled white blood cells in stool[25,26]. Relatively simple and more practical these days are faecal measurements of stable white blood cell protein products, such as alpha-1 antitrypsin[27–29], lactoferrin[30,31], and, recently most promising, the neutrophil calcium-binding protein, calprotectin[26,32,33].

The third group of clinical laboratory investigative markers of Crohn's disease activity comprises urinary levels of inflammatory indicators like neopterin[34,35] or F2-isoprostanes[36]. Indeed, it is hard to open any month's journals of gastroenterology without coming across some newly proposed laboratory markers of disease activity, but, if I had to venture a prediction of the most promising among them today, I would favour faecal calprotectin concentration for its sensitivity and its relative ease of measurement in spot samples[37].

CLINICAL TRIALISTS

Probably the greatest investment of time and effort in the study of activity markers in Crohn's disease has been stimulated by the need for quantitative, consistent and reproducible outcome measures for *clinical trials*. Indeed, a forthcoming review of clinical trial endpoints has already occupied the considerable energies of a 'blue-ribbon' joint task force of the Crohn's and Colitis Foundation of America (CCFA), the Crohn's and Colitis Foundation of Canada (CCFC), the Groupe d'Etude Thérapeutique des Affections Inflammatoires Digestives (GETAID), and the International Organization for the Study of Inflammatory Bowel Disease (IOIBD).

Of course, there is little doubt that the most widely used instrument for measuring Crohn's disease activity in clinical trials is the CDAI, or Crohn's Disease Activity Index, developed in the 1970s for the purposes of the National Cooperative Crohn's Disease Study[38,39]. Latter-day critiques of the CDAI have been abundant throughout the subsequent decades[40,41]. The best known effort to simplify it has been the Harvey-Bradshaw Index[42], with somewhat less well-known modifications proposed by Clamp and Softley and colleagues in 1984[43] and by Wright *et al.* in 1985[44]. These latter indices are all variations on the same CDAI theme, so it is not surprising that they correlate with each other[40] and that they offer few advantages over each other, except perhaps for the refreshing ease of calculation of the Harvey-Bradshaw ('Simple') Index, whose bibliographical citation is unique in consisting of a single page[41].

Another widely cited alternative to the CDAI is the van Hees or Dutch Index[45]. It is puzzling that this index is often alluded to as relying much more on laboratory values than the CDAI. In fact, while the CDAI has only one laboratory component (haematocrit) out of eight items, the van Hees Index has only two (albumin and erythrocytic sedimentation rate) out of nine – hardly a statistically significant difference! Nonetheless, the van Hees Index correlates poorly with the CDAI, the Harvey-Bradshaw Index, the Softley–Clamp OMGE Index, or Wright's Cape Town Index[40], and it is rarely used today in clinical trials.

However, reference to the laboratory components of the various indices does bring us to further discussion of the use of more-or-less 'routine' laboratory tests for another clinical investigative purpose besides therapeutic trials; namely, to *predict or define relapses* of Crohn's disease. I have reviewed this topic elsewhere[46], so the details need not be repeated here. Suffice it to say that concerted efforts have been made to predict[47] or define[48] relapses of Crohn's disease on the basis of formulas constructed retrospectively from masses of laboratory data on hundreds if not thousands of patients.

Of course, it comes as no surprise to clinicians that such simple blood tests as haemoglobin, haematocrit, white blood cell count, platelet count, or serum albumin provide non-specific indications of inflammation. When it comes to correlations with global clinical assessment of 'disease activity', however, three of the laboratory tests that seem to perform particularly well, albeit far from perfectly, in Crohn's disease are the erythrocytic sedimentation rate, or ESR[29,32,47,49,50]; the C-reactive protein, or CRP[29,32,47,51,52]; and the serum alpha-1 acid glycoprotein, or orosomucoid[29,47,53].

Evaluation of many of these clinical indices and laboratory tests has been the subject of a number of recent reviews[54,55]. Special considerations must be undertaken when assessing disease activity in children[55]. In all cases, moreover, it is essential to take into account the influences on these measurements that are exerted by recent treatment status, prior surgery, or anatomic extent, distribution, and clinical pattern of disease[46].

OTHER MEDICAL SPECIALISTS

Clearly, each diagnostic or therapeutic specialty will bring its own skills, interests, and concerns to bear on the process of measuring disease activity. The *pathologist*, for example, will focus on gross[56] or histological[57–59] scoring systems for severity of microscopic inflammation and macroscopic tissue injury. Similarly, the *surgeon* will want to know the initial disease location, as categorized in the Vienna Classification[60], as well as the operative history, which is incorporated in broad outline in the Rome Classification[61] and in much more anatomic detail in the short-lived but ingenious SICK-SLICE system proposed by Best and Lee[56]. More specifically, the colorectal surgeon who is studying perianal Crohn's disease will most likely adopt Irvine's five-item Perianal Crohn's Disease Activity Index, or PDAI[62].

The *radiologist* has a broad array of imaging techniques available for disease assessment. The principal nuclear methods comprise scintigraphy of radionuclide-labelled white blood cells with either ^{111}indium[63], or more recently with ^{99m}technetium hexamethyl propylene amine oxime, or HMPAO[64,65]. More traditional methods include assessments of disease status and activity by ultrasound[66,67] or magnetic resonance imaging[68,69]. Complementary to radiological imaging, of course, is *endoscopy*, The most scholarly endoscopists and their colleagues in France and Belgium have developed and validated two highly useful scoring systems: for colonic lesions, the Crohn's Disease Endoscopic Index of Severity, or CDEIS[70]; and for recurrent pre-anastomotic disease in the neoterminal ileum, the Rutgeerts Index[71].

HEALTH POLICY ADMINISTRATORS

If life's only certainties are death and taxes, then health policy workers are surely well-justified in focusing attention on mortality, morbidity, and costs. The related disciplines of cost–utility calculation, decision analysis, and pharmacoeconomics all come into play when addressing health policy issues in Crohn's disease related to medical therapy[72–75], surgery[76,77], colonoscopic surveillance for cancer[78], nutritional support[79], and nursing strategies[80].

PATIENTS

In the last analysis, of course, it is the patients who have the greatest stake in wise decision-making regarding management of their disease, but it is not a favourable number or an index or a score they seek. They just want to feel well. It is the effort to gauge our success as a profession in helping them meet this goal that has led us to devise instruments to measure 'quality of life'. Reviews and assessments of these various instruments can and do fill volumes, but, with respect to Crohn's disease, the two most highly developed and widely applied tools are the Rating Form of IBD Patient Concerns[81] and the Inflammatory Bowel Disease Questionnaire (IBDQ), which exists both as a full 32-question form[82] and in a shorter 10-item version[83]. Whatever an individual practitioner may feel about the practicality and utility of such instruments, there can be no argument about the importance of the entities they seek to measure.

TREATING PHYSICIANS

It is the treating physicians who have the closest personal relationships with patients, gather the most clinical and laboratory data on them, and bear the heaviest responsibility for their medical care, yet they rely the *least* on quantitative indices and scoring systems to guide them in their management. Advocates of 'evidence-based medicine' decry the aversion of practitioners for systematic and quantitative approaches to medical decision-making, but, as treating physicians, we are often flying in what Davidoff has called 'the teeth of the evidence'[84]. We incorporate history, physical examination, laboratory data, histology, radiology and endoscopy, as well as economic, cultural and psychosocial factors, into the process of making life-altering decisions and recommendations, yet we do this with little more consciousness of the cognitive steps we are taking than when we drive a car or catch a baseball.

Perhaps it is for all these reasons, as well as on account of the heterogeneity of Crohn's disease and the unpredictability of the human condition, that our quest for the Holy Grail of one 'best measure of disease activity' still remains today, in Korelitz's words of fifteen years ago, 'a need unfulfilled'[85].

References

1. de Dombal FT. Measures of disease activity. In: Bayless TM, editor. Current Management of Inflammatory Bowel Disease. Toronto and Philadelphia, B.C. Dekker Inc. 1989;1–8.
2. Hodgson HJF. Inflammatory cytokines, naturally occurring regulators of inflammation, and inflammatory bowel disease. Eur J Gastroenterol Hepatol. 1995;7:1021–3.
3. Hyams JS, Fitzgerald JE, Wyzga N, Treem WR, Justinich CJ, Kreutzer DL. Characterization of circulating interleukin-1 receptor antagonist expression in children with inflammatory bowel disease. Dig Dis Sci. 1994;39:1893–9.
4. Propst A, Propst T, Herold M, Vogel W, Judmaier G. Interleukin-1 receptor antagonist in differential diagnosis of inflammatory bowel diseases. Eur J Gastroenterol Hepatol. 1995;7:1031–6.
5. Lobo AJ, Evans SW, Jones SC *et al.* Plasma interleukin-6 in inflammatory bowel disease. Eur J Gastroenterol Hepatol. 1992;4:367–72.
6. Louis E, Belaiche J, van Kemseke C *et al.* A high serum concentration of interleukin-6 is predictive of relapse in quiescent Crohn's disease. Eur J Gastroenterol Hepatol. 1997;9:939–44.
7. Kjeldsen J, Schafflitsky de Muckadell OB, Junker P. Seromarkers of collagen I and III metabolism in active Crohn's disease: relation to disease activity and response to therapy. Gut. 1995;37:805–10.
8. Zielen S, Bender SW, Krenz W, Posselt HG, Solem F, Scharrer L. Crohn's disease activity: assessment by factor VIII coagulation proteins. J Pediatr Gastroenterol Nutr. 1985;4:730–4.
9. Hudson M, Wakefield AJ, Hutton RA *et al.* Factor XIIIA subunit and Crohn's disease. Gut. 1993;34:75–9.
10. Nielsen OH, Langholz E, Hendel J, Brynskov J. Circulating soluble intercellular adhesion molecule-1 (sICAM-1) in active inflammatory bowel disease. Dig Dis Sci. 1994;39:1918–23.
11. Arber N, Berliner S, Hallak A *et al.* Increased leucocyte adhesiveness/aggregation is a most useful indicator of disease activity in patients with inflammatory bowel disease. Gut. 1995;37:77–80.
12. Seegert D, Rosenstiel P, Pfahler H, Pfefferkorn P, Nikolaus S, Schreiber S. Increased expression of IL-16 in inflammatory bowel disease. Gut. 2001;48:326–32.
13. Kanai T, Watanabe M, Okazawa A, Sato T, Hibi T. Interleukin-18 and Crohn's disease. Digestion. 2001;63 (Suppl 1):37–42.
14. Arnott ID, Drummond HE, Ghosh S. Gut mucosal secretion of interleukin 1beta and interleukin 8 predicts relapse in clinically inactive Crohn's disease. Dig Dis Sci. 2001;46:402–9.

15. Plevy SE, Landers CJ, Prehn J *et al.* A role for TNF-alpha and mucosal T helper-1 cytokines in the pathogenesis of Crohn's disease. J Immunol. 1997;159:6276–82.
16. Schreiber S, Nikolaus S, Hampe J. Activation of nuclear factor Kappa B in inflammatory bowel disease. Gut. 1998;42:477–84.
17. Maratka Z. Crohn's disease activity indexes: need for distinguishing activity from severity. Hepato-gastroenterology. 1981;28:187–8.
18. Miki K, Moore DJ, Butler RN, Southcott E, Couper RT, Davidson GP. The sugar permeability test reflects disease activity in children and adolescents with inflammatory bowel disease. J Pediatr. 1998;133:750–4.
19. Arnott ID, Kingstone K, Ghosh S. Abnormal intestinal permeability predicts relapse in inactive Crohn disease. Scand J Gastroenterol. 2000;35:1163–9.
20. Irvine EJ, Marshall JK. Increased intestinal permeability precedes the onset of Crohn's disease in a subject with familial risk. Gastroenterology. 2000;119:1740–4.
21. Jorgensen J, Ranlov PJ, Bjerrum PJ, Diemer H, Bisgaard K, Elsborg L. Is an increased intestinal permeability a valid predictor of relapse in Crohn disease? Scand J Gastroenterol. 2001;36: 521–7.
22. Vermeire S, Peeters M, Vlietinck R *et al.* Anti-Saccharomyces cerevisiae antibodies (ASCA), phenotypes of IBD, and intestinal permeability: a study in IBD families. Inflamm Bowel Dis. 2001;7:8–15.
23. Choudari CP, O'Mahony S, Brydon G, Mwantembe O, Ferguson A. Gut lavage fluid protein concentrations: objective measures of disease activity in inflammatory bowel disease. Gastroenterology. 1993;104:1064–71.
24. Roberts WG, Simon TJ, Berlin RG *et al.* Leukotrienes in ulcerative colitis: results of a multicenter trial of a leukotriene biosynthesis inhibitor, MK-591. Gastroenterology. 1997;112:725–32.
25. Saverymuttu SH, Peters AM, Lavender JP. Quantitative fecal indium-111 labeled leukocyte excretion in the assessment of disease activity in Crohn's disease. Gastroenterology. 1983;85:1333–9.
26. Roseth AG, Schmidt PN, Fagerhol MK, Roseth AG, Schmidt PN, Fagerhol MK. Correlation between faecal excretion of indium-111-labelled granulocytes and calprotectin, a granulocyte marker protein, in patients with inflammatory bowel disease. Scand J Gastroenterol. 1999;34: 50–4.
27. Karbach U, Ewe K, Bodenstein H. Alpha 1 antitrypsin, a reliable endogenous marker for intestinal protein loss and its application in patients with Crohn's disease. Gut. 1983;24:718–23.
28. Meyers S, Wolke A, Field SP, Feuer EJ, Johnson JW, Janowitz HD. Fecal alpha 1-antitrypsin measurement: an indicator of Crohn's disease activity. Gastroenterology. 1985;89:13–18.
29. Cellier C, Sahmoud T, Froguel E *et al.* Correlations between clinical activity, endoscopic severity, and biological parameters in colonic or ileocolonic Crohn's disease: a prospective multicentre study of 121 cases. Gut. 1994;35:231–5.
30. Sugi K, Saitoh O, Hirata I, Katsu K. Fecal lactoferrin as a marker for disease activity in inflammatory bowel disease: comparison with other neutrophil-derived proteins. Am J Gastroenterol. 1996;91:927–34.
31. Fine KD, Ogunji F, George J, Niehaus MD, Guerrant RL. Utility of a rapid fecal latex agglutination test detecting the neutrophil protein, lactoferrin, for diagnosing inflammatory causes of chronic diarrhea. Am J Gastroenterol. 1998;93:1300–5.
32. Tibble J, Sigthorsson G, Bridger S, Fagerhol MK, Bjarnason I. Surrogate markers of intestinal inflammation are predictive of relapse in patients with inflammatory bowel disease. Gastroenterology. 2000;119:15–22.
33. Limburg P, Ahlquist D, Sandborn W, Mahoney DW, Devens ME, Harrington JJ. Fecal calprotectin levels predict colorectal inflammation among patients with chronic diarrhea referred for colonoscopy. Am J Gastroenterol. 2000;95:2831–7.
34. Prior C, Bollbach R, Fuchs D *et al.* Urinary neopterin, a marker of clinical activity in patients with Crohn's disease. Clin Chim Acta. 1986;155:11–21.
35. Judmaier G, Meyersbach P, Weiss G, Wachter H, Reibnegger G. The role of neopterin in assessing disease activity in Crohn's disease: classification and regression trees. Am J Gastroenterol. 1993;88:706–11.
36. Cracowski JL, Stanke-Labesque F, Souvignet C, Bessard G. Isoprostanes: new markers of oxidative stress in human diseases. (Article in French) Presse Med. 2000;29:604–10.
37. Tibble J, Teahon K, Thjodleifsson B *et al.* A simple method for assessing intestinal inflammation in Crohn's disease. Gut. 2000;47:506–13.

38. Best WR, Becktel JM, Singleton JW, Kern F, Jr. Development of a Crohn's disease activity index. National Cooperative Crohn's Disease Study. Gastroenterology. 1976;70:439–44.
39. Best WR, Becktel JM, Singleton JW. Rederived values of the eight coefficients of the Crohn's Disease Activity Index (CDAI). Gastroenterology. 1979;77:843–6.
40. de Dombal FT, Softley A. IOIBD report no. 1: observer variation in calculating indices of severity and activity in Crohn's disease. Gut. 1987;28:474–81.
41. Korelitz BI. Is the Crohn's Disease Activity Index outdated? Yes. Is it the gold standard that clinicians should use? No. Inflamm Bowel Dis. 1999;5:139–43.
42. Harvey RF, Bradshaw JM. A simple index of Crohn's disease activity. Lancet. 1980;1:514.
43. Myren J, Bouchier IA, Watkinson G, Softley A, Clamp SE, de Dombal FT. The OMGE multinational inflammatory bowel disease survey 1976–1982: a further report in 2,657 cases. Scand J Gastroenterol. Suppl. 1984;95:1–27.
44. Wright JP, Marks IN, Parfitt A. A simple index of Crohn's disease activity – the Cape Town index. S Afr Med J. 1985;68:502–3.
45. van Hees PA, van Elteren PH, van Lier HJJ, van Tongeren JHM. An index of inflammatory activity in patients with Crohn's disease. Gut. 1980;21:279–86.
46. Sachar DB. Predicting relapses of Crohn's disease: clouds in the crystal ball (editorial). Dig Dis Sci. 1897;32:206–8.
47. Wright JP, Young GO, Tigler-Wybrandi N. Predictors of acute relapse of Crohn's disease: a laboratory and clinical study. Dig Dis Sci. 1987;32:164–70.
48. André C, Descos L, André F, Vignal J, Landais P, Fermanian J. Biological measurements of Crohn's disease activity – a reassessment. Hepatogastroenterology. 1985;32:135–7.
49. Sachar DB, Smith H, Chan S, Cohen LB, Lichtiger S, Messer J. Erythrocytic sedimentation rate as a measure of clinical activity in inflammatory bowel disease. J Clin Gastroenterol. 1986;8:647–50.
50. Sachar DB, Luppescu NE, Bodian C, Shlien TD, Fabry TL, Gumaste VV. Erythrocytic sedimentation rate as a measure of Crohn's disease activity: opposite trends in ileitis versus colitis. J Clin Gastroenterol. 1990;12:643–6.
51. Pepys MB, Baltz BL. Acute phase proteins with special reference to C-reactive protein and related proteins (pentraxins) and serum amyloid A protein. Adv Immunol. 1983;34:141–212.
52. Fagan EA, Dyck RF, Maton PN *et al.* Serum levels of C-reactive protein in Crohn's disease and ulcerative colitis. Eur J Clin Invest. 1982;12:351–9.
53. Kjeldsen J, Lauritsen K, De Muckadell OB. Serum concentrations of orosomucoid: improved decision-making for tapering prednisolone therapy in patients with active inflammatory bowel disease? Scand J Gastroenterol. 1997;32:933–41.
54. Nielsen OH, Vainer B, Madsen SM, Seidelin JB, Heegard NH. Established and emerging biological activity markers of inflammatory bowel disease. Am J Gastroenterol. 2000;95:1849–50.
55. Otley A, Loonen H, Parekh N, Corey M, Sherman PM, Griffiths AM. Assessing activity of pediatric Crohn's disease: which index to use? Gastroenterology. 1999;116:527–31.
56. Best WR, Lee ECG. A system for anatomical coding of Crohn's disease involvement. In: de Dombal FT, Myren J, Bouchier IAD, Watkinson G, editors, Inflammatory Bowel Disease: Some International Data and Reflections. Oxford, England: Oxford University Press, 1986:286.
57. Keren DF, Appelman HD, Dobbins WO III *et al.* Correlation of histopathologic evidence of disease activity with the presence of immunoglobulin-containing cells in the colons of patients with inflammatory bowel disease. Hum Pathol. 1984;15:757–63.
58. Korelitz BI, Sommers SC. Response to drug therapy in Crohn's disease: evaluation by rectal biopsy and mucosal cell counts. J Clin Gastroenterol. 1984;6:123–7.
59. D'Haens GR, Geboes K, Peeters M, Baert F, Penninckx F, Rutgeerts P. Early lesions of recurrent Crohn's disease caused by infusion of intestinal contents in excluded ileum. Gastroenterology. 1998;114:262–7.
60. Gasché C, Scholmerich J, Brynskov J *et al.* A simple classification of Crohn's disease: report of the Working Party for the World Congresses of Gastroenterology, Vienna 1998. Inflamm Bowel Dis. 1999;6:8–15.
61. Sachar DB, Andrews HA, Farmer RG *et al.* Proposed classification of patient subgroups in Crohn's disease. Gastroenterol Int. 1992;5:141–54.
62. Irvine EJ, for the McMaster IBD Study Group. Usual therapy improves perianal Crohn's disease as measured by a new disease activity index. J Clin Gastroenterol. 1995;20:27–32.

63. Saverymuttu SH, Camilleri M, Rees H, Lavender JP, Hodgson HJF, Chadwick VS. Indium 111-granulocyte scanning in the assessment of disease extent and disease activity in inflammatory bowel disease: a comparison with colonoscopy, histology and fecal indium-111 granulocyte excretion. Gastroenterology. 1986;90:1121–8.
64. Schölmerich J, Schmidt E, Schumichen C, Billman P, Schmidt H, Gerok W. Scintigraphic assessment of bowel involvement and disease activity in Crohn's disease using technetium 99m-hexamethyl propylene amine oxime as leucocyte label. Gastroenterology. 1988;95:1287–93.
65. Sciaretta G, Furno A, Mazzoni M, Basile C, Malaguti P. Technetium-99m hexamethyl propylene amine oxime granulocyte scintigraphy in Crohn's disease: diagnostic and clinical relevance. Gut. 1993;34:1364–9.
66. Futagami Y, Haruma K, Hata J *et al.* Development and validation of an ultrasonographic activity index of Crohn's disease. Eur J Gastroenterol Hepatol. 1999;11:1007–12.
67. Haber HP, Busch A, Ziebach R, Stern M. Bowel wall thickness measured by ultrasound as a marker of Crohn's disease activity in children (letter). Lancet. 2000;355:1239–40.
68. Maccioni F, Viscido A, Broglia L *et al.* Evaluation of Crohn disease activity with magnetic resonance imaging. Abdom Imaging. 2000;25:219–28.
69. Schunk K, Kern A, Oberholzer K *et al.* Hydro-MRI in Crohn's disease: appraisal of disease activity. Invest Radiol. 2000;35(7):431–7.
70. Mary JY, Modigliani R, for GETAID. Development and validation of an endoscopic index of the severity for Crohn's disease: a prospective multicentre study. Gut. 1989;30:983–9.
71. Rutgeerts P, Geboes K, Vantrappen G, Kerremans R, Coenegrachts JL, Coremans G. Natural history of recurrent Crohn's disease at the ileocolonic anastomosis after curative surgery. Gut. 1984;25:665–72.
72. Kennedy ED, Detsky AS, Llewellyn-Thomas HA *et al.* Can the standard gamble be used to determine utilities for uncertain health states? An example using postoperative maintenance therapy in Crohn's disease. Med Decis Making. 2000;20:72–8.
73. Feagan BG. Economic issues in Crohn's disease – assessing the effects of new treatments on health-related quality of life (review article). Aliment Pharmacol Ther. 1999;13(Suppl 4):29–37.
74. Ward FM, Bodger K, Daly MJ, Heatley RV. Clinical economics review: medical management of inflammatory bowel disease. Aliment Pharmacol Ther. 1999;13:15–25.
75. Trallori G, Messori A. Drug treatments for maintaining remission in Crohn's disease. A lifetime cost–utility analysis. Pharmacoeconomics. 1997;11:444–53.
76. Sardinha TC, Wexner SD. Laparoscopy for inflammatory bowel disease: pros and cons. World J Surg. 1998;22(4):370–4.
77. Sonnenberg A, Gavin MW. Timing of surgery for enterovesical fistula in Crohn's disease: decision analysis using a time-dependent compartment model. Inflamm Bowel Dis. 2000;6:280–5.
78. Solomon MJ, Schnitzler M. Cancer and inflammatory bowel disease: bias, epidemiology, surveillance, and treatment. World J Surg. 1998;22:352–8.
79. Malone M. Quality of life of patients receiving home parenteral or enteral nutrition support. Pharmacoeconomics. 1994;5:101–8.
80. Nightingale AJ, Middleton W, Middleton SJ, Hunter JO. Evaluation of the effectiveness of a specialist nurse in the management of inflammatory bowel disease (IBD). Eur J Gastroenterol Hepatol. 2000;12:967–73.
81. Drossman DA, Leserman J, Li ZM, Mitchell CM, Zagami EA, Patrick DL. The rating form of IBD patient concerns: a new measure of health status. Psychosom Med. 1991;53:701–12.
82. Guyatt G, Mitchell A, Irvine EJ *et al.* A new measure of health status for clinical trials in inflammatory bowel disease. Gastroenterology. 1989;96:804–10.
83. Irvine EJ, Zhou Q, Thompson AK. The Short Inflammatory Bowel Disease Questionnaire: a quality of life instrument for community physicians managing inflammatory bowel disease. CCRPT Investigators. Canadian Crohn's Relapse Prevention Trial. Am J Gastroenterol. 1996;91:1571–8.
84. Davidoff F. In the teeth of the evidence: the curious case of evidence-based medicine. Mt Sinai J Med. 1999;66:75–83.
85. Korelitz BI. An indicator of Crohn's disease activity – a need unfulfilled. J Clin Gastroenterol. 1986;8:220–2.

Section II
Paediatrics in IBD

6
Severe ulcerative colitis in a toddler: a complicated course

F. VIOLA, C. PACCHIAROTTI, G. DI NARDO, M. PORCELLI, L. DITO, A. L. GRANDINETTI and S. CUCCHIARA

Inflammatory bowel disease (IBD) includes two major entities, ulcerative colitis (UC) and Crohn's disease (CD), and a third form, known as indeterminate colitis, that is when the traditional diagnostic tools do not allow a clear differentiation between UC and CD[1]. Approximately 25–30% of CD patients and 20% of those with UC have their onset of disease before the age of 20 years. Recently, it has been shown that the incidence of IBD among children and adolescents is increasing over time. For UC, various studies[2–6] have reported the incidence in children to be 1.5–10 cases per 10^5 head of population per year; the prevalence appears to be 18 to 30 per 10^5. For CD[6], the incidence in children seems to be 3.11 cases per 10^5 population per year; the prevalence is 20 per 10^5. Males and females are equally affected.

Diagnosis of IBD in childhood rests upon the exclusion of systemic and infectious disorders and upon the same investigative tools as in adult gastroenterology. Classical clinical features are similar to those described in adults; however, impairment of nutritional status and linear growth as well as pubertal delay characterize IBD in children[7]. Even if IBD during the paediatric age is more frequently detected in adolescents, recent data indicate that is not unusual to see young children with UC and that the latter can also be observed during the first year of age[8].

We describe a case of UC in a toddler, characterized by a complicated clinical course due to refractoriness to conventional anti-inflammatory therapy. The case is of interest because it raises several comments.

CASE REPORT

A 17-month-old male child was referred to our Unit for diarrhoea with mucus and streaks of blood in the stools by the age of 12 months, when his weight and height were 10.450 kg and 75 cm, with a weight/height ratio at 75th percentile.

Table 1 Main diagnostic hypotheses in a toddler with diarrhoea and haematochezia

- Infectious colitis
- Food allergy colitis
- Post-antibiotic colitis
- Inflammatory bowel disease
- Autoimmune enteropathy
- Colitis in immunodeficiency
- Enterocolitis in Hirschsprung's disease

The family history was positive for ulcerative colitis (mother affected) and negative for atopic disorders. He was breast fed for 4 months, then cow's milk was introduced into his diet. Weaning started at 6 months of age. Growth was regular and stools were normal for the first 12 months of life.

At the age of 13 months, he presented with colicky abdominal pain, poor caloric intake, and a marked weight failure (weight was 9.500 kg). Cow's milk allergy was suspected but, despite administration of a casein-hydrolysed formula, there was no symptomatic improvement. At the age of 14 months, his weight was at the 10th percentile (9.350 kg). Subsequently, he was fed with rice flour, lyophilized lamb and olive oil. However, haematochezia, diarrhoea and failure to thrive persisted. At the age of 16 months, he was admitted to a paediatric unit of a general Hospital. Rectosigmoidoscopy demonstrated rectal inflammation, with erosions, and diffuse small ulcerations. Inflammatory and nutritional activity indices (ESR, RCP, haemoglobin, serum iron and ferritin) were abnormal. Stool bacteria and parasites were negative. Subsequently, he was referred to our Unit at the age of 17 months (weight: 10.600 kg, height: 80 cm, with a weight/height ratio at 25th percentile) for a more extensive diagnostic work up (Table 1).

At admission to our Unit, he was ill, pale and febrile, with abdominal distension and reduced muscle trophism. He underwent nutritional activity and absorption tests, as well as assessment of immunological status. On the basis of the investigative work-up, we excluded immunodeficiency, infectious colitis, and post-antibiotic colitis, and failure to detect anti-enterocyte antibodies made a diagnosis of autoimmune enteropathy unlikely. A colonoscopy showed a diffuse inflammation of all segments of the colon whereas the ileum was apparently normal. Histology of the colon revealed a picture strongly suggestive of ulcerative colitis with a diffuse lymphoplasmacellular infiltrate, crypt distortion and abscesses, cryptitis and mucus depletion. He was treated with steroids (starting with 40 mg of methylprednisolone, given i.v. for one week and then followed by oral administration, according to the widely agreed therapeutic protocols reported in the literature) and sulphasalazine (75 $mg\,kg^{-1}\,day^{-1}$). After a transient improvement during the first two weeks of treatment, haematochezia, loose stools and colicky abdominal pain reappeared. Cyclosporine (Cya) was then given i.v. for one week (4 $mg\,kg^{-1}\,day^{-1}$), followed by oral administration (6 $mg\,kg^{-1}\,day^{-1}$). Azathioprine (1.5 $mg\,kg^{-1}\,day^{-1}$), and 5-ASA (50 $mg\,kg^{-1}\,day^{-1}$) were also introduced as

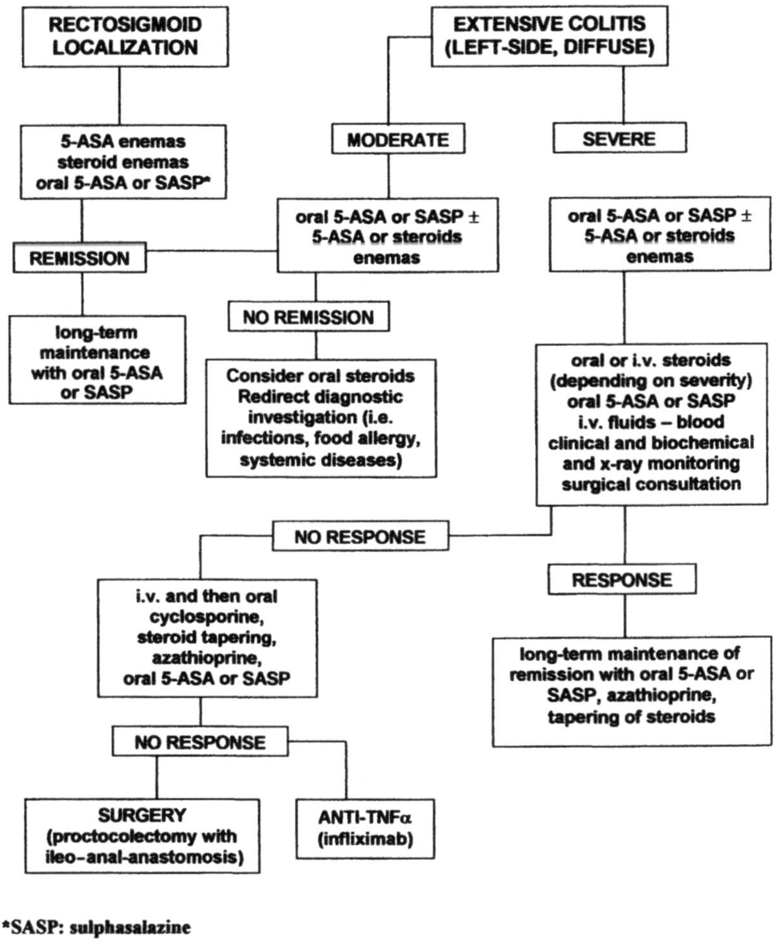

Figure 1 Therapeutic approach to children with ulcerative colitis

antibiotic prophylaxis for infections. Cya was planned for three months with a gradual tapering of steroids. During the first four weeks of treatment, a dramatic improvement in the clinical course was observed, with normalization of stools, reduction of serum activity indices, and weight gain. However, diarrhoea, abdominal pain and haematochezia reappeared after four weeks of treatment. He was admitted to our Unit at the age of 20 months: he was pale, dehydrated and ill. He underwent colonoscopy, which showed a picture of severe diffuse inflammation of all the colonic regions, with friability, erosions and ulcerations of the mucosa. This clinical condition prompted us to plan a proctocolectomy with stapled ileal J-pouch anal anastomosis. Proctocolectomy was successfully performed at the age of 21 months in one stage without a temporary ileostomy. After two weeks, a sudden occlusive episode requiring laparotomy occurred: an internal hernia of a proximal jejunal loop was detected. The subsequent clinical course was uneventful and, six weeks later, bowel movements with normal stools and improvement in caloric intake and weight gain (25th percentile) were observed. Blood activity indexes were normal. The patient was seen as an outpatient at 24 months of age: he appeared well without any gastrointestinal symptoms. He had 2 daily passages of stools of normal consistency. His weight and height were 12.400 kg and 87 cm, respectively, with a weight/height ratio at 50th percentile.

DISCUSSION

This case is worth describing because it raises several points of interest. Firstly, the young age of onset of UC in our patient. Paediatricians are becoming familiar with IBD cases occurring throughout the paediatric age range; however, there are recent reports that emphasize the occurrence of UC in the first year of age[7,8]. This has several diagnostic implications since a careful differential diagnosis should be done with different entities which are typical of the first months of age and mimic UC. In particular, food allergy colitis and infectious colitis must be excluded. Clinical history showed unresponsiveness to a cow's milk extensive hydrolysed formula, and stool cultures were repeatedly negative for the commonest pathogenic organisms. The endoscopic picture, by showing diffuse severe ulcerations of the large bowel mucosa, made the diagnosis of food allergy colitis unlikely, whereas histology strongly suggested UC[9]. Other entities which typically occur during the first months of age were excluded through an exhaustive diagnostic work up; in particular, failure to detect anti-enterocyte antibodies allowed us to exclude an autoimmune enteropathy[10].

The positive family history supported a diagnosis of IBD in our patient. It is well known that the major risk factor for developing an IBD is an affected first-degree relative: it has been calculated that the risk is increased by a factor of 10–15 compared with the general population[11]. Genetic anticipation has been suggested as a possible explanation for an early age at onset and severity of the course as the disease is passed through generations. However, the concept of genetic anticipation in IBD has been challenged due to several methodological biases[12]. It is possible that, as in polygenic disorders, a younger age at onset could be the consequence both of a heavier genetic load in families as compared with sporadic cases and of early exposure to environmental factors[12].

The clinical course was characterized by unresponsiveness to steroids that were given intravenously according to the widely agreed therapeutic protocols[13] (Figure 1). Reappearance of haematochezia and diarrhoea with abdominal pain was evident during oral administration of steroids at full dose. Oral corticosteroids are mainly indicated to induce remission in the acute phases of the disease; they have no place in maintenance therapy and are not efficacious in preventing relapse of UC[14]. In severe acute cases, steroids are usually given intravenously at high doses for a few days followed by oral administration together with other anti-inflammatory drugs.

Cyclosporine is considered a medical alternative to colectomy in severe steroid-refractory UC in adults as well as children[15–17]. The introduction of cyclosporine for use in patients with severe steroid-refractory UC has provided an effective medical alternative to patients previously faced with only the surgical option. Cyclosporine inhibits IL-1-stimulated production of IL-2 and IL-2 receptors by T-cells[18]. Thus it inhibits the induction of cytotoxic T-cells, with relative sparing of suppressor T-cells. It also inhibits the production of B-cell-activating factors and IFN-γ. Therefore, it blunts the cellular immunoresponse. The initial rate of response to cyclosporine has been reported to range from 20% to 80% with either oral or intravenous administration. Response usually occurs within 1–2 weeks of the beginning of treatment; unfortunately, relapses requiring colectomy occur within 1 year in 70–100% of initial responders, either during or after discontinuation of cyclosporine[15–17]. It has been shown that azathioprine (or 6-mercaptopurine), if added early, is useful in maintaining a cyclosporine-induced remission. This is of importance because, without azathioprine (or 6-mercaptopurine), cyclosporine tapering often causes relapse of the disease, and in view of the fact that cyclosporine at low doses is unable to maintain remission[19,20].

Due to relapse of the disease while on therapy with cyclosporine and azathioprine, the child was considered a candidate for surgery. However, the administration of intravenous infliximab was considered. Infliximab is a monoclonal antibody to TNFα, which has been identified as a key mediator in the pathogenesis of IBD, acting early in the cytokine cascade at the level of intestinal mucosa[21]. Whereas infliximab has been widely used in severe refractory Crohn's disease, both in adults and children[22], its use in UC is limited[23,24] and more extensive studies are warranted. Furthermore, there were some concerns about the use of infliximab in this patient due to his young age and to the risk of infection in a subject already treated with immunosuppressive drugs. The child was then referred to the Pediatric Surgical Unit of our University where he successfully underwent one-stage proctocolectomy with ileo-pouch–anal anastomosis without temporary ileostomy.

This case is worth reporting for the following reasons: the young age at onset of the disease (in the first year of age); the importance of a diagnostic work-up aimed at excluding several entities which mimic UC and characteristically occur in infancy; the severe course characterized by refractoriness to systemic steroids and cyclosporine; and, finally, the successful operation with a one-stage proctocolectomy. To our knowledge, this is the smallest child described in the literature who has been subjected to surgical removal of the colon due to severe unresponsive UC.

References

1. Hyams JS. Inflammatory bowel disease. Pediatr Rev. 2000;21:291–5.
2. Olafsdottir EJ, Fluge G, Haug K. Chronic inflammatory bowel disease in children in western Norway. J Pediatr Gastroenterol Nutr. 1989;8:454–8.
3. Binder V, Both H, Hansen TK *et al.* Incidence and prevalence of UC and CD in the County of Copenhagen 1962–1978. Gastroenterology. 1982;83:563–8.
4. Hildebrand H, Fredrikzon B, Holmquist L *et al.* Chronic inflammatory bowel disease in children and adolescents in Sweden. J Pediatr Gastroenterol Nutr. 1991;13:293–7.
5. Barton JR, Gillon S, Ferguson A. Incidence of inflammatory bowel disease in Scottish children between 1968 and 1983: marginal fall in ulcerative colitis, three-fold rise in Crohn's disease. Gut. 1989;30:618–22.
6. Cosgrove M, Al-Atia RF, Jenkins HR. The epidemiology of pediatric inflammatory bowel disease. Arch Dis Child. 1996;74:460–1.

7. Gryboski JD. Ulcerative colitis in children 10 years old or younger. J Pediatr Gastroenterol Nutr. 1993;17:24–31.
8. Dady IM, Thomas AG, Miller V, Kelsen AJ. Inflammatory bowel disease in infancy: an increasing problem? J Pediatr Gastroenterol Nutr. 1996;23:569–76.
9. Bischoff SC, Mayer JH, Manns MP. Allergy and the gut. Int Arch Allergy Immunol. 2000;121:270–83.
10. Russo PA, Brochu PA, Seidman EG, Roy CC. Autoimmune enteropathy. Pediatr Dev Pathol. 1999;2:65–71.
11. Yang H, Rotter JI. The genetics of ulcerative colitis and Crohn's disease. In: Kirsner JB, ed. Inflammatory Bowel Diseases. Philadelphia: Saunders, 2000;250–79.
12. Peeters M, Cortot A, Vermeire S, Colombel JF. Familial and sporadic inflammatory bowel disease: different entities? Inflamm Bowel Dis. 2000;6:314–20.
13. Hanauer SB. Medical therapy for ulcerative colitis. In: Kirsner JB, ed. Inflammatory Bowel Disease. Philadelphia: Saunders, 2000;529–56.
14. Present DH. How to do without steroids in inflammatory bowel disease. Inflamm Bowel Dis. 2000;6:48–57.
15. Benkov KJ, Rosh JR, Schwerenz AH *et al.* Cyclosporine as alternative to surgery in children with inflammatory bowel disease. J Pediatr Gastroenterol Nutr. 1994;19:290–4.
16. Treem WR, Cohen J, Davis PM *et al.* Cyclosporin for the treatment of fulminant ulcerative colitis in children. Dis Colon Rectum. 1995;38:474–9.
17. Cohen RD, Stein R, Hanauer SD. Intravenous cyclosporin in ulcerative colitis: a five year experience. Am J Gastroenterol. 1999;94:1587–92.
18. Sandborn WJ, Tremaine WJ. Cyclosporine treatment of inflammatory bowel disease. Mayo Clin Proc. 1992;67:981–90.
19. Ramakrishna J, Langhans N, Calenda K, Grand RJ, Verhave M. Combined use of cyclosporine and azathioprine or 6-mercaptopurine in pediatric inflammatory bowel disease. J Pediatr Gastroenterol Nutr. 1996;22:296–302.
20. Lobo AJ, Juby LD, Rothwell J *et al.* Long-term treatment of Crohn's disease with cyclosporine: the effect of a very low dose on maintenance of remission. J Clin Gastroenterol. 1991;13:42–5.
21. Sands BE. Biologic therapy for inflammatory bowel disease. Inflamm Bowel Dis. 1997;3: 95–113.
22. Hyams JS, Markowitz J, Wyllie R. Use of infliximab in the treatment of Crohn's disease in children and adolescents. J Pediatr. 2000;137:192–6.
23. Sands BE, Tremaine WJ, Sandborn WJ *et al.* Infliximab in the treatment of severe, steroid-refractory ulcerative colitis: a pilot study. Inflamm Bowel Dis. 2001;7:83–8.
24. Chey WY. Infliximab for patients with refractory ulcerative colitis. Inflamm Bowel Dis. 2001;7:S30–3.

7
Paediatrics in IBD – epidemiology and risk factors

A. EKBOM

Inflammatory bowel diseases (ulcerative colitis and Crohn's disease) are diseases which emerged during the 20th century. These two epidemics are closely linked both genetically and probably also environmentally; populations with high incidence or mortality of Crohn's disease are characterized with a high incidence or mortality of ulcerative colitis and *vice versa*. However, it is worth pointing out that a shift from a low incidence area to a high incidence area in ulcerative colitis usually precedes a similar shift in Crohn's disease with a time lag of about 15–20 years[1].

Paediatric inflammatory bowel disease has, in most descriptive epidemiological studies, been regarded as an outlier in the age-specific incidence, which peaks between the ages of 20 and 40 years in high-incidence areas. Retrospective and prospective incidence studies have shown stable incidence rates in younger age groups over time until the 1980s[1]. In the 1980s, there was a first report from Scotland of a dramatic increase in the incidence of Crohn's disease among paediatric patients with a three-fold increase from 0.7 per 100 000 per year in 1968 to 2.3 in 1983[2]. This increase was present both in males and females and the incidence of ulcerative colitis remained unchanged during this time-period. In a follow-up study through 1992, this increase continued with a reported incidence of 2.8 per 100 000 per year for 1990 to 1992[3]. Similar findings have been reported from Wales[4] where an increase in incidence from 1.3 per 100 000 per year during the period 1983 to 1988 should be compared with an annual incidence of 3.1 per 100 000 per year for the period 1989 to 1993. Similar to the results from the Scottish studies, the incidence of ulcerative colitis remained unchanged and, both in Scotland and Wales, Crohn's disease had a higher annual incidence than ulcerative colitis during the latter time-periods.

The increase in incidence in Scotland was due to an increase in older children, especially among those 12–16 years of age. No such analysis was possible in the data from Wales as the study consisted of only 21 cases of Crohn's disease. This small number is also a good illustration of inherent problems any researcher is facing trying to study temporal trends in paediatric inflammatory bowel disease.

The small number of cases on a yearly basis makes such studies vulnerable to variations caused by chance.

The predominance of Crohn's disease in a paediatric inflammatory bowel disease has recently been confirmed in a survey of childhood inflammatory bowel disease in the British Isles[5]. The authors used a prospective design in order to identify all newly diagnosed cases of inflammatory bowel disease during a period of 13 months (1 June 1998 to 30 June 1999). A total of 739 cases were identified, giving an overall incidence of 5.2 per 100 000 per year, with an incidence of Crohn's disease of 3.1, of ulcerative colitis of 1.4 and indeterminate colitis of 0.6 per 100 000 per year. The highest incidence of Crohn's disease was found in Scotland (4.2); Scotland also has a somewhat higher incidence of ulcerative colitis compared with the rest of the British Isles (1.8 per 100 000 per year). For a subset consisting of about 75% of all patients, it was possible to ascertain details of maternal and paternal ethnicity. Those with an Afro-Caribbean background did not differ from those with an Anglo-Saxon background whereas those with an Asian background had a 50% increased relative risk compared with those with an Anglo-Saxon background. This is in line with a previous small study which also demonstrated an increased incidence among those with an Asian background[6]. This is of special interest as data from the Asian continent indicate a very low incidence of inflammatory bowel disease. These findings therefore strongly indicate the presence of an interaction between environmental and genetic factors.

Results from studies from the United Kingdom have repeatedly been contrasted to data from Scandinavia[7,8], especially Sweden, where the incidence of paediatric inflammatory bowel disease has been stable since the 1960s and with a predominance of ulcerative colitis[1]. However, in a Swedish study which in a population-based setting covered a substantial part of Sweden, there was a rise in incidence between 1984 and 1995[9] from 4.6 per 100 000 per year in the period 1984–1986 to be compared to 7.0 for 1993–1995. In contrast to the figures for the United Kingdom, this was entirely due to an increase in ulcerative colitis (from 1.4 to 3.2 per 100 000 per year) and the annual incidences of Crohn's disease and indeterminate colitis remained unchanged. However, these trends are not representative for all parts of Sweden. In Stockholm[10], there was an overall increase in the incidence of inflammatory bowel disease during the 1990s due to an increase in the incidence of Crohn's disease from 2.4 in 1990–1992 to 5.4 in 1996–1998, and preliminary data from 1999 indicate an even higher incidence. There were also cases in Stockholm of children below the age of five years who were diagnosed during the later part of the study period.

Although one cannot rule out that an increasing awareness of paediatric inflammatory bowel disease, especially Crohn's disease, may be the underlying reason for the increasing trend, the consistency of the findings in Stockholm, Scotland and Wales argues against such a bias. It is therefore not unlikely that we are facing a new phase in the epidemiology of inflammatory bowel disease. This especially affects paediatric Crohn's disease as there are no signs of a decrease in the incidence in the older age groups and the increase can therefore not be explained by an earlier diagnosis. If such an increase is confirmed in other populations, this could be interpreted as meaning that paediatric inflammatory bowel disease, especially Crohn's disease, does not constitute an outlier of an age-specific incidence but is a specific disease entity.

Very little is known to what extent specific clinical characteristics in paediatric inflammatory bowel disease compare to patients who later develop the disease. However, in at least two studies of patients with ulcerative colitis with an onset of disease before the age of 16 years[11,12], this patient group has been found to have an especially high cumulative risk of a malignant transformation of the colorectal tract. It remains unknown whether this is a characteristic which can be causally attributed to an early onset or whether these patients constitute a 'pure' group of patients with IBD. It is, however, obvious that paediatric inflammatory bowel disease patients, especially those with ulcerative colitis, should receive clinical work-up on a regular basis. It has also been shown that patients with an early onset of ulcerative colitis more frequently have extensive disease and proctitis is a rarity. In the case of Crohn's disease, there are scarce data showing to what extent clinical presentation differs from that of other age groups with Crohn's disease.

No special risk factor has been implicated for paediatric inflammatory bowel disease compared with those with onset at an older age. Smoking or former smoking is a non-issue due to the age but exposure to passive smoking has been implicated as a risk factor for both paediatric Crohn's disease and ulcerative colitis[13]. However, there is only one report on this association with a somewhat questionable study design. There have also been reports of genetic anticipation in inflammatory bowel disease, i.e. a stronger family history link with paediatric inflammatory bowel disease compared with other inflammatory bowel disease[14]. However, such studies are hampered by methodological difficulties and there is presently no consensus on the extent to which genetic anticipation exists.

Finally, appendectomy for appendicitis is a protective factor for ulcerative colitis but the extent to which this has a special impact on paediatric inflammatory bowel disease has not been analysed. It is, however, of interest that, in some studies, there are strong indications that the protective effect against ulcerative colitis of an appendectomy for appendicitis is confined to an early appendectomy, i.e. before the age of 20[15].

In conclusion, although no specific characteristics of paediatric inflammatory bowel disease compared with other inflammatory bowel disease have been identified, there are strong indications that we are currently facing a new phase in the temporal trends of Crohn's disease in children. The underlying reasons for this remain an enigma but could, in the future, provide a biological domain where new aetiological factors could be identified.

References

1. Ekbom A, Helmick C, Zack M, Adami HO. The epidemiology of inflammatory bowel disease: a large, population-based study in Sweden. Gastroenterology. 1991;100(2):350–8.
2. Barton JR, Gillon S, Ferguson A. Incidence of inflammatory bowel disease in Scottish children between 1968 and 1983; marginal fall in ulcerative colitis, three-fold rise in Crohn's disease. Gut. 1989;30(5):618–22.
3. Armitage E, Drummond H, Ghosh S, Ferguson A. Incidence of juvenile-onset Crohn's disease in Scotland. Lancet. 1999;353(9163):1496–7.
4. Cosgrove M, Al-Atia RF, Jenkins HR. The epidemiology of paediatric inflammatory bowel disease. Arch Dis Child. 1996;74(5):460–1.
5. Sawczenko A, Sandhu BK, Logan RF *et al.* Prospective survey of childhood inflammatory bowel disease in the British Isles. Lancet. 2001;357(9262):1093–4.

6. Probert CS, Jayanthi V, Rampton DS, Mayberry JF. Epidemiology of inflammatory bowel disease in different ethnic and religious groups: limitations and aetiological clues. Int J Colorectal Dis. 1996;11(1):25–8.
7. Olafsdottir EJ, Fluge G, Haug K. Chronic inflammatory bowel disease in children in western Norway. J Pediatr Gastroenterol Nutr. 1989;8(4):454–8.
8. Hildebrand H, Fredrikzon B, Holmquist L, Kristiansson B, Lindquist B. Chronic inflammatory bowel disease in children and adolescents in Sweden. J Pediatr Gastroenterol Nutr. 1991;13(3): 293–7.
9. Lindberg E, Lindquist B, Holmquist L, Hildebrand H. Inflammatory bowel disease in children and adolescents in Sweden, 1984–1995. J Pediatr Gastroenterol Nutr 2000;30(3):259–64.
10. Askling J, Grahnquist L, Ekbom A, Finkel Y. Incidence of paediatric Crohn's disease in Stockholm, Sweden. Lancet. 1999;354(9185):1179.
11. Devroede GJ, Taylor WF, Sauer WG, Jackman RJ, Stickler GB. Cancer risk and life expectancy of children with ulcerative colitis. N Engl J Med. 1971;285(1):17–21.
12. Ekbom A, Helmick C, Zack M, Adami HO. Ulcerative colitis and colorectal cancer. A population-based study. N Engl J Med. 1990;323(18):1228–33.
13. Lashner BA, Shaheen NJ, Hanauer SB, Kirschner BS. Passive smoking is associated with an increased risk of developing inflammatory bowel disease in children. Am J Gastroenterol. 1993; 88(3):356–9.
14. Polito JM 2nd, Childs B, Mellits ED, Tokayer AZ, Harris ML, Bayless TM. Crohn's disease: influence of age at diagnosis on site and clinical type of disease. Gastroenterology. 1996; 111(3):580–6.
15. Andersson RE, Olaison G, Tysk C, Ekbom A. Appendectomy and protection against ulcerative colitis. N Engl J Med. 2001;344(11):808–14.

8
The diagnosis of paediatric inflammatory bowel disease

M. C. DUBINSKY and A. DOVER

INTRODUCTION

Inflammatory bowel disease (IBD) has become an increasingly important diagnostic consideration in the paediatric age group. Approximately 20–25% of patients with Crohn's disease (CD) and ulcerative colitis (UC) are diagnosed before the age of 20 years. Although functional disorders are much more common, the incidence and prevalence of IBD, particularly CD, has notably increased over the last 2 decades[1–3]. To date, much of the epidemiological information reported in children has come from European databases[2–5]. Although the reasoning behind the observed rising incidence in children remains unclear, many have hypothesized that physicians caring for young children are getting better at recognizing the disease and thus making the appropriate diagnosis earlier in the disease course. However, despite rising incidence rates, the recognition of paediatric-onset IBD continues to pose somewhat of a diagnostic challenge to primary care and subspecialty physicians alike. Although adult-onset and paediatric-onset IBD share many common features, for instance aetiology, disease location, major clinical features and response to therapy, there are many features unique to the paediatric age group that pose additional clinical challenges. In an attempt to address the issue of whether or not 'children are just little adults', this chapter will highlight these unique features and other important diagnostic considerations that should be taken into account when caring for children with suspected IBD.

APPROACH TO THE RECOGNITION AND DIAGNOSIS OF EARLY-ONSET IBD

As for adult-onset IBD, there are essentially three diagnostic levels or tiers that clinicians may use when evaluating a child with suspected IBD (Figure 1). In this chapter, emphasis will be given to the first level of diagnosis given the aforementioned potential challenges of recognizing IBD in children. Level II,

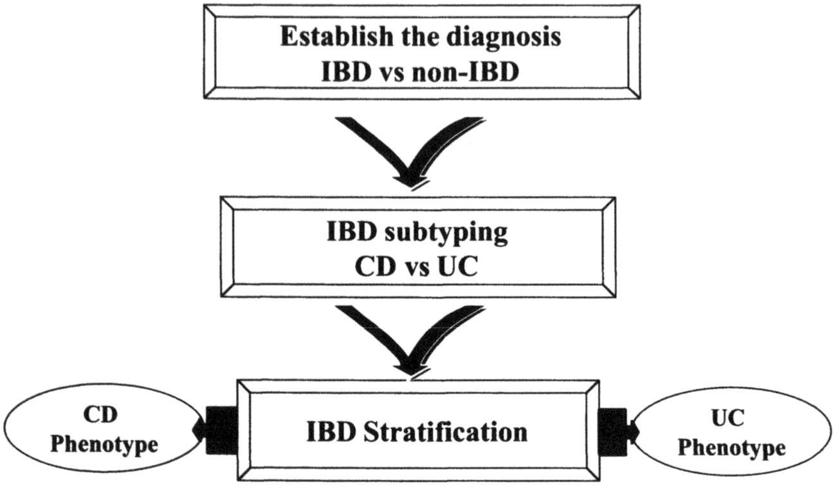

Figure 1 A tiered approach to the diagnosis of IBD

the differentiation of CD from UC, and Level III, stratifying patients based on disease behaviours, will be discussed elsewhere. This first level involves establishing a diagnosis, and hence the recognition and differentiation of IBD from non-IBD disorders. The differential diagnosis of IBD is dependent upon the presenting signs and symptoms. For instance, in patients presenting with colitis-like symptoms, infectious enterocolitis should be excluded, and patients presenting with periumbilical abdominal pain should be evaluated for organic diseases as well as non-organic or functional disorders which are common in the younger age group. At this level, clinicians rely on a thorough clinical history and physical examination as well as, in most circumstances, routine laboratory (serological and stool) tests in order to decide which patients should undergo further diagnostic evaluation in order to confirm their clinical suspicion. Although a gold standard for the diagnosis of IBD does not exist, currently employed diagnostic criteria are based on confirmatory endoscopic, histopathological and radiological findings[6]. This step in the decision process is typically straightforward when the clinical presentation is unambiguous. This is particularly so for patients presenting with so-called 'classic' symptoms and physical signs, such as abdominal pain, diarrhoea, haematochezia, enterocutaneous fistulas and weight loss. However, a substantial proportion of children with IBD, early-onset CD in particular, present with 'non-classic'/non-specific intestinal (intermittent right lower quandrant abdominal pain and loose stools) and extra-intestinal (growth and pubertal delay, arthralgias, fevers) symptoms often delaying the recognition and diagnosis of IBD. In some cases, growth delay may be the only clinical presentation, in the absence of any digestive signs or symptoms[7]. A report from the Hospital for Sick Children in Toronto observed that approximately 20% of CD patients presented with 'non-classic' signs and symptoms upon initial evaluation[8]. This delay is usually a byproduct of the insidious nature of many of these symptoms and the frequency of misdiagnoses, in particular of a functional bowel disorder. A recent report demonstrated that the median time delay from onset of symptoms to recognition and established diagnosis was 7.1 months for CD and 6.7 months for UC[9]. Interestingly, patients with indeterminate colitis (IC) had the longest diagnostic delay of 14 months. Conversely, due to the ambiguity and overlapping nature of these symptoms with the functional bowel disorders in particular, physicians may rely heavily on standard invasive testing to differentiate IBD from non-IBD disorders when faced with diagnostic uncertainty. Unfortunately, suspicion of IBD commonly results in extensive diagnostic investigations of paediatric patients who are indeed ultimately found to have a functional bowel disorder.

Given these diagnostic challenges the search has intensified for a marker or a combination of non-invasive tests that may enable clinicians to accurately screen for IBD, hence aiding the prompt recognition of those patients requiring invasive diagnostic testing and minimizing diagnostic delay. Similarly, sensitive non-invasive screening aids may allow the confident elimination of IBD from diagnostic consideration without the necessity for costly invasive testing with the attendant inconvenience, discomfort and risk. The advent of a tool that maximizes the likelihood that a patient undergoing a complete diagnostic evaluation truly has the disease is very appealing to most clinicians, paediatric gastroenterologists in particular, who often seek to minimize the use of invasive testing. Although the differential diagnoses are similar for adults and children, a number of organic diseases are less frequent among the younger age group, malignancy and premalignant lesions in particular, and thus avoiding endoscopy may be more justified.

The ideal diagnostic screening test must be both sensitive and specific in order to detect all patients with IBD and to exclude all others. Invasive endoscopy and radiology remain the diagnostic standard to which all non-invasive tests must be compared and thus is regarded as the ‘gold standard’. A number of candidate non-invasive markers have been evaluated in the literature. Faecal markers such as faecal lactoferrin have recently been shown to be elevated in patients with IBD compared with healthy controls or those with irritable bowel syndrome (IBS), thus suggesting that this marker is sensitive to inflammation. However, whether it is specific to inflammatory colitis and not infectious colitis remains to be seen[10,11]. Since faecal lactoferrin was not elevated in IBS patients, it may well prove useful to differentiate IBD from non-IBD disorders. Recent studies have suggested that abdominal ultrasound (U/S) may be useful, not only for generating a diagnosis but also in localizing disease and defining extent of inflammation[12]. A positive abdominal U/S was highly predictive of inflammation but lacked the necessary sensitivity to serve as a screening tool. It has been suggested that routine serological tests may be valuable in the selection of children presenting with non-specific gastrointestinal symptoms who require endoscopic assessment. Beattie *et al.* evaluated the sensitivity and specificity of haemoglobin, platelet count, erythrocyte sedimentation rate (ESR), C reactive protein (CRP) and serum albumin in 93 children in whom the diagnosis was uncertain and who underwent a complete diagnostic work-up for IBD[13]. Overall, no child with CD had all normal screening investigations and only one child with UC had normal investigations despite classic symptoms (Table 1). Ninety-one per cent of children with normal endoscopy and 88% with polyps had all normal tests. A

Table 1 The prevalence of normal and abnormal routine laboratory tests in patients with IBD and non-IBD

	CD ($n=26$)	*UC* ($n=13$)	*Polyps* ($n=8$)	*Normal* ($n=37$)	*Others* ($n=7$)
Haemoglobin <10 g/dl	16	30	12	6	28
ESR >25 mm	85	23	0	0	25
Albumin <36 g/dl	35	15	0	0	14
Platelets >400 × 10^9/L	88	70	12	6	42
CRP	100	60	0	0	42
All normal	0	8	88	91	28

Adapted from ref. 13.

similar study performed in adults suggested that CRP and ESR elevation was 100% specific for IBD and concluded that normal investigations may be useful in identifying those patients with chronic GI disorders who may thus avoid invasive testing[14]. Despite these interesting findings, in general, routine blood tests are sensitive biological markers of inflammation, yet lack disease specificity. Similarly, diagnostic scoring models for organic and non-organic GI disease have been less than satisfactory and thus not widely used in routine clinical practice[15]. As alluded to earlier the ideal screening test must be both disease sensitive and disease specific. Few markers possess the disease-specific characteristics of anti-*Saccharomyces cerevisiae* antibodies (ASCA IgA and IgG) for CD and perinuclear anti-neutrophil cytoplasmic antibodies (pANCA) for UC. IBD-associated pANCA is produced in the colonic mucosa and reacts with a nuclear envelope protein of the neutrophil, probably recognizing the histone H1 antigen. It has been suggested that pANCA reflects a distinct mucosal inflammatory process[16]. ASCA was discovered in the course of studies designed to search for putative dietary antigens involved in the pathogenesis of IBD[17–19]. CD-associated ASCA reacts to yeast cell was phosphopeptidomannans[20]. One or both of these antibodies characterize approximately a half to two thirds of IBD patients[21,22]. Traditionally, ASCA and pANCA serodiagnostic assays have been adapted to maximize disease specificity and accurately confirm a diagnosis of IBD when positive and differentiate CD from UC. However, these highly specific confirmatory assays are insufficiently sensitive to serve as ideal non-invasive screening tests, in particular for patient populations with a low prevalence of disease. Recent research has focused on maximizing the sensitivity and hence the screening capability of these novel serological diagnostic markers. The challenge lies in maintaining the high disease specificity that distinguishes these diagnostic antibody markers from the routine serological markers. There are essentially two mechanisms by which such high diagnostic standards may be achieved. The first would be the development of a panel of serological antibody markers that characterize all patients with IBD, thus, in essence uncovering the antibody responses in patients who are ASCA and pANCA seronegative. Two novel antibodies reactive to bacterial proteins, outer membrane protein C (OmpC) and I2, have recently been reported in patients with CD[23]. These antibodies may

Table 2 The prevalence of IBD-specific antibody markers in CD, UC and non-IBD

Marker	*CD* (%)	*UC* (%)	*Non-IBD* ($n = 8$)
ASCA	15	65	<5
pANCA	60	5	<5
PAB	31	4	0
OmpC	38	2	<5
I2	54	10	19

represent the host response to a pathogenic organism or perhaps reflect a subgroup of CD patients whose inflammation is perpetuated by luminal bacteria. I2 has been shown to be present in 12% of CD patients who are ASCA and pANCA negative and OmpC has been observed in approximately 10% of seronegative CD patients[22]. Autoantibodies against exocrine pancreas (PAB) have been found in approximately 30% of patients with CD and have been touted as a specific marker for CD[21,24]. The prevalence of IBD-specific antibody markers is illustrated in Table 2[22]. The search continues for the ultimate antibody panel such that all patients with IBD are characterized serodiagnostically. As this endeavour continues, our group recently published an article on the use of sequential diagnostic testing using modified ASCA/pANCA assays in combination with the traditional IBD-specific assays as an alternative mechanism to optimize IBD screening in a group of children presenting with non-specific signs and symptoms suggestive of, but not classic for, IBD[25]. The modifications to currently existing assays rendered these antibody diagnostic markers more sensitive and less expensive than the traditional marker assays[26]. Essentially, the cut-off values for the modified assays were recalculated to optimize sensitivity in order to facilitate early detection of disease. Based on the improved sensitivity of the modified assay and the high specificity of the confirmatory traditional assay, a diagnostic testing strategy was proposed. In the proposed testing sequence all positive modified assay results were confirmed by the traditional assay. Such a diagnostic serological testing sequence is not unlike that which is currently employed for the evaluation of systemic lupus erythematosus. In this scenario the antinuclear antibody assay, a sensitive screening test with a high negative predictive value, is followed by a more specific confirmatory test, the anti-double stranded DNA antibody assay. The purpose of this study, however, was to see whether sequential antibody marker testing would have accurately identified which patients did or, perhaps more importantly, did not, have IBD, and could therefore have avoided unnecessary invasive testing had these results been known at the time of initial evaluation. This testing strategy was accurate in differentiating IBD from non-IBD in 84% of cases. Had this testing sequence been performed upon initial presentation, 95% of the confirmed non-IBD patients would have been correctly identified in the absence of invasive testing. Only 3 patients with a false positive serology result would have undergone an unnecessary invasive work-up. Had the modified assay been applied independently rather than in sequence with the confirmatory assay, the overall accuracy would have decreased to 76% and 21 as opposed to 3 patients would have had false positive serology, potentially resulting in unnecessary and costly invasive testing. Thus, sequential serodiagnostic testing was proposed as an alternative mechanism to screen children for IBD, improving the quality of care. As novel antibody markers are introduced and the screening panel is developed, the need for sequential testing will diminish and clinicians will probably be able to rely on a single test, possessing both the sensitivity and specificity standards necessary to screen for IBD. The goal of such a tool would be to maximize diagnostic accuracy and to minimize both the diagnostic delay and the use of unnecessary invasive testing. Although the potential screening capabilities of other tools will be investigated in the future, emphasis will be placed on IBD-specific antibodies given their potential utility in other areas of IBD diagnosis. The two areas in particular that enhance the utility of these antibody markers are their demonstrated capability to differentiate CD from UC[27–30] with a great degree of certainty and the stratification of CD and perhaps UC into immunologically homogeneous subgroups with distinct disease behaviours[31].

APPROACH TO THE RECOGNITION OF UNIQUE PRESENTATIONS OF EARLY-ONSET IBD

Physical growth

Although there are many presenting features common to both adult- and paediatric-onset IBD, there are also distinctive differences that need to be highlighted. The effect of IBD, particularly CD, on physical growth is different among children as compared with adults. The profound effect of disease on growth can be attributed to the timing of disease onset, such that IBD often occurs at a time when a child is undergoing significant physical change. The three primary aspects of physical growth that are adversely affected by chronic inflammation and resultant malnutrition are body weight, linear growth and sexual maturity. Weight loss is the most common presenting sign of the three and can be seen in up to 90% and 65% of children with CD and UC, respectively[32]. There are many concomitant factors that contribute to a state of malnutrition in children with IBD. Although increased intestinal losses, malabsorption, increased energy and nutrient requirements and psychological factors contribute to the nutritional disturbances, reduced intake remains the principal reason for continued weight loss. Anorexia is most likely due to the inflammatory process itself; however, voluntary refusal as well as perhaps the appetite suppressive effect of certain cytokines may contribute to reduced intake. In addition to weight loss, a proportion of children will present with linear growth impairment and delayed sexual maturity as a result of the chronic malnutrition. Pubertal delay typically accompanies growth impairment. Growth failure is more often seen in children with CD than UC. However, approximately 6–10% of children with UC have been reported to develop growth failure over the course of their disease[32,33]. When focusing on children with CD, the reported incidence of growth failure at the time of diagnosis varies between 7% and 88%[7,34–37]. This variability is probably attributable to the different definitions of growth failure employed in the various studies as well as the different populations evaluated. As mentioned earlier, one study demonstrated that linear growth impairment may precede the onset of intestinal symptoms[7]. Males may be at higher risk of growth impairment than females since they go through a growth spurt later on in the stages of normal pubertal development and this growth period tends to persist for a greater period of time than their female counterparts. It is very important to recognize IBD, CD in particular, early on in the course of disease, to maximize physical growth at this very vulnerable and dynamic stage of a child's development. Early identification of growth failure will enable clinicians to maximize both nutritional and medical therapies to ensure maximal catch-up growth and avoid persistent stunted growth into adulthood.

Psychosocial growth and development

Psychosocial growth and development is a critical yet underdeveloped area of research in paediatric IBD. Chronic diseases in general cause significant psychological stresses to both the children and their families. Chronic inflammatory bowel diseases are no different such that it has been estimated that some form of psychopathology exists in approximately 40–70% of either adults or children with IBD[38–40]. A recent meta-analysis confirmed that children with IBD have more psychological disturbances than age-matched groups with other chronic illnesses[41]. It is not surprising that the psychological stresses of IBD challenge the psychosocial resources of both the affected child and his/her family. Disrupted education, limited physical activities and social interactions as well as delayed growth and puberty pose the biggest challenges. These stressors may appear insurmountable to the adolescent dealing with many other psychological stressors associated with that time in their development. Depression is a common emotional problem and it remains unclear whether this is an emotional reaction to being diagnosed with the disease, is part of the disease process, is due to genetic predisposition or is a result of certain treatments. One study demonstrated that up to 60% of children with CD were depressed as compared with 10% of healthy children[42]. Similarly, another study found that CD children had a higher frequency of depression compared with their unaffected siblings[43]. Other emotional problems observed among children with CD include separation anxiety, social withdrawal, relationship problems, lowered self-esteem and problems with body image[44–48]. Many of these psychological stresses are manifested clinically by intestinal symptomatology. At times, it is hard to discover which symptoms are related to the underlying disease process as opposed to the functional overlay.

The psychological impact of IBD is not limited to the affected child but tends to permeate to the parents and siblings as well. The child relies heavily on the parents for support and mechanisms of dealing with life stressors, in particular the stress of disease. Thus a well-functioning family unit is critical for the affected child. It has been shown, however, that parents of children with CD have an increased frequency of psychopathology themselves[44,47,49,50]. Family dysfunction has been reported to be higher among families of children with IBD than in families with diabetic or healthy children[49,51]. IBD may have a psychological impact on the unaffected siblings in the family as well. It has been reported that siblings of children with IBD had poorer peer relations, more mood disturbances and lower self-esteem[52]. In addition to fearing for their ill sibling's well being, it is not uncommon for siblings to express their fear of developing the disease themselves[52,53].

Given the significant impact of IBD on both physical and psychological growth and development, it is critical for clinicians caring for young children with suspected or diagnosed IBD to address these pertinent issues at the time of evaluation. A thorough caloric intake history, serial anthropometric evaluations, pubertal assessment, bone age determination and detailed family history are some of the tools clinicians may employ to maximize the recognition of the physical growth effects of IBD. Similarly, inquiring about daily activities, school attendance, family functioning, mood and anxiety disturbances as well as overall quality of life in affected children and their families is an important aspect of the evaluation of a child with IBD. A multidisciplinary team approach is warranted in patients with early-onset IBD as all areas of intervention, medical, surgical, nutritional and psychosocial, have a major impact on the long-term outcome of this chronic disease.

RECOGNIZING THE PROGNOSIS OF EARLY-ONSET IBD

We have come to understand that there is great diversity in the types of IBD and that this variation goes beyond the broad categorization of just CD or UC. Thus, CD and UC are themselves very heterogeneous groups that are composed of many different phenotypic subgroups. It has become clear that this spectrum of IBD phenotypes is a result of diverse patterns of immune imbalances triggered by certain environmental factors in a genetically susceptible individual. It is this unique immune response that translates clinically into specific disease behaviours. Attempts have been made to try to characterize these patients based on their clinical and perhaps immune similarities into more homogeneous subgroups. Currently, disease location is often used to stratify patients with UC, for instance those with proctitis, left-sided colitis or pancolitis. For CD, the classification system has become a little more sophisticated with the advent of the Vienna classification which proposes to stratify patients based on age of onset (<40 vs. >40 years), disease location (small bowel only vs. small and large bowel vs. large bowel only) and disease behaviour (inflammatory vs. stricturing vs. penetrating). However, even within each of these categories, there exist many different phenotypes. Researchers have focused their attention on uncovering markers or predictors of certain disease behaviours and disease characteristics. The goal is to identify certain prognostic factors such that known interventions may be employed to try to alter the natural history of the disease. It has been suggested that one such predictor is diagnosis of IBD when less than 20 years old. An important study from the group at Johns Hopkins concluded that early age of onset is associated with more complicated disease and a greater likelihood of having affected relatives (Table 3)[54]. This suggests that the genetic influences on patients with early-onset disease are different from those on patients who are diagnosed after the age of 20 years. The key is in finding those haplotypes or perhaps candidate genes that give rise to this genetic heterogeneity. It has been suggested recently that the MHC Class III Notch 4 haplotype is associated with

Table 3 Influence of age at diagnosis on disease characteristics including disease site and disease behaviour

	<20 y	*20–39 y*	*>40 y*
Family history (%)	30	19	14
Site			
Small bowel (%)	89	78	58
Large bowel (%)	70	65	85
Disease behaviour			
Stricturing (%)	46	34	29
Inflammatory (%)	34	45	55
Surgery (%)	71		56

younger age of onset and fibrostenosing disease behaviour in patients with CD[55]. As the search for the gene that predicts specific disease phenotypes continues, recent research has focused on the potential role of ASCA and pANCA as representative markers of Crohn's disease behaviours[31]. The results of this study demonstrated that certain disease behaviours and clinical features could be linked to the presence *and* levels of ASCA and pANCA. Interestingly, high ASCA titres were independently associated with early-onset CD (<13 years) and fibrostenosing disease behaviour. Thus, in this study, it appeared that ASCA characterizes a subgroup of patients with a more aggressive form of small bowel CD. Conversely, high pANCA levels were associated with older age of onset CD and ulcerative colitis-like disease behaviour. It can be suggested that perhaps those patients described in the earlier study conducted at Johns Hopkins expressed ASCA as a subclinical marker of their disease behaviour. It is these kinds of studies that will help to uncover whether antibody markers may provide a tool linking genotype to a particular phenotype. Knowledge of the association between certain immune markers, antibodies in particular, and specific disease behaviours may enable clinicians to use this information as a prognostic factor such that appropriate intervention may be implemented early in order to alter the natural history of the disease course in at-risk populations. For instance, in a patient at risk for more aggressive disease behaviours, earlier and more aggressive immunosuppressive therapy may avoid predictable complications in a subgroup of patients. Prospective studies are needed to determine whether the presence of certain immune markers at the time of diagnosis is predictive of specific disease phenotypes and whether early intervention does indeed alter the natural history of the disease.

CONCLUSIONS

Although there are many similarities between early-onset and late-onset IBD, clearly there are features unique to the younger age group. These unique clinical presentations probably reflect a unique genotype and resultant immune response specific to this age group. The three main challenges highlighted in this chapter are certainly unique to this population. They included: (1) the recognition of

IBD in children presenting with subtle or non-specific symptoms; (2) the recognition of unique clinical presentations, such as impaired physical and psychosocial growth; and (3) the recognition of the prognosis of early-onset IBD. In order to address these diagnostic challenges, clinicians caring for young children with suspected or diagnosed IBD may employ a goal-oriented approach. The goals of recognizing IBD early in the course of disease of patients with non-specific symptoms and accurately discriminating disease from non-disease are to minimize diagnostic delay, maximize diagnostic accuracy and minimize unnecessary invasive testing. The goal of recognizing the unique complications of early-onset disease is to minimize any growth delay and maximize psychosocial development. Lastly, by recognizing the potential impact of early-onset IBD on the disease prognosis, clinicians may choose to employ alternative therapeutic interventions in order to alter the natural history of the disease. Studies are needed to further delineate the features unique to patients across all age groups. The question of whether or not children are just little adults should perhaps be rephrased to more accurately reflect the changing views of IBD classification, such that the question in the future may read 'how does early-onset IBD differ from late-onset IBD?'

References

1. Loftus EV Jr., Silverstein MD, Sandborn WJ *et al.* Crohn's disease in Olmsted county, Minnesota, 1940–1993: Incidence and prevalence, and survival. Gastroenterology. 1998;114:1161–8.
2. Olafsdottir EJ, Fluge G, Haug K. Chronic inflammatory bowel disease in children in western Norway. J Pediatr Gastroenterol Nutr. 1989;8:454–8.
3. Hildebrand H, Fredrikzon B, Holmquist L *et al.* Chronic inflammatory bowel disease in children and adolescents in Sweden. J Pediatr Gastroenterol Nutr. 1991;13:293–7.
4. Barton JR, Gillon S, Ferguson A. Incidence of inflammatory bowel disease in Scottish children between 1968 and 1983: Marginal fall in ulcerative colitis: Three-fold rise in Crohn's disease. Gut. 1989;30:618–22.
5. Stewenius J, Anderhill I, Ekelund G *et al.* Ulcerative colitis and indeterminate colitis in the city of Malmo, Sweden – a 25 year study. Scand J Gastroenterol. 1995;30:38.
6. Lennard-Jones JE. Classification of inflammatory bowel disease. Scand J Gastroenterol. 1989;24 (suppl 170):2–6.
7. Hildebrand H, Karlberg J, Kristiansson B. Longitudinal growth in children and adolescents with inflammatory bowel disease. J Pediatr Gastroenterol Nutr. 1994;18:165–73.
8. Griffiths AM. Crohn's disease. In: David TJ, editor, Recent Advances in Paediatrics No.10, Edinburgh, UK: Churchill Livingstone, 1992.
9. Heikenen JB, Werlin SL, Brown CW, Balint JP. Presenting symptoms and diagnostic lag in children with inflammatory bowel disease. Inflamm Bowel Dis. 1999;5:158–60.
10. Kane S, Sandborn WJ, Rufo P *et al.* Fecal lactoferrin is a sensitive and specific marker for chronic inflammatory bowel diseases. Gastroenterology. 2001;120(suppl):A276.
11. Fine KD, Ogunji F, George J *et al.* Utility of rapid fecal latex agglutination test detecting neutrophil protein, lactoferrin, for diagnosing inflammatory causes of chronic diarrhea. Am J Gastroenterol. 1998;93:1300–5.
12. Holerbach S, Geissler A, Schiegl H *et al.* The accuracy of abdominal ultrasound in the assessment of bowel disorders. Scand J Gastroenterol. 1998;33:1201–8.
13. Beattie RM, Walker Smith JA, Murch SH. Indications for investigation of chronic gastrointestinal symptoms. Arch Dis Child. 1995;73:354–5.
14. Shine B, Berghouse L, Lennard-Jones JE *et al.* C-reactive protein as an aid in the differential diagnosis of functional and inflammatory disorders. Clin Chim Acta. 1985;148:105–9.
15. Starmans R, Muris JWM, Fijten G *et al.* The diagnostic value of scoring models for organic and non-organic gastrointestinal disease, including the irritable-bowel syndrome. Med Decis Mak. 1994;14:208–16.

16. Targan SR, Landers CJ, Cobb L *et al.* Perinuclear anti-neutrophil cytoplasmic antibodies are spontaneously produced by mucosal B cells of ulcerative colitis patients. J Immunol. 1995;155: 3262–7.
17. Main J, McKenzie H, Yearman GR *et al.* Antibody to *Saccharomyces cerevisiae* (baker's yeast) in Crohn's disease. Br Med J. 1988;297:1105–6.
18. McKenzie H, Main J, Pennington CR *et al.* Antibody to selected strains of *Saccharomyces cerevisiae* (baker's and brewer's yeast) and *Candida albicans* in Crohn's disease. Gut. 1990;31:536–8.
19. Giaffer MH, Clark A, Holdsworth CD. Antibodies to *Saccharomyces cerevisiae* in patients with Crohn's disease and their possible pathogenic importance. Gut. 1992;33:1071–5.
20. Sendid B, Colombel JF, Jacquinot PM *et al.* Specific antibody response to oligomannosidic epitopes in Crohn's disease. Clin Diag Lab Immunol. 1996;3:219–26.
21. Sandborn W, Loftus EV, Colombel JF *et al.* Utility of perinuclear anti-neutrophil cytoplasmic antibodies (pANCA), anti-*Saccharomyces cerevisiae* (ASCA), and anti-pancreatic antibodies (APA) as serologic markers in a population based cohort of patients with Crohn's disease (CD) and ulcerative colitis (UC). Gastroenterology. 2000;118(4) Suppl 2:A106.
22. Rutgeerts P, Vermieire S. Serological diagnosis of inflammatory bowel disease. Lancet. 2000;356:2117.
23. Abreu MT, Vasiliauskas EA, Kam LY, Dubinsky MC. Use of serologic tests in Crohn's disease. Clin Perspect Gastroenterol. 2001;155–64.
24. Seibold F, Mork H, Tanza S *et al.* Pancreatic autoantibodies in Crohn's disease: a family study. Gut. 1997;40:481–4.
25. Dubinsky MC, Ofman JJ, Urman M *et al.* Clinical utility of serodiagnostic testing in suspected paediatric inflammatory bowel disease. Am J Gastroenterol. 2001:96;758–65.
26. Rose S, Lentz J, Walsh M. Clinical evaluation of a new immunodiagnostic assay system for inflammatory bowel disease. Am J Gastroenterol. 1998;93:A597.
27. Ruemmele FM, Targan SR, Levy G, Dubinsky M, Braun J, Seidman EG. Diagnostic accuracy of serological assays in paediatric inflammatory bowel disease. Gastroenterology. 1998;115:822–9.
28. Quinton JF, Sendid B, Reumaux D *et al.* Anti-*Saccharomyces cerevisiae* mannan antibodies combined with antineutrophil cytoplasmic autoantibodies in inflammatory bowel disease: prevalence and diagnostic role. Gut. 1998;42:788–91.
29. Duerr RH, Targan SR, Landers CJ, Sutherland LR, Shanahan F. Anti-neutrophil cytoplasmic antibodies in ulcerative colitis. Comparison with other colitides/diarrheal illnesses. Gastroenterology. 1991:100:1590–6.
30. Saxon A, Shanahan F, Landers C, Ganz T, Targan S. A distinct subset of antineutrophil cytoplasmic antibodies is associated with inflammatory bowel disease. J Allergy Clin Immunol. 1990;86:202–10.
31. Vasiliauskas EA, Kam LY, Karp LC, Gaiennie J, Yang HY, Targan SR. Marker antibody expression stratifies Crohn's disease into immunologically homogeneous subgroups with distinct clinical characteristics. Gut. 2000;47:487–96.
32. Griffiths AM, Nguyen P, Smith C, MacMillan JH, Sherman PH. Growth and clinical course of children with Crohn's disease. Gut. 1993;34:939–43.
33. Markowitz JF, Grencher K, Rosa J, Aiger H, Daum F. Growth failure in paediatric inflammatory bowel disease. J Pediatr Gastroenterol Nutr. 1993;16:373–80.
34. Kanof ME, Lake AM, Bayless TM. Decreased height velocity in children and adolescents before the diagnosis of Crohn's disease. Gastroenterology. 1988;95:1423–527.
35. Kirschner BS. Growth and development in chronic inflammatory bowel disease. Acta Pediatr Scand (Suppl). 1990;366:98–104.
36. Lindquist BL, Jarnerot G, Wickbom G. Clinical and epidemiological aspects of Crohn's disease in children and adolescents. Scand J Gastroenterol. 1984;19:502–6.
37. Gryboski J, Hileimeier C. Inflammatory bowel disease in children. Med Clin N Am. 1980;64:1185–202.
38. Helzer JE, Chammas S, Norland CC *et al.* A study of the association between Crohn's disease and psychiatric illness. Gastroenterology. 1984;86:324–9.
39. McKegney F, Gordon R, Levine S. A psychosomatic comparison of patients with ulcerative colitis and Crohn's disease. Psychosom Med. 1970;32:155–66.
40. Whybrow P, Kane F, Lipton M. Regional ileitis and psychiatric disorder. Psychosom Med. 1968;30:209–21.
41. Lavigne J, Faier-Rueteman J. Psychosocial adjustment to paediatric physical disorders: A meta-analytic review. J Pediatr Psychol. 1992;17:133–57.

42. Engstrom I. Mental health and psychological functioning in children and adolescents with inflammatory bowel disease: A comparison with children having other chronic illness and with healthy children. J Child Psychol Psychiatry. 1992:33:563–82.
43. Wood B, Watkins JB, Boyle JT *et al.* Psychological functioning in children with Crohn's disease and ulcerative colitis: Implications for models of psychobiological interaction. J Am Acad Child Adolesc Psychiatry. 1987;26:774–81.
44. Szajnberg N, Krall V, Davis P *et al.* Psychopathology and relationship measures in children with inflammatory bowel disease and their parents. Child Psychiatry Hum Dev. 1993;23: 215–32.
45. Steinhausen H-C, Kies H. Comparative studies of ulcerative colitis and Crohn's disease in children and adolescents. J Child Psychol Psychiatry. 1982:23:33–42.
46. Raymer D, Weininger O, Hamilton J. Psychological problems in children with functional abdominal pain. Lancet. 1984;1:439–40.
47. Engstrom I. Parental distress and social interaction in families with children with inflammatory bowel disease. J Am Acad Child Adolesc Psychiatry. 1991;30:904–12.
48. Ruhland J, Tennenbaum F, De Tichey C. Approche de l'image du corps chez les adolescents atteints de recto-colite hemorragique ou de maladie de Crohn par le conte de la fourmi. Psychol Med. 1992;24:1143–8.
49. Engstrom I. Inflammatory bowel disease in children and adolescents: Mental health and family functioning. J Pediatr Gastroenterol Nutr. 1999;28:528–33.
50. Burke PM, Kocoshis S, Neigut D *et al.* Maternal psychiatric disorder in paediatric inflammatory bowel disease and cystic fibrosis. Child Psychiatry Hum Dev. 1994;25:45–52.
51. Engstrom I. Family interaction and locus of control in children and adolescents with inflammatory bowel disease. J Am Acad Child Adolesc Psychiatry. 1991;33:563–82.
52. Engstrom I. Psychological problems in siblings of children and adolescents with inflammatory bowel disease. Eur Child Adolesc Psychiatry. 1992;1:24–33.
53. Akobeng AK, Suresh-Babu MV, Firth D *et al.* Quality of life in children with Crohn's disease. J Pediatr Gastroenterol Nutr. 1999;28:S37–9.
54. Politi JM, Childs B, Mellitis ED *et al.* Crohn's disease: Influence of age at diagnosis on site and clinical type of disease. Gastroenterology. 1996;111:5580–6.
55. Taylor KD, Kam LY, Lin YC *et al.* Specific clinical and immunologic features in Crohn's disease patients are associated with the MHC Class III Marker Notch 4. Gastroenterology. 2000;118 (suppl):A869.

9
Growth failure in children with IBD

H. A. BÜLLER

INTRODUCTION

Childhood inflammatory bowel disease is frequently complicated by impaired linear growth and retardation of pubertal development[1–4]. The percentage of growth failure found in children with inflammatory bowel disease (IBD) depends on which method was used and what is considered normal or abnormal. For example, many studies use height for age below the 3rd percentile as abnormal. Height for age below the 3rd percentile will only identify severely affected children but not other subnormal growing individuals. Recently, the important introduction of standard deviation scores (Z-scores) which give height for age relative to the population, allows us to identify subtle changes and is very useful for longitudinal and comparative studies[5]. Z-scores provide a number instead of a percentage. However, the most sensitive measurement of growth in children is height velocity. Measurement of height velocity allows the identification of very subtle changes and is most important for the individual child[4,6]. Motil *et al.* showed that, using these different measurement options, the percentage of growth failure in IBD varies depending upon the method employed[5]. They found that 39% of a paediatric IBD population had a height for age below the 3rd percentile at diagnosis. This occurred twice as often in patients with Crohn's disease as in patients with ulcerative colitis. However, if they analysed the same population of children for Z-scores, they found that 23% of the children had a Z-score >-1.64. Using height velocity defined as less than 4 cm/year, they identified 24% of the children within the same population.

Much more important than growth failure at diagnosis is the permanent growth failure at the end of puberty. Kirschner found, in her IBD population, a severely short adult stature in 17% of the paediatric IBD patients[1]. Markowitz *et al.* found permanent growth failure as measured by bone age, parental height (growth potential), height-for-age percentile and chronological age in 31% of adult IBD patients with onset in the paediatric age range[7]. Interestingly, in this study, age at diagnosis, age at cessation of linear growth and site of disease did not differ between impaired and normal growth in these children. It is, however, important to state that, in comparing the different studies on permanent growth failure, one should know the age of onset exactly because children with onset of disease during late puberty will most likely differ in final height from those with onset before puberty.

Griffiths *et al.* showed that weight loss in children with IBD at diagnosis is, as expected, very prevalent[8]. They found 85% of Crohn's disease and 65% of ulcerative colitis patients had moderate to severe weight loss. The pivotal study of Motil *et al.* in which 69 IBD patients were followed up for an extended period of time showed for the first time that there was no association between growth failure and the use of steroids or surgery[5]. The major factor influencing growth failure was disease activity. In addition, in a retrospective study, Griffiths *et al.* found 22% permanent growth failure in 100 Crohn's disease patients[8]. Similarly to Motil *et al.*, they also identified no effect of surgery on final height. They correctly pointed out that attention should be paid particularly to patients who are stunted at diagnosis. These patients have the greatest likelihood of permanent growth failure in adulthood. Moreover, both studies concluded that the severity of IBD symptoms is the major factor influencing linear growth velocity[5,8].

Apart from growth failure, pubertal delay is another important aspect of IBD in children. Walker Smith found compared to controls an approximately 13 month delay in the onset of puberty in girls while this was 14 months in boys[4]. Failure to identify delayed puberty is often the result of inadequate follow up of patients at clinical visits and simply of not determining pubertal stage. It is important to realize that growth retardation or delayed puberty occurring during treatment signals inadequate therapy. Savage *et al.* showed, in a recent study, that intestinal resection in Crohn's disease should preferably be performed before puberty[9]. They found that height velocity before and after surgery in pubertal stages 4 and 5 only increased by approximately 1 cm/year while for surgery in pubertal stages 1, 2 and 3, the increase in height velocity before and after intestinal resection was 5–8 cm/year. On the other hand, it is quite disappointing to see that recording of growth and sexual development in children with IBD in a recent study by Ghosh *et al.* is hardly ever performed by gastroenterologists, surgeons and paediatricians alike[10]. This paper showed that, during clinical visits, height and weight are measured regularly but sexual staging and bone age assessment are hardly ever assessed. Unfortunately, these authors had already reported in an earlier paper, approximately a decade ago, the serious underrecording of these growth variables.

Thus, growth retardation is commonly found in paediatric IBD patients, varying from 20% to 40% depending on which measurement is used and what definition is applied. It is clear that growth retardation is found more often in Crohn's disease than in ulcerative colitis, approximately by a factor 2. Of the three most used measurements of growth, height for age, Z-scores and growth velocity, it has been established that growth velocity is the most sensitive measurement of growth retardation. Furthermore, catch-up growth or restoration of growth to normal levels depends primarily on adequate treatment of inflammation, timed surgery and the age of onset and thus stage of puberty.

MECHANISM OF GROWTH FAILURE

The three major mechanisms of growth failure in IBD are: (1) inadequate caloric intake, (2) disease activity, and (3) daily steroids[1–3,11]. Inadequate caloric intake is the major factor resulting in malnutrition and growth failure. Some have poor dietary intakes because of diminished taste acuity for salt, sugar and acid foods. Often, patients may be unwilling to eat because of increased diarrhoea accompanying the ingestion of food or because of exacerbation of abdominal pain following meals. It is the combination of anorexia, early satiety, and poor nutrient intake during acute flares of chronic diseases that ultimately leads to poor growth[2–4,8,9]. Disease activity, in other words chronic intestinal inflammation, leads to the release of all kinds of inflammatory mediators, such as TNFα, of which it has been suggested that it interferes with growth plate kinetics[3,11,12]. There is also a possible role of increased IL-6 mediating IGF (insulin-like growth factor) decrease resulting in growth failure[13]. Daily steroids, certainly when given in high doses for long periods of time, is a factor influencing growth failure. However, it is thought that growth failure is much more often a reflection of severe disease activity than that the steroids themselves cause the major effect on growth. Kirschner found that paediatric IBD patients consume approximately 50–60% of the recommended daily intake of food[1]. She stated that a reversal of growth failure could be accomplished by increasing the RDA by 40–50% or 80–90 $kCal\,kg^{-1}\,day^{-1}$. Although the relationship between malnutrition and IBD is still somewhat unclear, several factors can be identified. Primarily, as stated before, there is an inadequate intake of calories. It should be emphasized that this is the major factor in malnutrition and IBD. Furthermore, excessive intestinal losses depend on the extent and severity of the disease. Steatorrhoea only occurs in extensive IBD. Similarly, protein-losing enteropathy is only found in active and extensive IBD. Another factor that may play a role in malnutrition is the occurrence of bacterial overgrowth which has been suggested to occur in 30% of patients. Another area of important research is energy expenditure and IBD[14]. It is unclear what role the resting energy expenditure plays in the development of malnutrition and growth retardation. In the elegant studies by Azcue *et al.* and Zoli *et al.*, it was established that resting energy expenditure (REE) per kilogram fat-free mass in inactive Crohn's disease is similar to that of normals[15,16]. However, resting energy expenditure increases during active disease. Compared with patients with anorexia nervosa who also have malnutrition, it seems that patients with Crohn's disease are unable to reduce their resting energy expenditure. Most of these children are malnourished themselves and thus fail to adapt their REE per unit lean body mass and thus this inadequate high REE contributes to malnutrition. Unfortunately the increased energy expenditure during active disease is not accompanied by an increase in energy intake. Therefore, even during active disease, therapy should be aimed at increasing caloric intake to maximize growth potential.

SURGERY

Many studies on surgery in paediatric IBD conclude that there was a good effect on growth[17–19]. However, most of these studies lack an adequate comparison with medical therapy and most do not look at final height but at catch-up growth one or two years after surgery. For example, El-Baba *et al.* published a retrospective study in 32 children[19]. The indications for surgery were growth failure, failure of medical therapy and complications. They report 47% complete relief after surgery and good catch-up growth. However, no comparison was performed with other therapeutic options nor was final adult height reported. It should be stated that surgery is always an option in IBD and clearly it may produce long-standing remission. Surgery should be a part of the treatment of IBD patients from the beginning. It should be considered when there is failure of medical treatment and especially in localized disease[1,4,5,8]. It is important that surgery is performed, if indicated, before the adolescent growth spurt in order to achieve the maximum effect on growth potential. The restoration of growth may be very limited or even impossible when the operation is performed during late puberty or after puberty has been completed[17]. Surgery for growth failure *per se* remains controversial. Surgery is indicated when there is failure to induce remission when, on an adequate dose of medical therapy, no effect has been obtained with extensive nutritional therapy, or long-standing dependency on steroids even when steroid-sparing treatment with azathioprine or methotrexate has been used[4,18]. Right hemicolectomy, limited small bowel resection, stricturoplasty, and subtotal or total colectomy with ileostomy or anal repair are all surgical options.

MANAGEMENT OF GROWTH FAILURE IN IBD

The management of growth failure in IBD depends primarily on the combination of adequate treatment of intestinal inflammation and the provision of sufficient calories. It is of interest to know that Voitk *et al.*, in 1973, were the first to demonstrate the effect of nutrition on IBD[20]. In this surgical study, 13 IBD patients were reported who, before undergoing major surgery for IBD, were pretreated with an elemental diet because of their poor nutritional status. To their surprise, they noted that the indication for surgery resolved in some patients due to nutritional as well as clinical improvement. They wondered if this represented a primary therapeutic effect of the elemental diet or the natural course of the disease. The dietary management of growth failure in IBD should be aimed at different levels[1–3,21,22]. First of all, there should be an increase in calories, particularly protein, at least up to the level of the recommended daily allowances. It is possible to use liquid dietary supplements but attention should be paid to replacement of regular food intake. In general, dietary instructions are needed and the diet may be adjusted according to the patient's wishes. It is now well established that nutritional support as an adjunctive therapy forms a cornerstone in the overall treatment of children with IBD, especially those with malnutrition or poor growth[21–24]. There is still controversy regarding the use of nutrition in IBD as primary therapy. Studies by Wilschanski *et al.* and Belli *et al.* have shown the positive effect of nutrition as adjunctive therapy in IBD to correct or avoid malnutrition and to facilitate growth[25,26]. Both studies were able to show normalization of linear growth either with oral or enteral nutrition, often nocturnal nasogastric tube infusion. It is important to start adjunctive therapy prior to completion of puberty in order to optimize the growth effects of adjunctive nutritional therapy. The use of nutrition as a primary therapy, mainly as exclusive enteral therapy, is still a matter of debate[27]. It is obvious that there is a treatment benefit; however, it does not seem to be superior to the use of steroids. Most studies have been performed in adults and only a few in children. From the paediatric studies, it seems clear that enteral primary treatment is better when disease is in the small intestine rather than in the large intestine[27]. The major problem is the relapse rate of up to 60–70% after stopping enteral therapy. Some studies have shown a positive effect of intermittent nocturnal treatment to maintain remission. It should be stated that it is much more important to supply adequate calories in children with IBD than in adults because of the growth potential.

The possible mode of action of enteral nutrition has not been established[3]. However, alteration in the intestinal microbial flora or elimination of dietary antigens have been suggested. Furthermore, a low fat content might affect inflammatory mediators. The most important effect is probably the overall nutritional repletion and the provision of nutrients to the diseased mucosa. There seems to be no benefit for elemental vs. non-elemental formulas in the enteral feeding approach.

In summary, growth retardation in paediatric IBD depends greatly on the definitions used. In general, growth failure is present in about 40% at diagnosis, while approximately 25% show permanent short stature as adults. It is much more common to see growth failure in Crohn's disease than ulcerative colitis. An important clinical aspect of IBD during treatment is pubertal delay. Growth retardation and pubertal delay together signal inadequate therapy. The major cause of growth failure is ongoing intestinal inflammation combined with inadequate caloric intake. It has been found that disease activity and not the use of steroids is the major factor influencing linear growth. There seems to be no extra effect of surgery on growth and adult height. In the management of growth failure, therefore, the emphasis should be placed on controlling the intestinal inflammation, possibly with a combination of the different drugs available. Nutritional studies, either as primary or adjunctive therapy, with adequate and proper control treatments, such as steroids in combination with azathioprine, are needed to identify the possible role of nutritional therapy as a primary option. In all this, it is essential to realize that, in the treatment of paediatric IBD, there is only a short therapeutic window to treat growth retardation before puberty is completed.

References

1. Kirschner BS. Growth and development in chronic inflammatory bowel disease. Acta Paediatr Scand. 1990;366(suppl):98–104.
2. Ferry GD, Büller HA. Mechanisms of growth retardation, drug therapy and nutritional support in pediatric inflammatory bowel disease: a workshop sponsored by the North American and European Societies for Pediatric Gastroenterology and Nutrition. Inflamm Bowel Dis. 1995;1:313–30.
3. Griffiths AM. Inflammatory bowel disease. Nutrition. 1998;14(10):788–91.
4. Walker-Smith JA. Management of growth failure in Crohn's disease. Arch Dis Childh. 1996;75:351–4.
5. Motil KJ, Grand RJ, Davis-Kraft L, Ferlic LL, O'Brian Smith E. Growth failure in children with inflammatory bowel disease: A prospective study. Gastroenterology. 1993;105:681–91.
6. Kanof ME, Lake AM, Bayless TM. Decreased height velocity in children and adolescents before the diagnosis of Crohn's disease. Gastroenterology. 1988;95:1523–7.
7. Markowitz J, Grancher K, Rosa J, Aiges H, Daum F. Growth failure in pediatric inflammatory bowel disease. J Ped Gastroenterol Nutr. 1993;16:373–80.

8. Griffiths AM, Nguyen P, Smith C, MacMillan JH, Sherman PM. Growth and clinical course of children with Crohn's disease. Gut. 1993;34:939–43.
9. Savage MO, Beattie RM, Camacho-Hübner C, Walker-Smith JA, Sanderson IR. Growth in Crohn's disease. Acta Paediatr. 1999;428(suppl):89–92.
10. Ghosh S, Drummond HE, Ferguson A. Neglect of growth and development in the clinical monitoring of children and teenagers with inflammatory bowel disease: review of case records. Br Med J. 1998;317:120–1
11. Kirschner BS, Sutton MM. Somatomedin-C levels in growth-impaired children and adolescents with chronic inflammatory bowel disease. Gastroenterology. 1986;91:830–6.
12. Murch SH, Lamkin VA, Savage MO, Walker-Smith JA, MacDonald TT. Serum concentrations of tumour necrosis factor α in childhood chronic inflammatory bowel disease. Gut. 1991; 32:913–17.
13. Benedetti F de, Alonzi T, Moretta A *et al.* I Interleukin 6 causes growth impairment in transgenic mice through a decrease in IGF-1. J Clin Invest. 1997;99(4):643–50.
14. Varille V, Cezard JP, Lagausie de P *et al.* Resting energy expenditure before and after surgical resection of gut lesions in pediatric Crohn's disease. J Pediatr Gastroenterol Nutr. 1996; 23:13–19.
15. Azcue M, Rashid M, Griffiths A, Pencharz PB. Energy expenditure and body composition in children with Crohn's disease: effect of enteral nutrition and treatment with prednisolone. Gut. 1997;41:203–8.
16. Zoli G, Katelaris PJ, Gasbarrini G, Farthing MJG. Increased energy expenditure in growing adolescents with Crohn's disease. Dig Dis Sci. 1996;41(9):1754–9.
17. Nicholls S, Vieira MC, Majrowski H, Shand WS, Savage MO, Walker-Smith JA. Linear growth after colectomy for ulcerative colitis in childhood. J Pediatr Gastroenterol Nutr. 1995;21:82–6.
18. Patel HI, Leichtner AM, Colodny AH, Shamberger RC. Surgery for Crohn's disease in infants and children. J Pediatr Surg. 1997;32:1063–8.
19. El-Baba M, Lin CH, Klein M, Tolia V. Outcome after surgical intervention in children with chronic inflammatory bowel disease. Am Surg. 1996;62(12):1014–17.
20. Voitk AJ, Echave V, Feller JH, Brown RA, Gurd FN. Experience with elemental diet in the treatment of inflammatory bowel disease. Arch Surg. 1973;107:329–33.
21. Beattie RM, Bentsen BS, MacDonald TT. Childhood Crohn's disease and the efficacy of enteral diets. Nutrition. 1998;14:345–50.
22. Sanderson IR, Udeen S, Davies PSW, Savage MO, Walker-Smith JA. Remission induced by an elemental diet in small bowel Crohn's disease. Arch Dis Childh. 1987;61:123–7.
23. Thomas AG, Holly JMP, Taylor F, Miller V. Insulin like growth factor-I, insulin like growth factor binding protein-1, and insulin in childhood Crohn's disease. Gut. 1993;34:944–7.
24. Thomas AG, Taylor F, Miller V. Dietary intake and nutritional treatment in childhood Crohn's disease. J Pediatr Gastroenterol Nutr. 1993;17:75–81.
25. Wilschanski M, Sherman P, Pencharz P, Davis L, Corey M, Griffiths A. Supplementary enteral nutrition maintains remission in paediatric Crohn's disease. Gut. 1996;38:543–8.
26. Belli DC, Seidman E, Bouthiller L, Weber AM, Roy CC, Plentincx M. Chronic intermittent elemental diet improves growth failure in children with Crohn's disease. Gastroenterology. 1988;94:603–10.
27. Griffiths AM, Ohlsson A, Sherman PM, Sutherland LR. Meta-analysis of enteral nutrition as a primary treatment of active Crohn's disease. Gastroenterology. 1995;108:1056–67.

10
Medical management of IBD: children versus adults

J. F. MARKOWITZ

"Children are not just little adults." This is a common theme in paediatrics and an especially important concept underlying the medical management of children and adolescents with IBD. This chapter will outline those factors which distinguish children with IBD from adults with the same conditions. By describing the 'natural history' of IBD in children and the resultant morbidity expected in this population, this review will focus on an approach to the medical management of children with IBD which at times differs significantly from that generally utilized in adults.

'NATURAL HISTORY' OF IBD IN CHILDREN

Extent and activity of disease

Both Crohn's disease and ulcerative colitis tend to be characterized by active disease courses in paediatric patients. Children with Crohn's disease commonly have extensive disease at the time of presentation, with 40–75% demonstrating ileocolonic disease, 20–30% diffuse small bowel disease and up to 40% demonstrating gastroduodenal involvement[1–3]. Data from a geographically derived incidence cohort from Denmark diagnosed between 1962 and 1987 reveal that 83% of children have moderate or high disease activity at presentation[4]. Only about 50% of the population maintains remission during each year of follow-up over the course of the first decade of disease, and 20–30% per year experience periods of moderate–severe disease activity. Similar rates of disease severity were noted in a parallel cohort of adults[4,5].

Children with ulcerative colitis also have extensive disease and experience significant periods of disease activity. In contrast to adult populations in whom there is a predominance of proctosigmoiditis, at presentation, 40–75% of children have pancolitis and only 10–25% proctosigmoiditis[1,4,6]. Children with initial evidence of proctosigmoiditis appear to be at high risk for proximal extension of disease over time, with 29–58% demonstrating inflammatory changes proximal to the sigmoid over the first 5–10 years of follow-up[7,8]. This contrasts with only 10–30% of adults who demonstrate similar proximal extension of disease[9,10]. Moderate to severe disease activity is present in 57–74% of children at presentation, and over the first 10 years of disease only 50–60% are in remission during any successive year of follow-up[4,6].

Duration of disease

When children develop IBD, a normal life span can mean a disease duration of as long as 60–80 years. This extended duration of illness potentially puts children with IBD at high lifetime risk for complications. One particular complication which has received attention is the development of colorectal cancer. The primary risk factors for the development of colorectal carcinoma in UC are duration of illness and anatomic extent of disease[11,12]. These two factors combine in the child with UC, resulting in a significant lifetime risk of developing colorectal cancer. Population-based data from Sweden reveal that relative risk for colorectal cancer increases with decreasing age at diagnosis, such that children less than 15 years of age at diagnosis of UC have the highest relative risk of all age groups, with a standardized incidence ratio of 118, and a cumulative risk of colorectal cancer of 40% after 35 years of illness[13]. While a recent meta-analysis estimates a somewhat lower cumulative risk of colorectal cancer (11% at 20 years, 16% at 30 years) for patients with onset of colitis during childhood, the risk remains significantly greater than in patients with adult-onset disease and similar duration of colitis[14]. Similar trends are also evident for children with Crohn's colitis[15].

Prolonged duration of illness probably also increases the risk of other complications of IBD. Among children with a fibrostenosing phenotype of Crohn's disease, prolonged duration of disease may heighten the lifetime risk for recurrent episodes of bowel obstruction and the need for recurrent surgery. While strictureplasty has limited the need for bowel resection[16], the risk of short bowel syndrome from repeated bowel resection remains. Similarly, individuals with recurrent fistula formation also suffer significant morbidity, and potentially undergo multiple surgeries when their illness begins in childhood. The fact is that children with Crohn's disease commonly require surgery. Studies from paediatric populations around the world report cumulative rates of surgery of 32–60%[17,18]. In one study, among the children who required major surgery for Crohn's disease, 59% required second surgery within 5 years, and 85% required second surgery within 10 years of initial surgery[17].

Corticosteroid dependency and resistance

Although never subjected to a controlled clinical trial in children, corticosteroids have traditionally been considered the treatment of choice for children with moderate and severe IBD. Despite the known potential toxicity of corticosteroids, its acute efficacy in inducing remission serves to perpetuate its use. The efficacy of corticosteroids in children with IBD has increasingly been questioned, however, especially with the realization that the 'natural history' data summarized above, drawn from clinical experience in the 1970s and 1980s, by and large reflects the effect (or lack of effect) of corticosteroid therapy. Despite the fact that commonly accepted clinical practice advocates only a brief course of corticosteroids, the persistence or frequent recurrence of active disease often results in children accumulating very significant corticosteroid exposure.

While the frequency of corticosteroid dependence and resistance in children with UC is not known, a controlled experience with the use of corticosteroids in the treatment of newly diagnosed children with Crohn's disease is available[19]. The data come from observations made on a group of children enrolled in a study designed to evaluate the effect of treatment with a combination of 6-MP and prednisone. The control group of 28 children received a standardized regimen of prednisone plus 'placebo 6MP'. In this group, the dose and duration of prednisone therapy was determined by the change in a subject's disease activity score, in a fashion designed to mimic clinical practice. In these previously untreated children, prednisone therapy alone resulted in 79% experiencing a partial or complete response after 1 month, and 89% experienced a clinical remission by 3 months. However, 31% of these children relapsed within 3 months of discontinuing the corticosteroid, and 57% relapsed by 1 year. Overall clinical response to prednisone could therefore be characterized as prolonged remission in only 50%, while corticosteroid dependence developed in 39% and corticosteroid resistance in 11%. Similar data are reported by Munkholm *et al.*[20] in a Danish population of 109 adults with Crohn's disease. In this population, 80% experienced a complete or partial remission within 1 month of initiating corticosteroid therapy, but 45% of initial responders had a disease relapse or were corticosteroid dependent within 1 year. In this group, 44% experienced a prolonged response to a course of corticosteroid but 36% became corticosteroid dependent and 20% corticosteroid resistant.

Growth impairment

Growth failure represents a problem unique to children which impacts directly on medical management. At the time of initial diagnosis, up to 88% of children with Crohn's disease have decreased height velocity[21] and 30–40% have absolute height deficiencies manifested by diminished height percentiles for age[22–24]. Among children who develop Crohn's disease before puberty, 60% demonstrate a drop of two or more major height percentiles for age at some time prior to the end of adolescence[24]. Permanent deficits of adult stature have been reported in 7–35% of young adults who developed IBD before puberty, depending upon what method was used to predict expected adult stature[24]. The result is that young adults with childhood-onset IBD are often significantly shorter than the general population. Fifty per cent have adult heights less than the tenth percentile for the general population, and 25% are shorter than the fifth percentile[22,24]. Although all children with IBD eventually mature, those with impaired growth also have associated delayed sexual development.

The aetiology for growth failure is multifactorial. Chronic undernutrition due to poor caloric intake is an important factor[25]. Poor nutrition results in decreased serum levels of insulin-like growth factor-I (IGF-I), the mediator of growth hormone's effects, and nutritional restitution improves both IGF-I and growth[26,27]. Increased levels of circulating cytokines, such as interleukin-6

(IL-6) and tumour necrosis factor-α (TNF-α), are associated with inadequate control of disease activity, and are likely to result directly in impaired bone growth[23,28]. However, minimizing disease activity through chronic corticosteroid use is counterproductive as corticosteroid use is itself growth inhibitory. Corticosteroid therapy has been shown to be associated with decreased type I procollagen production[29] and to directly interfere with the effect of growth hormone and its mediators[30].

Quality of life

IBD results in social as well as physical morbidity in the child and adolescent. Seventy-five per cent of children miss significant amounts of school[31]. In a survey of young adults with childhood-onset Crohn's disease, 57% reported at least one absence of 2 months or more at some time during their school years, and 8% reported involuntary unemployment after school due to active Crohn's disease[32]. One half to two thirds of children experience difficulty playing sports, and many others report that the symptoms of IBD interfere with common social activities, such as staying over at friends' homes and going on family vacations[31–33]. The impact of disease activity on the lives of these youngsters and the resulting social morbidity are important factors influencing medical therapy.

MEDICAL THERAPY

As summarized above, children and adolescents with IBD tend to have extensive disease, frequent relapses, and a high likelihood of corticosteroid dependence or resistance (Table 1). Their many decades of ongoing disease put them at increased risk for complications, including growth failure, colorectal cancer and recurrent surgery. Recognition of these facts has focused attention on the inadequacies of therapy with traditional agents such as 5-aminosalicylates and corticosteroids. While differences in emphasis exist between North American and European practice, increasingly, paediatric gastroenterologists on both continents are utilizing a combination of nutritional approaches, coupled with the early and more widespread use of immunomodulatory and biological agents to

Table 1 'Natural history' of IBD in the child: factors which affect medical therapy

Disease activity
• Extensive anatomic disease
• Frequent relapses
Disease duration
• Colorectal cancer
• Surgery
Corticosteroid dependence and resistance
Growth impairment
Impaired quality of life

more successfully control the morbidity and resulting complications of IBD in children.

Nutrition as primary therapy

Nutritional approaches to the control of IBD in children are conceptually appealing given the impact these illnesses have on growth and development. While no nutritional therapy has been shown to be of benefit in the primary control of UC in children, there are data to support such an approach in children with Crohn's disease. Parenteral nutrition, both total and as a supplement to oral dietary intake, can suppress active disease symptoms, promote positive nitrogen balance, induce remission and enhance growth[34]. Enteral feeding, delivered orally or via nasogastric or gastrostomy tube, also appears to be effective. A number of small paediatric trials have demonstrated that enteral feeding results in lessening of gut permeability and reduction of mucosal inflammation[35–37]. Small paediatric studies, both uncontrolled and controlled, have suggested that enteral nutrition with elemental, semielemental and whole protein formulae lessens Crohn's disease activity[38–40]. While the largest controlled trial in adults[41] as well as meta-analyses of adult experience[42–44] have concluded that corticosteroids are superior to enteral nutrition for induction of remission in active Crohn's disease, a recent meta-analysis of paediatric trials suggests that enteral nutrition and corticosteroids are comparably effective for inducing remission in children[45].

Given that both enteral nutrition and corticosteroids induce remission in children with active Crohn's disease, the choice between these modalities must be made based on other factors. Neither therapy maintains remission once discontinued. The advantages of corticosteroid therapy are rapidity of effect (usually less than 10 days) and ease of administration. By contrast, the advantages of nutritional management relate to the avoidance of steroid-related side effects, including cosmetic changes, drug-induced bone disease and interference with linear bone growth. Given the frequency of growth failure in children with Crohn's disease, nutritional management offers the potential to induce remission and promote, rather than interfere with, future growth. In centres committed to such an approach, patients and their families have a high degree of acceptance for such an intervention, even when a nasogastric or gastrostomy tube is necessary. In fact, less than 10% of children enrolled in published trials are unable to complete a course of enteral therapy[45]. As newer, more palatable formulae become available, the number of children and families accepting nutritional therapy is likely to increase even more, as oral rather than tube administration of the formula will become practical[37].

Immunomodulatory agents

The adverse effects attributable to corticosteroids, especially the cosmetic and growth-suppressive effects, are of great concern to children and adolescents, as well as to their parents. As physicians have recognized that chronic corticosteroid therapy offers no benefit in terms of maintenance of remission, treatment regimens designed to minimize or eliminate the use of corticosteroids have become central to the management of IBD in the paediatric population. The potential for extensive, active disease and consequent severe morbidity has led to more aggressive medical intervention than even a decade ago.

One of the most dramatic changes in the treatment of children with IBD has been the increasing use of immunomodulatory medications. Surveys of the physician members of the North American Society for Pediatric Gastroenterology and Nutrition in 1990 and 2000 have documented the extent of this change[46]. Over the decade, the surveys documented a twenty point increase (from 73% in 1990 to 93% in 2000; $p < 0.0001$) in the percentage of survey respondents who agreed with the statement that immunosuppressive agents 'are effective therapies for children and adolescents with IBD'[46]. Clinicians increased use of immunomodulatory agents for all of the major forms of IBD, more commonly prescribed immunomodulators for a variety of indications, and extended the use of these medications to even the youngest of patients, including those under 5 years of age.

This change in attitude regarding the use of immunomodulatory therapy has been based on broadening clinical experience and a few controlled clinical trials. 6-Mercaptopurine and azathioprine are by far the two most commonly prescribed immunomodulatory agents for paediatric IBD. The initial use of these agents was restricted to children and adolescents with corticosteroid-resistant or -dependent Crohn's disease. Retrospective reports of clinical experience demonstrated results similar to those noted in adult populations, with about two thirds of patients having a significant response or remission following institution of immunomodulatory treatment[47,48]. As use of these agents broadened, paediatric safety data emerged. In a summary of the experience from the paediatric gastroenterology service of the University of Chicago, Kirschner[49] reported that, overall, 82% of children and adolescents tolerated 6-MP or azathioprine well, and most successfully reduced or eliminated their concomitant steroid use. Fifty-four per cent had no adverse reactions, and 28% had mild side effects, including an increase in aminotransferase levels, which responded to dose reduction or improved spontaneously. Only 18% of patients required discontinuation of therapy because of recurrent fever, pancreatitis, gastrointestinal intolerance, recurrent infections, or neutropenia[49]. These data are comparable to the safety profile for these agents in adults[50].

The initial encouraging paediatric efficacy and safety data for 6-MP and azathioprine led to a realization that restricting the use of these agents to corticosteroid-dependent children with IBD potentially allowed preventable morbidity to develop. As a consequence, the earlier use of immunomodulators in children has been investigated in a multicentre placebo-controlled trial[19]. Newly diagnosed children with moderate–severe Crohn's disease activity received as their initial IBD treatment either 6-MP or placebo, in conjunction with a standardized regimen of prednisone in both groups. Prednisone induced remission in 89% of both treatment groups within the first three months of therapy. However, when followed over the next 18 months, 91% of the 6-MP group who achieved remission remained well compared with only 53% of corticosteroid-treated controls (p=0.007). At the same time, the 6-MP group required significantly less cumulative corticosteroid than controls. Mild leukopenia was seen in 22% of 6-MP-treated subjects, but only 1 subject was withdrawn for an absolute neutrophil count less than 1250/mm^3. Mild elevations of aminotransferases were seen in the first three months of treatment in 15% of 6-MP-treated subjects but no concomitant evidence of liver dysfunction was noted and the abnormal aminotransferases normalized in 3 of 4 subjects without change in 6-MP therapy.

Indications for the use of immunomodulators in paediatric Crohn's disease continue to expand. 6-MP and azathioprine have been shown to promote improvement in 75% of children with chronic perianal Crohn's disease[51]. 6-MP has also been shown to limit recurrence of Crohn's disease following intestinal resection when introduced in the perioperative period[52]. In a small paediatric trial, none of 5 children treated with 6-MP and a 5-aminosalicylate medication had a postoperative relapse in a mean of 32.6 ± 18.4 months of follow-up. By contrast, 3 of 5 children treated only with 5-aminosalicylates postoperatively relapsed a mean of 3.7 ± 1.2 months after surgery[52]. It has also been observed that relapse after intestinal resection is particularly rapid if a child receiving 6-MP or azathioprine preoperatively is not continued on the medication postoperatively[53].

The value of immunomodulators in the treatment of ulcerative colitis in children has also been recognized. Fifty to 80% of children with fulminant colitis avoid imminent colectomy when treated with either intravenous cyclosporine[54] or oral tacrolimus[55]. However, remission is only rarely maintained unless 6-MP or azathioprine is added to the therapeutic regimen[56]. Children with chronic, severe, corticosteroid-dependent ulcerative colitis also respond to 6-MP and azathioprine. In a review of clinical experience from the Children's Hospital of Philadelphia, 75% of patients discontinued corticosteroids after a mean of 8.4 months of immunomodulator therapy, and two thirds of these had a prolonged remission[57].

These reports are reflected in a fundamental change in the attitude of North American paediatric gastroenterologists regarding the use of immunomodulators in UC. As evidenced by the 1990 and 2000 surveys of the membership of NASPGN[46], in 1990, 55% of respondents did not prescribe immunomodulators for UC. Nearly half of those, or 27% of all respondents, reported that they preferred colectomy to the use of immunomodulatory agents for a child with severe colitis. By contrast, in 2000, over 90% of respondents had prescribed immunomodulators for children with UC, leaving colectomy as the preferred therapy for only 6% of respondents ($p<0.0001$). The increased preference for medical over surgical therapy for severe colitis was associated with only a minimum number of respondents expressing concern that the use of immunomodulators might promote the development of dysplasia or cancer (1.4% in 1990, 0.4% in 2000; $p=\text{NS}$).

Infliximab

The role of infliximab and other anti-TNF monoclonal antibodies in the treatment of children with IBD is just beginning to be systematically studied. Despite this, the commercial availability of this agent in the US since the end of 1999 has made a major impact on clinical practice. Current published experience is limited to two open-label treatment trials of children with intractable Crohn's disease[58,59]. In both studies, safety and efficacy of one or more 5-mg/kg infusions were similar to data reported in adults[60–62]. Of the 34 children included in the two reports, 33 had significantly decreased disease activity (PCDAI) scores within 4 weeks of the initial infusion, and most were also able to reduce or eliminate concomitant corticosteroid use. While beneficial clinical effects tended to wane 6–12 weeks after the infusion in many of those treated, repeat infusions often resulted in restitution of clinical response. A few patients were noted to have quite prolonged response after a single infusion, however, which in one study was seen exclusively in children who had been diagnosed with Crohn's disease less than 2 years prior to the infliximab infusion[59]. Whether the use of infliximab early in the course of Crohn's disease is capable of fundamentally changing the natural course of the illness remains to be determined.

Despite the limited published data, North American paediatric gastroenterologists have apparently rapidly adopted the use of infliximab in clinical practice. As judged by responses to a recent survey of the membership of NASPGN, 157 physicians (59% of respondents representing 22% of the society's physicians) had prescribed infliximab in the first year of the therapy's commercial availability[63]. Respondents reported using infliximab to treat an estimated 720 children and adolescents with Crohn's disease, 32 with ulcerative colitis and 21 with indeterminate colitis, primarily for intractable IBD symptoms (66%), intractable perianal disease (61%) and chronic non-perianal fistulae (40%). If infliximab induced remission, 53% of respondents added or continued 6-mercaptopurine or azathioprine to maintain remission, 34% added/continued 5-aminosalicylates, and 14% added/continued corticosteroids. Repeated infliximab infusions were used to maintain remission by 34% of respondents to the survey. Efficacy and toxicity was judged comparable to published adult clinical experience.

Aminosalicylates

There is extensive clinical experience with sulphasalazine and mesalamine in children, which, by and large, has mirrored adult efficacy and safety data[64]. Small open-label or double-blind paediatric trials, as well as a retrospective analysis of 10 years clinical experience with Eudragit coated 5-aminosalicylate preparations have reported therapeutic benefits in active ulcerative colitis, active Crohn's colitis, and active small bowel Crohn's disease[65–68]. The only paediatric study to compare the efficacy of different 5-aminosalicylate preparations found that, in children with mildly to moderately active ulcerative colitis, 79% of those treated with sulphasalazine (60 mg kg^{-1} day^{-1}) demonstrated clinical improvement compared with only 39% of those treated with olsalazine (30 mg kg^{-1} day^{-1})[69]. There are no paediatric studies evaluating balsalazide, a 5-aminosalicylate which has just been commercially released in the US, nor any data on the use of rectal 5-aminosalicylate preparations in children. There are also no paediatric studies assessing maintenance of remission with any aminosalicylate preparation in either ulcerative colitis or Crohn's disease, nor in preventing disease recurrence after surgery in Crohn's disease. The usefulness of aminosalicylates is limited in many children because of the lack of liquid preparations and the fact that the enteric coatings on a number of the products makes it impossible to crush the tablets without loss of efficacy. Adverse reactions to all of the 5-aminosalicylate preparations have been described, requiring discontinuation in 5–15% of cases. The more serious complications reported in children have included pancreatitis, nephritis, exacerbation of disease, and sulpha- or salicylate-induced allergic reactions.

Corticosteroids

Given their lack of efficacy for maintaining remission, and their potential for inducing toxicity such as growth suppression, osteopenia, and ocular toxicity, corticosteroids have a limited role in the management of children and adolescents with IBD. However, in the setting of acute, severe disease, corticosteroids are useful in the treatment of both Crohn's disease and ulcerative colitis in children. When steroid therapy is initiated, however, it should be with the intention of controlling the inflammation acutely, serving as a bridge to the use of less-toxic remission-maintaining therapy. For children with severe Crohn's disease, either 6-MP or azathioprine is the best agent to maintain remission, although methotrexate can be used for patients intolerant of 6-MP[70]. For children with active ulcerative colitis, aminosalicylate medications can be used successfully in some cases, although, for most children with moderate–severe UC, an immunomodulator will be required. While oral forms of budesonide have the potential to deliver the beneficial effects of corticosteroid with less systemic toxicity (e.g. less growth suppression), no paediatric studies evaluating this agent in IBD have been published.

Guidelines for the treatment of children with IBD

Figures 1–4 propose algorithms based on the data described above. They represent guidelines for the treatment of children and adolescents with IBD derived, as much as possible, from evidence-based data.

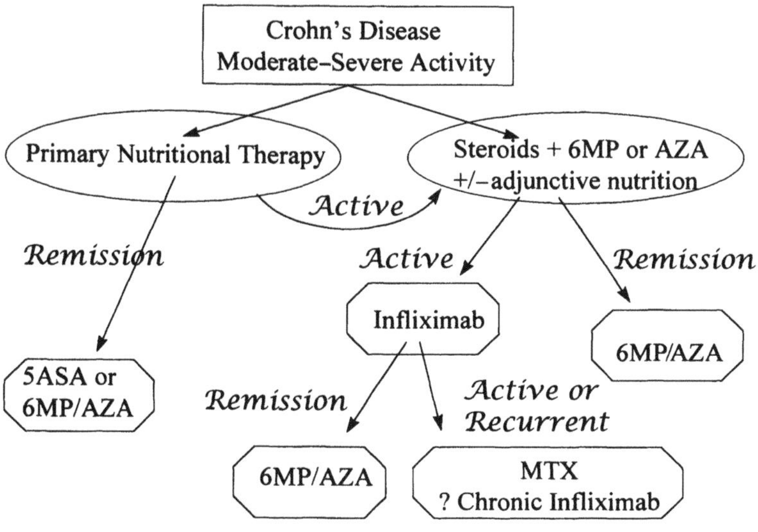

Figure 1 Recommended treatment algorithm for children and adolescents with moderate–severe Crohn's disease

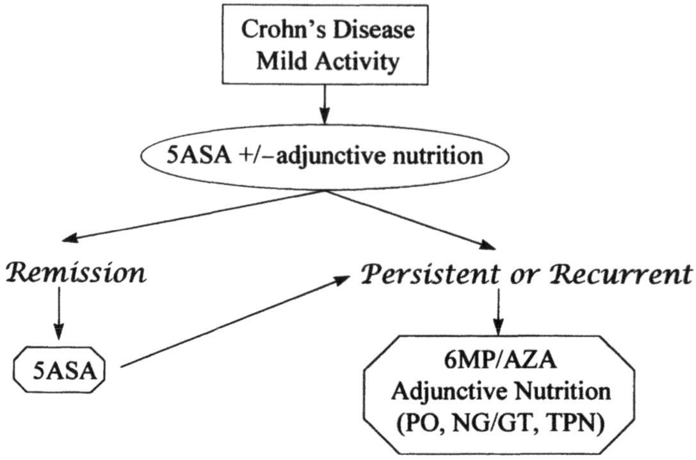

Figure 2 Recommended treatment algorithm for children and adolescents with mild Crohn's disease

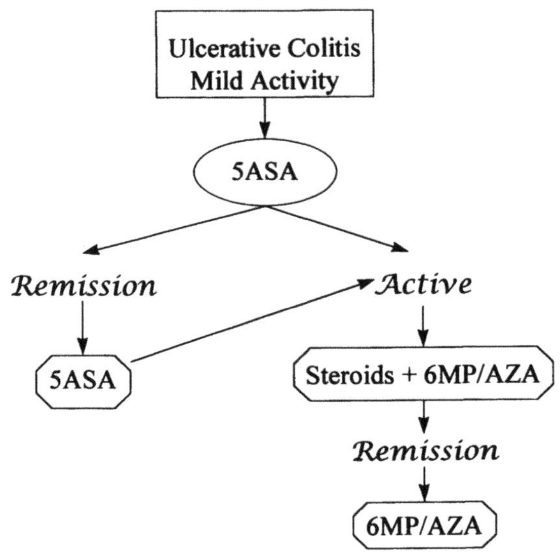

Figure 3 Recommended treatment algorithm for children and adolescents with mild ulcerative colitis

Key to abbreviations in Figures 1–4:

6MP	6-Mercaptopurine	PO	Per os
AZA	Azathioprine	NG	Nasogastric
5ASA	5-Aminosalicylate	GT	Gastrostomy
MTX	Methotrexate	TPN	Total parenteral nutrition

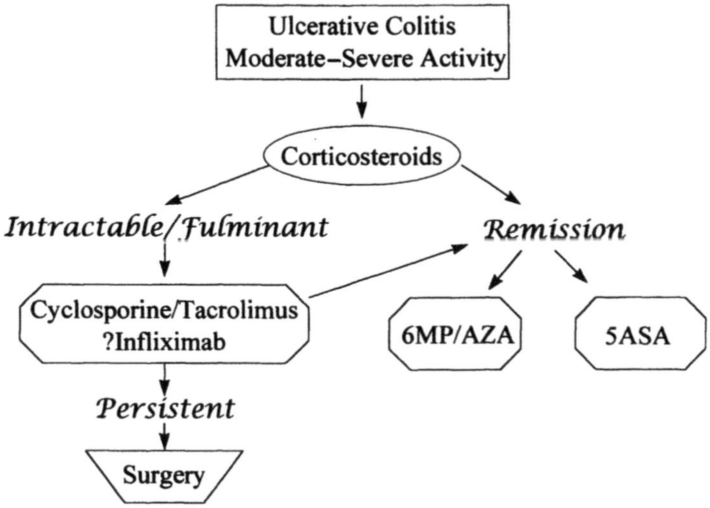

Figure 4 Recommended treatment algorithm for children and adolescents with moderate–severe ulcerative colitis

References

1. Ferguson A, Sedgwick DM. Juvenile-onset inflammatory bowel disease: predictors of morbidity and health status in early adult life. J R Coll Phys London. 1994;28:220–7.
2. Puntis J, McNeish AS, Allen RN. Long term prognosis of Crohn's disease with onset in childhood and adolescence. Gut. 1984;25:329–36.
3. Mashako MNL, Cezard JP, Navarro J *et al.* Crohn's disease lesions in the upper gastrointestinal tract: correlation between clinical, radiological, endoscopic, and histological features in adolescents and children. J Pediatr Gastroenterol Nutr. 1989;8:442–6.
4. Langholz E, Munkholm P, Krasilnikoff PA, Binder V. Inflammatory bowel diseases with onset in childhood. Clinical features, morbidity and mortality in a regional cohort. Scand J Gastroenterol. 1997;32:139–47.
5. Binder V, Hendriksen C, Kreiner S. Prognosis in Crohn's disease based on results from a regional patient group from the county of Copenhagen. Gut. 1985;26:146–50.
6. Hyams JS, Davis P, Grancher K, Lerer T, Justinich CJ, Markowitz J. Clinical outcome of ulcerative colitis in children. J Pediatr. 1996;129:81–8.
7. Hyams J, Davis P, Lerer T *et al.* Clinical outcome of ulcerative proctitis in children. J Pediatr Gastroenterol Nutr. 1997;25:149–52.
8. Mir-Madjlessi SH, Michener WM, Farmer RG. Course and prognosis of idiopathic ulcerative proctosigmoiditis in young patients. J Pediatr Gastroenterol Nutr. 1986;5:570–5.
9. Farmer RG. Long-term prognosis for patients with ulcerative proctosigmoiditis (ulcerative colitis confined to the rectum and sigmoid colon). J Clin Gastroenterol. 1979;1:47–50.
10. Powell-Tuck J, Ritchie JK, Lennard-Jones JE. The prognosis of idiopathic proctitis. Scand J Gastroenterol. 1977;12:727–32.
11. Devroede GJ, Taylor WF, Sauer WG, Jackman RJ, Stickler GB. Cancer risk and life expectancy of children with ulcerative colitis. N Engl J Med. 1971;285:17–21.
12. Sugita A, Sachar DB, Ribeiro MB, Aufses AH Jr, Greenstein AJ. Colorectal cancer in ulcerative colitis: influence of anatomical extent and age at onset on colitis–cancer interval. Gut. 1991;32: 167–9.
13. Ekbom A, Helmick C, Zack M, Adami H-O. Ulcerative colitis and colorectal cancer: a population based study. N Engl J Med. 1990;323:1228–33.
14. Eaden JA, Abrams KR, Mayberry JF. The risk of colorectal cancer in ulcerative colitis: a meta-analysis. Gut. 2001;48:526–35.

15. Ekbom A, Helmick C, Zack M, Adami H-O. Increased risk of large-bowel cancer in Crohn's disease with colonic involvement. Lancet. 1990;336:357–9.
16. Oliva L, Wyllie R, Alexander F *et al.* The results of strictureplasty in pediatric patients with multifocal Crohn's disease. J Pediatr Gastroenterol Nutr. 1994;18(3):306–10.
17. Sedgwick DM, Barton JR, Hamer-Dodges DW, Nixon SJ, Ferguson A. Population-based study of surgery in juvenile onset Crohn's disease. Br J Surg. 1991;78:171–5.
18. Griffiths AM. Factors that influence the postoperative recurrence of Crohn's disease in childhood. In: Hadziselimovic F, Herzog B, Burgin-Wolff A, eds. Inflammatory Bowel Disease and Coeliac Disease in Children. Boston: Kluwer Academic Publishers, 1990:131–6.
19. Markowitz J, Grancher K, Kohn N, Lesser M, Daum F, and the 6MP Collaborative Group. A multicenter trial of 6-mercaptopurine and prednisone in newly diagnosed children with Crohn's disease. Gastroenterology. 2000;119:895–902.
20. Munkholm P, Langholz E, Davidsen M, Binder V. Frequency of glucocorticoid resistance and dependency in Crohn's disease. Gut. 1994;35:360–2.
21. Kanof ME, Lake AM, Bayless TM. Decreased height velocity in children and adolescents before the diagnosis of Crohn's disease. Gastroenterology. 1988;95:1523–7.
22. Kirschner BS. Growth and development in chronic inflammatory bowel disease. Acta Pediatr Scand (Suppl). 1990;366:98–104.
23. Motil KJ, Grand RJ, Davis-Kraft L, Ferlic LL, O'Brian Smith E. Growth failure in children with inflammatory bowel disease: a prospective study. Gastroenterology 1993;105:681–91.
24. Markowitz J, Grancher K, Rosa J, Aiges H, Daum F. Growth failure in pediatric inflammatory bowel disease. J Pediatr Gastroenterol Nutr. 1993;16:373–80.
25. Kelts DG, Grand RJ, Shen G, Watkins JB, Werlin SL, Boehme C. Nutritional basis of growth failure in children and adolescents with Crohn's disease. Gastroenterology. 1979;76(4):720–7.
26. Thomas AG, Holly JMP, Taylor F, Miller V. Insulin like growth factor-I, insulin like growth factor binding protein-I, and insulin in childhood Crohn's disease. Gut. 1993;34:944–7.
27. Aiges H, Markowitz J, Rosa J, Daum F. Home nocturnal supplemental nasogastric feedings in growth-retarded adolescents with Crohn's disease. Gastroenterology. 1989;97:905–10.
28. Koniaris SG, Fisher SE, Rubin CT, Chawla A. Experimental colitis impairs linear bone growth independent of nutritional factors. J Pediatr Gastroenterol Nutr. 1997;25(2):137–41.
29. Hyams JS, Moore RE, Leichtner AM, Carey DE, Goldberg BD. Relationship of type I procollagen to corticosteroid therapy in children with inflammatory bowel disease. J Pediatr. 1988;112:893–8.
30. Hyams JS, Carey DE. Corticosteroids and growth. J Pediatr. 1988;113(2):249–54.
31. Rabbett H, Elbadri A, Thwaites R *et al.* Quality of life in children with Crohn's disease. J Pediatr Gastroenterol Nutr. 1996;23:528–33.
32. Ferguson A, Sedgwick DM, Drummond J. Morbidity of juvenile onset inflammatory bowel disease: effects on education and employment in early adult life. Gut. 1994;35:665–8.
33. Moody G, Eaden JA, Mayberry JF. Social implications of childhood Crohn's disease. J Pediatr Gastroenterol Nutr. 1999;28:S43–5.
34. Seidman EG. Nutritional management of inflammatory bowel disease. Gastroenterol Clin N Am. 1989;18(1):129–55.
35. Sanderson IR, Boulton P, Menzies I, Walker-Smith JA. Improvement of abnormal lactulose/rhamnose permeability in active Crohn's disease of the small bowel by elemental diet. Gut. 1987;28:1073–6.
36. Breese EJ, Michie CA, Nicholls SW *et al.* The effect of treatment on lymphokine-secreting cells in the intestinal mucosa of children with Crohn's disease. Aliment Pharmacol Ther. 1995;9:547–53.
37. Fell JME, Paintin M, Arnaud-Battandier F *et al.* Mucosal healing and a fall in mucosal pro-inflammatory cytokine mRNA induced by a specific oral polymeric diet in paediatric Crohn's disease. Aliment Pharmacol Ther. 2000;14:281–9.
38. Sanderson IR, Udeen S, Davies PSW, Savage MO, Walker-Smith JA. Remission induced by an elemental diet in small bowel Crohn's disease. Arch Dis Child. 1987;61:123–7.
39. Seidman E, Griffiths A, Jones A, Issenman R. Semi-elemental diet vs prednisolone in pediatric Crohn's disease (abstract). Gastroenterology. 1993;104:778.
40. Ruuska T, Savilahti E, Maki M, Ormala T, Visakorpi JK. Exclusive whole protein enteral diet versus prednisolone in the treatment of acute Crohn's disease in children. J Pediatr Gastroenterol Nutr. 1994;19:175–80.

41. Lochs H, Steinhardt HJ, Klaus-Wentz B *et al.* Comparison of enteral nutrition and drug treatment in active Crohn's disease: results of the European Cooperative Crohn's Disease Study IV. Gastroenterology. 1991;101:881–8.
42. Griffiths AM, Ohlsson A, Sherman P, Sutherland LR. Meta-analysis of enteral nutrition as primary treatment of active Crohn's disease. Gastroenterology. 1995;108:1056–67.
43. Fernandez-Banares F, Cabre E, Esteve-Comas M, Gassull MA. How effective is enteral nutrition in inducing clinical remission in active Crohn's disease? A meta-analysis of the randomized clinical trials. J Parenteral Enteral Nutr. 1995;19:356–364.
44. Messori A, Trallori G, D'Albasio G, Milla M, Vannozzi G, Pacini F. Defined-formula diets versus steroids in the treatment of active Crohn's disease: a meta-analysis. Scand J Gastroenterol. 1996;31:267–72.
45. Heuschkel RB, Menache CC, Megerian JT, Baird AE. Enteral nutrition and corticosteroids in the treatment of acute Crohn's disease in children. J Pediatr Gastroenterol Nutr. 2000;31:8–15.
46. Markowitz J, Grancher K, Kohn N. Immunomodulatory therapy for pediatric inflammatory bowel disease: changing patterns of use 1990–2000. J. Pediatr Gastroenterol Nutr. 2000;31(Suppl 2):S79.
47. Verhave M, Winter HS, Grand RJ. Azathioprine in the treatment of children with inflammatory bowel disease. J Pediatr. 1990;117(5):809–14.
48. Markowitz J, Rosa J, Grancher K, Aiges H, Daum F. Long term 6-mercaptopurine treatment in adolescents with Crohn's disease. Gastroenterology. 1990;99:1347–51.
49. Kirschner BS. Safety of azathioprine and 6-mercaptopurine in pediatric patients with inflammatory bowel disease. Gastroenterology. 1998;115:813–21.
50. Present DH, Meltzer SJ, Krumholz MP, Wolke A, Korelitz BI. 6-Mercaptopurine in the management of inflammatory bowel disease: short- and long-term toxicity. Ann Intern Med. 1989; 111(8):641–9.
51. Jeshion WC, Larsen KL, Jawad AF *et al.* Azathioprine and 6-mercaptopurine for the treatment of perianal Crohn's disease in children. J Clin Gastroenterol. 2000;30:295–8.
52. Kader HA, Raynor SC, Young R *et al.* Introduction of 6-mercaptopurine in Crohn's disease patients during the perioperative period: a preliminary evaluation of recurrence of disease. J Pediatr Gastoenterol Nutr. 1997;25:93–7.
53. Han PD, Lichtenstein GR, Jeshion WC *et al.* Preoperative therapy with 6-mercaptopurine predicts early recurrence following surgical resection for Crohn's disease in children. J Pediatr Gastroenterol Nutr. 1997;25:451(abstract).
54. Treem WR, Cohen J, Davis PM, Justinich CJ, Hyams JS. Cyclosporine for the treatment of fulminant ulcerative colitis in children. Dis Colon Rectum. 1995;38:474–9.
55. Bousvaros A, Kirschner BS, Werlin SL *et al.* Oral tacrolimus treatment of severe colitis in children. J Pediatr. 2000;137(6):794–9.
56. Ramakrishna J, Langhans N, Calenda K, Grand RJ, Verhave M. Combined use of cyclosporine and azathioprine or 6-mercaptopurine in pediatric inflammatory bowel disease. J Pediatr Gastroenterol Nutr. 1996;22(3):296–302.
57. Kader HA, Mascarenhas MR, Piccoli DA, Stouffer NO, Baldassano RN. Experiences with 6-mercaptopurine and azathioprine therapy in pediatric patients with severe ulcerative colitis. J Pediatr Gastroenterol Nutr. 1999;28:54–8.
58. Hyams J, Markowitz J, Wyllie R. Use of infliximab in the treatment of Crohn's disease in children and adolescents. J Pediatr. 2000;137:192–6.
59. Kugathasan S, Werlin SL, Martinez A, Rivera MT, Heikenen JB, Binion DG. Prolonged duration of response to infliximab in early but not late pediatric Crohn's disease. Am J Gastroenterol. 2000;95:3189–94.
60. Cohen RD, Tsang JF, Hanauer SB. Infliximab in Crohn's disease: first anniversary clinical experience. Am J Gastroenterol. 2000;95:3469–77.
61. Farrell RJ, Shah SA, Lodhavia PJ *et al.* Clinical experience with infliximab therapy in 100 patients with Crohn's disease. Am J Gastroenterol. 2000;95:3490–7.
62. Schaible TF. Long term safety of infliximab. Can J Gastroenterol. 2000;14 (Suppl C):29C–32C.
63. Markowitz J, Grancher K, Kohn N. Infliximab for IBD: A survey of NASPGN physicians' attitudes. J Pediatr Gastroenterol Nutr. 2000;31(Suppl 2):S79.
64. Leichtner AM. Aminosalicylates for the treatment of inflammatory bowel disease. J Pediatr Gastroenterol Nutr. 1995;21:245–52.
65. Tolia V, Massoud N, Klotz U. Oral 5-aminosalicylic acid in children with colonic inflammatory bowel disease: clinical and pharmacokinetic experience. J Pediatr Gastroenterol Nutr. 1989;8:333–8.

66. Barden L, Lipson A, Pert P, Walker-Smith JA. Mesalazine in childhood inflammatory bowel disease. Aliment Pharmacol Ther. 1989;3:597–603.
67. Griffiths A, Koletzko S, Sylvester F, Marcon M, Sherman P. Slow-release 5-aminosalicylic acid therapy in children with small intestinal Crohn's disease. J Pediatr Gastroenterol Nutr. 1993;17:186–92.
68. D'Agata ID, Vanounou T, Seidman E. Mesalamine in pediatric inflammatory bowel disease: a 10 year experience. Inflamm Bowel Dis. 1996;2:229–35.
69. Ferry GD, Kirschner BS, Grand RJ *et al.* Olsalazine versus sulfasalazine in mild to moderate childhood ulcerative colitis: results of the Pediatric Gastroenterology Collaborative Research Group Clinical Trial. J Pediatr Gastroenterol Nutr. 1993;17:32–8.
70. Mack DR, Young R, Kaufman SS, Ramey L, Vanderhoof JA. Methotrexate in patients with Crohn's disease after 6-mercaptopurine. J Pediatr. 1998;132(5):830–5.

11
Nutrition therapy in inflammatory bowel disease

M. A. GASSULL and E. CABRÉ

More than 15 years have elapsed since the first description by O'Morain *et al.* of a series of steroid-dependent Crohn's disease patients responding to the administration of an elemental diet with a decrease in the disease activity index comparable to that achieved by prednisolone[1]. This finding opened new perspectives in the treatment of these patients, offering them the possibility of a less aggressive therapy. Since then, persistent attempts have been made to introduce enteral nutrition as a primary therapy in Crohn's disease but without full success. The most likely reasons for this lack of interest in nutrition by the physicians in charge of these patients may be:

(1) Enteral nutrition is not seen as a 'true treatment';
(2) Lack of enough and proper clinical trials;
(3) More exigent outcomes in trials using enteral nutrition than those performed with drugs;
(4) The possibility that some subgroups of patients may respond better than others to this therapy.

In the following pages, these possibilities will be analysed.

ENTERAL NUTRITION IS NOT SEEN AS A 'TRUE TREATMENT'

Nutrition has been sought mainly as an adjuvant therapy in IBD. It was first thought that nutritional support would favour 'bowel rest' (a cornerstone for many years in the treatment of severe IBD) while supplying nutrients to otherwise fasted patients. Parenteral nutrition has been used for this purpose. However, various studies have shown that withholding nutrients from the gut during acute attacks of IBD does not influence disease outcome either in ulcerative colitis or in Crohn's disease[2–5].

A second reason for using parenteral nutrition as nutritional support in IBD patients was to diminish the antigenic load in the intestinal lumen, since it was believed that complex nutrients may act as antigens, thereby triggering or perpetuating the enhanced intestinal inflammatory response. In an attempt to reach a compromise for using the intestine as a nutritional route and at the same time diminishing the luminal antigenic load, the administration of amino-acid-based elemental enteral diets was proposed[1,6]. These diets would, theoretically, be easily absorbed with minimal metabolic needs (bowel rest) and would provide low antigenic nutrients. However, several trials and at least two meta-analyses have shown no differences in the outcome for Crohn's disease patients receiving elemental or whole protein based polymeric diets, with higher antigenic potential[7–10].

The third reason for considering nutritional support as an adjuvant therapy was to prevent (acute ulcerative colitis) or improve (especially in Crohn's disease) nutritional derangement which develops in up to 80% of severe cases[11]. The consequences of macronutrient (protein-energy malnutrition, fatty acid metabolism derangement)[11–16] and micronutrient (antioxidants)[17–20] deficiencies are still not completely understood in adulthood. However, nutritional derangement has proved to be a severe complication of IBD in childhood and adolescence, since it negatively influences linear growth, bone mass and sexual development[21]. In this population, enteral nutrition seems to be essential for treating these abnormalities[22].

LACK OF ENOUGH AND PROPER CLINICAL TRIALS

As mentioned above, O'Morain *et al.*'s observation that elemental diet was as effective as prednisolone in decreasing clinical and biological inflammatory activity in steroid-dependent patients with Crohn's disease[1] raised much hope about the possibility of using a non-aggressive therapeutic approach in these cases. Several trials have been performed since then, with different designs, in an attempt to reproduce these results with either elemental or polymeric diets[23–29] or to demonstrate that polymeric diets are as effective as elemental diets in inducing[30–38] or maintaining[39,40] remission in Crohn's disease. In fact, there are only a few well-designed randomized clinical trials to ascertain whether or not enteral nutrition can induce remission in active Crohn's disease. The answer to this question in the methodologically best designed trials is not consistent, either in the positive (i.e. therapeutically useful) or in the negative sense (i.e. therapeutically useless). In addition, the sample size in most trials was not large enough to reach solid conclusions. This, together with the qualitative and quantitative differences among trials in the composition of the formula diets used, generated great confusion to those physicians and surgeons lacking nutritional expertise, but interested in a less or non-aggressive approach to the treatment of Crohn's disease.

Three meta-analyses, almost simultaneously published[9,10,41], attempted to answer the question about the therapeutic effectiveness of enteral nutrition in IBD. All reached the same conclusions: Prednisolone was significantly more effective (80%) than any type of formula diet for enteral nutrition (60%) in inducing remission in adult active Crohn's disease. Although these figures, at first glance, may induce us to disregard the use of enteral nutrition as a first-choice therapy in active

Crohn's disease in adults, it is worth pointing out that a 60% remission rate is much more than a placebo effect.

Meta-analyses also showed that the source of nitrogen of the diet does not influence therapeutic outcome. That is, administering amino-acid-based elemental diets (low antigenicity) is not better than feeding polymeric diets (high antigenicity) as far as inducing remission is concerned. Thus, there is no rationale for using elemental diets to decrease intraluminal antigenic load in order to induce remission in Crohn's disease[9].

Finally, meta-analyses also disclosed that properly performed randomized clinical trials (RCT) in this field are very scarce. The quality scores of the RCT, as assessed by the investigators, looking blindly at the material and methods of the trials, yielded very low scores, ranging from 22 to 72 points (on a scale of 100 points) with a median 49.5. This low score was due, in general, to elemental defects in the design of the study (sample size, homogeneity of the groups, evaluation of the inflammatory activity, population not described, etc.) and because essential information was not given in the paper (type of diet administered, route of administration, reasons for drop out, etc.)[9]. It is astonishing that, when dealing with drug therapy, proper trials are usually designed and performed while this is very seldom found in nutritional trials.

MORE EXIGENT OUTCOMES IN NUTRITIONAL RCT THAN IN THOSE WITH DRUGS

The remission rate of placebo in controlled trials performed with drugs in CD ranges from 20% to 30%[42–45]. Thus, the 60% remission rate is 2–3 times that achieved by placebo in these studies. This suggests that, even when specially designed formula diets are not used, enteral nutrition has a primary therapeutic effect, at least in some patients (subgroups) with Crohn's disease. In addition, any formula diet for enteral nutrition appears to be at least as effective in inducing remission as some of the drugs used and accepted as treatment for Crohn's disease, namely: budesonide (9 mg/day), prednisolone (40 mg/day) or mesalamine (2 g/day)[45–51].

Moreover, in trials using enteral nutrition as primary therapy in Crohn's disease, the end point of the study is always 'disease remission', that is: the disease activity index used has to reach the level of 'inactivity' during the established period of treatment. The concept of 'response', meaning a certain arbitrarily agreed decrease in the IBD activity index used in a study (without reaching the inactivity level), has never been used in trials trying to find out the possible therapeutic effect of enteral nutritional formula diets in CD.

In spite of these facts, and the lack of side effects of the nutritional therapy compared with drug treatment, enteral nutrition is still not seen as a therapeutic tool by most physicians treating adult Crohn's disease patients. This is not so in paediatric and adolescent Crohn's disease, where enteral nutrition is used in most circumstances as the first-choice therapy, not only to prevent or overcome the severe nutritional derangements often seen in this population, but also to induce and maintain disease remission[21,22,52–54].

NOT ENOUGH DATA ABOUT THE TYPE OF ENTERAL NUTRITION USED

It is surprising that, in studies on the therapeutic effect of nutrition in CD, information about the formulation of the enteral diet administered to the patients is very seldom provided. In most publications, diets are only defined by the source of nitrogen, that is: it is an amino-acid-based elemental diet or a whole protein-based polymeric diet. This simplistic view, suggesting that the potential therapeutic effect of enteral nutrition can be related to the antigenic capacity of its nitrogen source has been, at least in adults, ruled out by the results of meta-analyses and by clinical experience. There is no difference in clinical outcome in patients treated with either elemental or polymeric diets[9]. Enteral diets contain other biologically active substrates, most of them involved in the mechanisms for the maintenance of the inflammatory/immunological homeostasis of the intestine, such as lipids, antioxidants, prebiotics (non-absorbed carbohydrates)[55], or in the repair mechanisms (growth factors)[56].

Null or scarce data still exist related to the anti-inflammatory therapeutic effect of antioxidants[57] and prebiotics[58] in humans. However, it is well known that lipids, in addition to being important contributors to the energy metabolism, are essential structural components of the cell membranes and, according to their degree of unsaturation, regulate the activity of membrane receptors, enzymes and transport systems and, as a consequence, intracellular signalling (e.g. transcription factors). Hence, cell membrane phospholipid composition influences the expression of molecules involved in the inflammatory process (cytokines, adhesion molecules, etc.). In addition, also in relation to their chemical structure and degree of fatty acid unsaturation, membrane lipids regulate the release of eicosanoids (prostaglandins, leukotrienes and thromboxanes), and other inflammatory mediators (diacyl-glycerol, PAF, phosphatidyl-inositol, etc.)[59–68]. Thus, cell membrane lipid composition represents a key factor modulating the expression or the synthesis of molecules involved in triggering and perpetuating the inflammatory process.

The literature provides several examples of the effect of dietary lipids on immune regulation. These go from the lower-than-expected prevalence of immune-related disease in the high dietary fish oil consuming communities like Greenland Eskimos[69,70] and increases in the annual incidence of both UC and CD in countries where qualitative changes in dietary fat took place because of public health reasons[71–73] or Western dietary influences[74] to many experimental and *in-vitro* studies[59–67]. Some clinical data also support the view that qualitative or quantitative manipulation of dietary fat may be therapeutically effective in CD[27,36,75,76]. Although, also in this case, the series published in adult CD are small in size and heterogeneous in both the type of patients included and the sources of dietary fat used, some of the studies show that dietary fat manipulation is able to induce clinical and biological remission in active CD to levels similar to those produced by full-dose prednisolone (1 mg/kg body weight)[27,36,77]. Other trials do not show such an effect. Differences in the predominant type of fatty acid, its chemical composition or the source where it is obtained may partly explain these discrepancies. The different chemical composition of the n-3 fatty acids may be one of the reasons why two similarly (although not equally) designed trials, aiming to evaluate the effect on maintaining remission in patients with CD, showed opposite outcomes[77,78].

In a study by Gonzalez-Huix *et al.*, it was shown that a polymeric enteral diet in which 30% of the total calories were provided by olive oil (75%) and MCT (25%) was as effective as 1 mg prednisone per kg body weight per day in inducing remission in moderate and severe active CD[27]. It was hypothesized that high n-6 fatty acids may enhance the inflammatory process and, conversely, that low n-6 or a high-monounsaturated fatty acid diet may be beneficial in the treatment of CD[76]. Later, Middleton *et al.*[36] suggested that it was the amount of long-chain fatty acids in the diet rather than the family (n-3, n-6, n-9, n-7) or the degree of unsaturation which, in fact, defines the anti-inflammatory response to enteral diets in CD. However, it is worth mentioning that, when the compositions of the diets in Middleton's study are carefully analysed, it can be observed that those diets with the highest remission rates are those with low fat contents or those where one third of the fat calories were administered as MCT. This fact was not mentioned in Middleton's paper.

On the other hand, although, in most cases, dietary fats from different sources have a predominant fatty acid, they also contain variable percentages of other fatty acids and non-fatty acid compounds. In an elegant experimental study, Sadeghi *et al.*[79] showed that the effect of different oils on the expression of different pro- and anti-inflammatory cytokines varies, not always according the predominant fatty acid. These findings suggest that, most probably, the modulatory effect of fat on the immune system may not be dependent on a particular predominant fatty acid but rather on a particular fatty acid mixture[80]. Also, it should be noted that the various immunomodulatory effects observed with different types of lipids may be related not only to its fatty acid composition but also to its non-fatty acid components[81,82].

SOME SUBGROUPS OF PATIENTS MAY RESPOND BETTER THAN OTHERS TO ENTERAL NUTRITION

One of the aspects still not clearly established is whether there might be a special subgroup(s) of patients with CD more likely to respond to nutritional therapy. Some data in the literature suggest that children and patients without colon involvement may respond better to this therapy[83]. As has been mentioned, the percentage of clinical and biological response in childrens with Crohn's disease is very high, between 75% and 90%. In addition, when pooling together randomized and non-randomized series of adult patients treated with either elemental (549 cases) or polymeric diets (124 cases), the mean remission rate was 79% and 70% respectively, very close to that with steroids[51], without taking into account the location of the disease. Only well-designed RCT may bring new data to this important question.

CONCLUDING REMARKS

Nutrition care has a crucial role in the prevention and treatment of nutritional derangements, often occurring in cases with acute or long-standing inflammatory bowel disease, especially in children and adolescents. However, it should no longer be considered only an adjuvant in the therapeutic armamentarium of such conditions. In the last 15 years, in spite of the lack of large enough good RCT, its use as primary therapy, at least in some subgroups of patients with Crohn's disease, is slowly but consistently being considered seriously, especially since this is a safe treatment without severe or long-lasting side effects. The mechanism(s) by which enteral nutrition may be effective in this condition is not completely understood, but it seems that it is not related to modifications in the nitrogen source, which have been used in an attempt to decrease their potential intestinal antigenic effect. It may be feasible that other components of the diet, such as fat, antioxidant and growth factors, may be of importance, influencing the inflammatory response and the intestinal mucosa repair mechanisms and leading to mucosal healing. It is possible that the therapeutic action of nutrients may not be explained by the action of a single substrate, but rather by the combination of a group of them[27,36,84]. Proper large clinical trials are ongoing in an attempt to clarify these questions. Moreover, the end points of these trials should be, as they always have been, 'disease remission' rather than a so-called arbitrarily agreed 'disease response'. Subgroup analysis should also be performed. Those interested may refer to recent reviews in this area[85–87].

It is, however, surprising that there is a lack of interest shown, after all these years, in exploring seriously this non-harming therapy for Crohn's disease. This may just represent a lack of pathophysiological knowledge among many GI doctors and surgeons and a lack of experience in performing RCT among nutritionists.

References

1. O'Morain C, Segal AW, Levi AJ. Elemental diet as primary treatment of acute Crohn's disease: A controlled study. Br Med J. 1984;228:1859–62.
2. Lochs H. Has total bowel rest been a beneficial effect in the treatment of Crohn's disease? Clin Nutr. 1983;2:61–4.
3. McIntyre PB, Powell-Tuck J, Wood SR *et al.* Controlled trial of bowel rest in the treatment of severe acute colitis. Gut. 1986;27:481–5.
4. Greenberg GR, Fleming CR, Jeejeebhoy KN, Rosenberg IH, Sales D, Tremaine WJ. Controlled trial of bowel rest and nutritional support in the management of Crohn's disease. Gut. 1988;29: 1309–15.
5. González-Huix F, Fernández Bañares F, Esteve M *et al.* Enteral versus parenteral nutrition as adjunct therapy in acute ulcerative colitis. Am J Gastroenterol. 1993;88:227–32.
6. Alun Jones V. Comparison of total parenteral nutrition and elemental diet in induction of remission of Crohn's disease: long-term maintenance of remission by personalized food exclusion diets. Dig Dis Sci. 1987;32:100S–107S.
7. Gassull MA, Fernández Bañares F, Cabré E, Esteve M. Enteral nutrition in inflammatory bowel disease. In: Rombeau JL, Rolandelli RH, editors. Clinical Nutrition. Enteral and Tube Feeding, 3rd edn. Philadelphia: W.B. Saunders Co., 1997:403–16.
8. Gassull MA, Fernández Bañares F. Nutrition inflammatory bowel disease. In: Payne-James J, Grimble, G, Silk DBA, editors. Artificial Nutrition Support in Clinical Practice, 2nd edn. London: Greenwich Medical Media, 2001:553–73.
9. Fernandez-Bañares F, Cabré E, Esteve-Comas M, Gassull MA. How effective is enteral nutrition in inducing remission in active Crohn's disease? A meta-analysis of the randomized clinical trials. J Parent Ent Nutr. 1995;19:356–64.
10. Griffiths AM, Ohlsson A, Sherman PM, Sutherland LR. Meta-analysis of enteral nutrition as a primary treatment of active Crohn's disease. Gastroenterology. 1995;108:1056–67.

11. Gassull MA, Abad A, Cabré E, González-Huix F, Giné JJ, Dolz C. Enteral nutrition in inflammatory bowel disease. Gut. 1986;27(Suppl. 1):76–80.
12. Esteve M, Ramírez M, Fernández-Bañares F *et al.* Plasma polyunsaturated fatty acid pattern in active inflammatory bowel disease. Gut. 1992;33:1365–9.
13. Esteve M, Núñez M, Fernández-Bañares F *et al.* Abnormal plasma polyunsaturated fatty acid pattern in non-active inflammatory bowel disease. Gut. 1993;34:1370–3.
14. Esteve M, Ramírez M, Fernández-Bañares F *et al.* Determinants of plasma fatty acid abnormalities in patients with active inflammatory bowel disease. A multivariate analysis. Inflamm Bowel Dis. 1995;1:95–100.
15. Esteve M, Navarro E, Klaassen J *et al.* Plasma and mucosal fatty acid pattern in colectomized ulcerative colitis patients. Dig Dis Sci. 1998;43:1071–8.
16. Fernández-Bañares F, Esteve M, Mañé J *et al.* Changes in mucosal fatty acid profile in inflammatory bowel disease and experimental colitis: a common response to bowel inflammation. Clin Nutr. 1997;16:177–83.
17. Cabré E, Fernández-Bañares F, Esteve M, Gassull MA. Micronutrients in inflammatory bowel disease. J Clin Nutr Gastroenterol. 1989;4:100–2.
18. Fernández-Bañares F, Abad A, Xiol X *et al.* Vitamin status in patients with inflammatory bowel disease. Am J Gastroenterol. 1989;84:744–8.
19. Fernández-Bañares F, Mingorance MD, Esteve M *et al.* Serum, zinc, copper and selenium levels in inflammatory bowel disease. Am J Gastroenterol. 1990;85:1584–9.
20. Abad A, Fernández-Bañares F, Cabré E *et al.* The effect of total enteral tube feeding on the vitamin status of malnourished patients with inflammatory bowel disease. Int J Vit Nutr Res. 1988;58:428–35.
21. Griffiths AM, Nguyen P, Smith C, MacMillan H, Sherman PM. Growth and clinical course of children with Crohn's disease. Gut. 1993;34:939–43.
22. Seidman E. Nutritional therapy for Crohn's disease: Lessons from the Ste. Justine Hospital experience. Inflamm Bowel Dis. 1997;3:49–53.
23. Teahon K, Bjarnason I, Pearson M, Levi AJ. Ten years' experience with an elemental diet in the management of Crohn's disease. Gut. 1990;31:1133–7.
24. Bodemar G, Nilsson L, Smedh K, Larson J. Nasogastric feeding with polymeric, whole protein low fat diet in Crohn's disease. J Clin Nutr Gastroenterol. 1991;6:75–83.
25. Coyle BL, Sladen GE. Whole protein diet in the treatment of acute uncomplicated Crohn's disease. J Hum Nutr Dietetics. 1989;2:25–30.
26. Gorard DA, Hunt JR, Payne-James JJ *et al.* Initial response and subsequent course of Crohn's disease treated with elemental diet and prednisolone. Gut. 1993;14:1198–202.
27. Gonzalez-Huix F, de Leon R, Fernandez-Bañares F *et al.* Polymeric enteral diets as primary treatment of active Crohn's disease; a prospective steroid controlled trial. Gut. 1993;34:778–82.
28. Okada M, Yao T, Takenaka K, Imamura K, Maeda K, Fujita K. Controlled trial comparing elemental diet with prednisolone in the treatment of active Crohn's disease. Hepato-Gastroenterology. 1990;37:72–80.
29. Ruuska T, Savilahti E, Maki M, Örmälä T, Visakorpi JK. Exclusive whole protein diet versus prednisolone in the treatment of acute Crohn's disease in children. J Pediatr Gastroenterol Nutr. 1994;19:175–80.
30. Royall D, Jeejeebhoy KN, Baker JP *et al.* Comparison of amino acid vs peptide based enteral diets in active Crohn's disease: clinical and nutritional outcome. Gut. 1994;35:783–7.
31. Giaffer MH, North G, Holdsworth CD. Controlled trial of polymeric versus elemental diet in the treatment of active Crohn's disease. Lancet. 1990;335:816–19.
32. Mansfield JC, Giaffer MH, Holdsworth CD. Controlled trial of oligopeptide versus amino acid diet in the treatment of active Crohn's disease. Gut. 1995;36:60–6.
33. Raouf AH, Hildrey V, Daniel J *et al.* Enteral feeding as sole treatment for Crohn's disease: controlled trial of whole protein *vs* amino acid based feed and a case study of dietary challenge. Gut. 1991;32:702–7.
34. Rigaud D, Cosnes J, Le Quintrec Y, René E, Gendre JP, Mignon M. Controlled trial comparing two types of enteral nutrition in treatment of active Crohn's disease: elemental vs polymeric diet. Gut. 1991;32:1492–7.
35. Hiwatashi N. Enteral nutrition for Crohn's disease in Japan. Dis Colon Rectum. 1997;40(Suppl): S48–S53.

36. Middleton SJ, Rucker JT, Kirby GA, Riordan AM, Hunter JO. Long-chain triglycerides reduce the efficacy of enteral feeds in patients with active Crohn's disease. Clin Nutr. 1995;14:229–36.
37. Verma S, Brown S, Kirkwood B, Giaffer MH. Polymeric versus elemental diet as primary treatment in active Crohn's disease: A randomized, double-blind trial. Am J Gastroenterol. 2000;95:735–9.
38. Matsui U, Ueki M, Yamada M *et al.* Indications and options of nutritional treatment for Crohn's disease: a comparison of elemental and polymeric diets. J Gastroenterol. 1995;30 (Suppl. 8):95–7.
39. Fakuda Y, Kosaka T, Okui M, Hirakawa H, Shimoyama T. Efficacy of nutritional therapy for active Crohn's disease. J Gastroenterol. 1995;30(Suppl. 8):83–7.
40. Wilschanski M, Sherman P, Pencharz P, Davis L, Corey M, Griffiths A. Supplementary enteral nutrition maintains remission in paediatric Crohn's disease. Gut. 1996;38:543–8.
41. Messori A, Trallori G, D'Albasio G, Milla M, Vannozzi G, Pacini F. Defined-formula diets versus steroids in the treatment of active Crohn's disease – A meta-analysis. Scand J Gastroenterol. 1996;31:267–72.
42. Summers RW, Switz DM, Sessions JT *et al.* National Cooperative Crohn's disease study: Results of drug treatment. Gastroenterology. 1979;77:847–69.
43. Malchow H, Eve K, Brandes JW *et al.* European Cooperative Crohn's Disease Study (ECCDS): Result of drug treatment. Gastroenterology. 1987;86:249–66.
44. Singleton JW, Hanauer SB, Gitnick GL *et al.* Mesalamine capsules for the treatment of active Crohn's disease: Results of a 16-week trial. Gastroenterology. 1993;104:1293–301.
45. Greenberg GR, Feagan BG, Martin F *et al.* Oral budesonide for active Crohn's disease. N Engl J Med. 1994;331:836–41.
46. Rutgeerts P, Löfberg R, Malchow H *et al.* A comparison of budesonide and prednisolone for active Crohn's disease. N Engl J Med. 1994;329:842–5.
47. Cesar I, Gross V, Roth M *et al.* Treatment of active and post-active colonic Crohn's disease with oral pH-modified-release budesonide. German budesonide group. Hepatogastroenterology. 1997;44:445–8.
48. Campieri M, Ferguson A, Doe W, Person T, Nilson LG. Oral budesonide is as effective as oral prednisolone in active Crohn's disease. The Global Budesonide Study Group. Gut. 1997;41:209–14.
49. Thompsen OO, Cortot A, Jewell D *et al.* A comparison of budesonide and mesalamine for active Crohn's disease. International Budesonide–Mesalamine Study group. N Engl J Med. 1998;339: 370–74.
50. Bar-Meier S, Chowers Y, Lavy A *et al.* Budesonide versus prednisone in the treatment of active Crohn's disease. Gastroenterology. 1998;115:835–40.
51. Gassull MA. Diet or steroids? In: Jewell DP, Mortensen N, Warren BF, editors. Challenges in Inflammatory Bowel Disease. Oxford: Blackwell Science, 2001:111–20.
52. Griffiths AM. Enteral nutrition: the neglected primary therapy of active Crohn's disease. J Pediatr Gastroenterol Nutr. 2000;31:3–5.
53. Heuschkel RB, Menache CC, Megerian JT, Baird AE. Enteral nutrition and corticosteroids in the treatment of acute Crohn's disease in children. J Pediatr Gastroenterol Nutr. 2000;31:8–15.
54. Ferguson A, Glen M, Ghoshi S. Crohn's disease: nutrition and nutritional therapy. Balliere's Clin Gastroenterol. 1998;12:93–114.
55. Green CJ. Fibre in enteral nutrition. Clin Nutr. 2001;20(Suppl. 1):23–39.
56. Playford RJ. Peptide therapy and the gastroenterologist: colostrum and milk derived growth factors. Clin Nutr. 2001;20(Suppl. 1):101–6.
57. Fernandez-Bañares F. Papel de los metabolitos de oxígeno reactivos en la patogenia de la enfermedad inflamatoria intestinal. Gastroenterol Hepatol. 1995;18:526–32.
58. Fernandez-Bañares F, Hinojosa J, Gomollón F, Sanchez-Lombraña JL, Rdariguez-Abascal J, Gassull MA and the Spanish Group for the Study of Crohn's Disease and Ulcerative Colitis. Randomised clinical trial of *Plantago ovata* (dietary fibre) as compared to mesalamine in maintaining remission in ulcerative colitis. Am J Gastroenterol. 1999;94:427–33.
59. De Caterina R, Cybysky MI, Clinton SK, Gimbrone M, Libby P. The omega-3 fatty acid docosahexaenoate reduces cytokine induced expression of proatherogenic and proinflammatory proteins in human endothelial cells. Arterioscler Thromb. 1994;14:1829–36.
60. Lee T, Hoover R, Williams J *et al.* Effect of dietary enrichment with eicosapentaenoic and docosahexaenoic acids on in vivo neutrophil and monocyte leucotriene generation and neutrophil function. N Engl J Med. 1985;312:1217–24.

61. Sanderson P, Calder PC. Dietary fish oil diminishes lymphocyte adhesion to macrophage and endothelial cell monolayers. Immunology. 1998;94:79–87.
62. De Caterina R, Libby P. Control of endothelial leucocyte adhesion molecules by fatty acids. Lipids. 1996;31(Suppl):S57–S63.
63. Yeh SL, Chang KY, Huang C, Chen WJ. Effect of n-3 and n-6 fatty acids on plasma eicosanoid and liver antioxidant enzymes in rats receiving total parenteral nutrition. Nutrition. 1997;13:32–6.
64. Miles EA, Calder PC. Modulation of immune function by dietary fatty acids. Proc. Nutr Soc. 1998;57:277–92.
65. Enders S. Messengers and mediators: Interactions among lipids, eicosanoids and cytokines. Am J Clin Nutr. 1993;57(Suppl):798S–800S.
66. Calder PC. N-3 polyunsaturated fatty acids and immune cell function. Adv Enzyme Regul. 1997;37:197–237.
67. Karsten S, Schäfer G, Schauder P. Cytokine production and DNA synthesis by human peripheral lymphocytes in response to palmitic, stearic, oleic, and linoleic acid. J Cell Physiol. 1994;161:15–22.
68. Fürst P, Kuhn KS. Fish oil emulsions: what benefits can they bring? Clin Nutr. 2000;19:7–14.
69. Kroman N, Green A. Epidemiological studies in the Upernavik district. Acta Med Scand. 1980;208:401–6.
70. Bang H, Dyerberg J, Hjorne N. The composition of food consumed by Greenland Eskimos. Acta Med Scand. 1976;200:69–73.
71. Guthy E. Morbus Crohn und Nahrundsfette; Hypothese zur Ätiologie der enteritis regionalis. Dtsch Med Wschr. 1982;107:71–3.
72. Guthy E. Ätiologie des Morbus Crohn: Was spright fur Fette als Moglishe Ursache. Dtsch Med Wschr. 1983;108:1729–33.
73. Nordenval B, Brostrom O, Hellers G. Entzundliche Darmkrankheiten und Nahrungsfette. Dtsch Med Wschr. 1982;107:1900.
74. Shoda R, Matsueda K, Yamato, Umeda N. Epidemiologic analysis of Crohn's disease in Japan: increased dietary intake of n-6 polyunsaturated fatty acids and animal protein relates to the increase of Crohn's disease in Japan. Am J Clin Nutr. 1996;63:741–5.
75. Roediger WEW, Giles A, Kaczmar A, Ali S. Does exclusion of enteral lipid assist remission in Crohn's disease? J Clin Gastroenterol. 1993;17:38–41.
76. Fernandez-Bañares F, Cabré E, Gonzalez-Huix F, Gassull MA. Enteral nutrition as primary therapy in Crohn's disease. Gut. 1994;35:S55–S59.
77. Belluzi A, Brignola C, Campieri M *et al.* Effect of an enteric-coated fish oil preparation on relapses in Crohn's disease. N Engl J Med. 1996;334:1557–60.
78. Lorenz-Meyer H, Bauer P, Nicolay C *et al.* for the German Crohn's Disease Study Group. Omega-3 fatty acids and low carbohydrate diet for maintenance of remission in Crohn's disease: a randomized controlled multicenter clinical trial. Scand J Gastroenterol. 1996;31:778–85.
79. Sadeghi S, Wallace FA, Calder PC. Dietary lipids modify cytokine response to bacterial lipopolysacharide in mice. Immunology. 1999;96:404–10.
80. Gassull MA. Dietary fat and inflammatory bowel disease. Curr Gastroenterol Rep. 2001;3:358–61.
81. Owen RW, Giacosa A, Hull WE *et al.* The antioxidant/anticancer potential of phenolic compounds isolated from olive oil. Eur J Cancer. 2000;36:1235–7.
82. Mangas-Cruz MA, Fernandez A, Albi T *et al.* Effects of minor constituents (non-glyceride compounds) of virgin olive oil on plasma lipid concentrations in male Wistar rats. Clin Nutr. 2001;20:211–15.
83. Griffits AM. Inflammatory bowel disease. Nutrition. 1988;14:788–91.
84. Fell JM, Paintin M, Arnoud-Battandier F *et al.* Mucosal healing and fall in mucosal pro-inflammatory cytokine mRNA induced by a specific polymeric diet in paediatric Crohn's disease. Aliment Pharmacol Ther. 2000;14:281–9.
85. Gassull MA. New insights in nutritional therapy in inflammatory bowel disease. Clin Nutr. 2001;20(Suppl. 1):113–21.
86. Cabre E, Gassull MA. Nutrition in inflammatory bowel disease: impact on disease and therapy. Curr Opin Gastroenterol. 2001;17:342–9.
87. Gassull MA, Cabré E. Nutrition in inflammatory bowel disease. Curr Opin Clin Nutr Metab Care. 2001:561–9.

Section III
Early vs late IBD

12
Early versus late IBD – clinical comments

S. G. M. MEUWISSEN and A. A. VAN BODEGRAVEN

In this introductory paper two case histories are presented, with the theme 'early versus late' IBD. Case I: the first patient was 24 years old ('*early IBD*'), had only a history of some weeks, was apparently in good health and had never been examined previously; she had a stable weight and did not take any drugs. At evaluation, however, biochemical abnormalities were considerable (raised ESR, C-reactive protein, low iron stores). Ultrasound and endoscopy showed Crohn's disease (CD) with localization in the distal ileum, caecum and sigmoid colon. The MRI showed stenotic areas in the ileum, with a fistula, which could be primary or secondary. The question arises whether she indeed was suffering from an early form of CD. The major radiological and MRI abnormalities, the anaemia of chronic origin, the chronicity of peri-umbilical pain, and the low weight were all arguments against an early course.

Case II: the second patient ('*late IBD*') was 11 years older and she had a long-standing history of Crohn's disease (15 years) and had had an ileocolonic resection 13 years previously. Some time after the first resection, she developed symptoms caused by duodenal localization (stenosis). Recent endoscopy showed narrowing of the ileocolonic anastomosis, moderate inflammation and narrowing of the duodenum. No data on smoking habits are given in the two presentations.

What is early CD; what is late CD? Some difficulties regarding providing a satisfactory definition are given in Table 1.

Table 1 Problems regarding a definition of early vs. late IBD

Is early related to the age of the patient at the onset of IBD symptoms?
Is early related to the short duration of IBD symptoms?
Is early related to minimal findings at evaluation (not extensive, limited stenosis, no fistulization)?
Is early IBD, when treated without delay, related to a better prognosis?
Are genetic factors related to early disease?

Major textbooks have given relatively little attention to the issue of age in relation to the clinical course and prognosis. In the textbook *Inflammatory Bowel Disease, From Bench to Bedside*, one chapter is devoted to the evidence for clinical subgroups[1]. Age-related problems, however, are mainly discussed for UC. More recently, in the textbook *Inflammatory Bowel Diseases*, a chapter is found on IBD in childhood[2] and, in the most recent textbook edited by Kirsner, in which subgroups are briefly discussed, the issue of age has hardly been mentioned[3]. Therefore, the clinician has to rely on other data from recent literature.

Is age, age of onset, or duration of symptoms of any clinical importance for the clinician in his decision making? In other words, which factors influence, in daily life, the management of patients with Crohn's disease? (See Table 2.) There are only limited data to be found in the literature, in which the clinical courses of younger CD patients are compared with those of older patients.

Which classification may be useful to unravel in detail the importance of 'age' in our patients? Let us review the literature in more detail. One of the first useful classifications was published by Sachar and colleagues[4]. *Anatomical location* was recognized as the main item (stomach/duodenum, jejunum, ileum, colon, rectum and perianal region). The *anatomical extent* differentiates between localized and diffuse disease, the *operative history* recognizes primary (unoperated) and recurrent disease. A most important item is new: *disease behaviour* (primary fibrostenotic, primary fistulizing and primary inflammatory types). Anatomic extent is a well-known major determinant for the clinical course of the disease: the classical studies performed in the seventies at the Cleveland clinic have shown that ileocolonic disease, for example, is the most likely to develop internal fistulae and abscesses with the highest likelihood of surgical intervention[5,6]. Therefore, anatomy determines the clinical course and clinicians should keep this aspect of the disease in mind. With regard to behaviour, previous studies have indeed suggested that the disease may have an indolent or more aggressive behaviour[7,8]. The present study proposes that disease behaviour should be a formal item in a classification[4], although Greenstein *et al.* already distinguished perforating from non-perforating CD patients[9]. Sachar *et al.* applied their criteria retrospectively in another study of a cohort of CD patients but found no differences with regard to postoperative recurrences between the fistulizing

Table 2 Factors which may or may not influence decision taking by the clinicians of patients with Crohn's disease

Known factors	*Unknown factors*
Location of disease	Age of patient?
Extent of disease	Age of onset?
Type of complications	Duration of symptoms?
Extra-intestinal manifestations	Gender?
Previous history	Family history and genetic aspects?
Drug efficacy	
Smoking	

(perforating) type and the obstructing type[10]. An Italian study could only observe differences between the inflammatory type and the combination of the fistulizing and stenotic types, because the latter two types did not differ, when compared, with regard to anatomical location, disease severity or surgical requirements[11]. In contrast, a Swiss study showed differences in recurrences between the fistulizing (perforating) type and non-perforating type[12]. In the Sachar classification, neither age of the patient nor age at onset has been an item. The latest classification, which can be used in the routine clinical evaluation of CD patients, is the Vienna classification[13]. *Age* is used as a factor but only to separate patients with regard to the time of diagnosis to below and above 40 years (A1 vs. A2). Age at onset and age at diagnosis were highly correlated. Other items in the Vienna classification are *location at time of diagnosis* (terminal ileum L1), colon (L2), ileocolon (L3) and upper GI (L4). Finally *behaviour*: non-stricturing, non-penetrating (B1), stricturing (B2) and penetrating (B3). Therefore, our first patient may be classified as A1, L3, B2 or 3 and the second patient also as A1, L3 and B2. These phenotypic characterizations, being almost identical in our two patients, give, however, no further insight into the clinical course of the disease, whether at an early or late stage. Several items are not included in this new classification: see Table 3.

Young age at the time of diagnosis may be an important issue, and, as stated by Gasché *et al.*[13], may be linked with genetic abnormalities. One of the few papers discussing the clinical course of the young adult included only patients who had started having symptoms before the age of 17[14]. Symptoms at the onset were compared with symptoms at the time of the interview, at a mean of 14 years later. In contrast to UC, CD patients, in particular female patients, showed continuing severe disease. A study from the Netherlands compared the clinical features from 347 patients between 16 and 40 years with those of patients older than 40 years[15]. In the older group, the mean time lag before establishing a diagnosis was shorter, they were found to undergo surgery earlier after onset of symptoms, and recurrences occurred earlier (3.7 vs. 5.8 years in the younger patients). Finally, the older patients had significantly fewer affected relatives than the younger patients. Another recent study (EC*IBD study group) looked at differences in symptoms between younger than 60 years and older than 60 years, excluding patients younger than 15 years of age[16]. The data are, however, not appropriate for an analysis in our patients; both were in their twenties. The data from the Netherlands are not completely in agreement with those of a retrospective study in a large CD cohort in Baltimore[17]. In the latter analysis of more than 500 patients, clinical features from younger CD patients (age at time of

Table 3 Items *not* included in the Vienna classification

Young age
Family history
Gender
Smoking
Ethnicity
Type of fistula (primary or secondary)

diagnosis less than 20 years) were compared with those of patients in the age group 20–39 years and older ones (age at diagnosis more than 40 years). The authors observed a greater prevalence of a family history of CD, greater small bowel involvement and a higher frequency of surgery. There was a clear difference in stricturing (more frequent in younger patients) vs. inflammatory types (more frequent in older patient groups). The observation that the youngest patient group had the highest frequency of positive family history was consistent with results of other studies[18,19]. Indeed, this study suggests that younger CD patients may run a more progressive and severe course than older CD patients. This important study should be repeated in a prospective fashion in primary as well as in referral centres, comparing clinical symptoms at onset, clinical course and complications in young adults with older patients. Such a study, which should have a long follow-up, does, to the best of our knowledge not yet exist, but could give a more detailed answer to the question of whether the clinical course of the early-onset CD patient is indeed a more severe one. It is still not clear whether referral bias may play a 'selection role' in the patient material from large tertiary referral centres; young CD patients with more severe clinical characteristics and an impressive genetic history may be referred more easily, but this point remains at present only speculative. In our two patients, no data are given on the family history: therefore, they should be considered as isolated cases without a special risk for a progressive course.

Another issue is the likelihood of developing recurrent disease after previous surgery and this feature applies to our second patient. There are few definite factors which promote early recurrence: only smoking has been shown to be an important risk factor and on these clinical data are not available[20,21]. Differences in recurrence rates between fibrostenotic disease and perforating type have, up to now, not been convincing[20,22]. Borley *et al.* write: 'at present, there is no clear indication that CD may be divided meaningfully into two forms according to speed and severity of recurrence'[20]. In the same review, the issue of age was also discussed. However, no influence of age on recurrences was found; length of history, which to some extent was related to age, did not show a relationship with the recurrence rate after surgery[10,20]. To our knowledge, only one study in 88 patients (limited to patients who had undergone at least two operations for their CD) has shown retrospectively that the perforating type (perforating indication) and a longer preoperative disease duration may be risk factors for earlier recurrence after initial surgery. There was no significant association between age at diagnosis or preoperative disease duration and indication for initial surgery[23].

Returning to the clinical course of our two patients: is there any convincing evidence that patients with early CD will run a different course when managed aggressively by immunosuppressive drugs or even infliximab? Can these drugs, when given early in the disease, prevent further progression of inflammation, stenosis or other complications? Up to now, no such data can be recovered from the literature. Even in the most recent practice guidelines publication by the American College of Gastroenterology, a conservative approach to CD management is given: guidelines are presented for mild–moderate active CD, moderate–severe disease and severe fulminant disease and finally for maintenance therapy of CD patients[24]. In this publication no reference is made to the age of the patient, length of clinical history, or previous complications. Additionally,

Table 4 Management of case I

5-Aminosalicylates: no ('one could try it')
Azathioprine: yes.
MTX not first choice
Prednisone: no. Place of budesonide?
Antibiotics: no
Infliximab: results 'top-down approach': not yet known
Surgery: unavoidable, at later date (symptoms of stenosis)

Table 5 Management of case II

5-Aminosalicylates: no
Azathioprine: yes
Prednisone: may be useful in duodenal CD. Place of budesonide in duodenal disease not known. Add proton pump antagonist. Dilatation of stenosis worth a trial
Infliximab: not indicated (likely to aggravate the stenosis)
Surgery: unavoidable, depending on symptoms

there is no reference to the family history of the patient, which theoretically might be of importance for the choice of drugs (more aggressive approach). According to this overview, infliximab should be given to patients not responding to steroids or other immunomodulators. However, the 'top down' approach, starting with infliximab, should be studied in prospective studies in different cohorts of younger and older patients as well as in patients classified as B1, B2 or B3 by the Vienna classification[13]. A final comment on the duodenal localization in the second patient: duodenal involvement (L4) remains a relatively rare localization in CD and most centres have only a few cases under their care. Patients have been treated with proton pump antagonists, steroids, dilatation of stenosis or surgery, clear guidelines, however, are not available[24]. In a recent study, 22 of 32 CD cases with upper GI involvement had a duodenal localization; 13 and 12 cases, respectively, received prednisone and azathioprine, usually with good success, but no further details are given[25]. A summary of our approach to the management of the two cases is given in Tables 4 and 5.

References

1. Peña AS, Meuwissen SGM. Evidence for clinical subgroups in IBD. In: Targan SSF, editor, IBD; From Bench to Bedside. Baltimore: Williams and Wilkins, 1994:272–8.
2. Evans C, Beattie R, Walker-Smith J. Inflammatory bowel disease in children. In: Allan R, Rhodes J, Hanuer S, Keighley M, Alexander-Williams J, Fazio V, editors, Inflammatory Bowel Diseases. New York, Edinburgh, London: Churchill Livingstone, 1997:647–71.
3. Lashner B. Clinical features, laboratory findings and course of Crohn's disease. In: Kirsner J, editor, Inflammatory Bowel Disease. Philadelphia, London, Toronto, Sydney: WB Saunders, 2000:305–15.
4. Sachar DB, Andrews HA, Farmer RG *et al.* Proposed classification of patient subgroups in Crohn's disease. Gastroenterol Int. 1992;5:141–54.

5. Farmer RG, Hawk WA, Turnbull RB, Jr. Clinical patterns in Crohn's disease: a statistical study of 615 cases. Gastroenterology. 1975;68:627–35.
6. Farmer RG, Hawk WA, Turnbull RB. Indications for surgery in Crohn's disease. An analysis of 500 cases. Gastroenterology. 1976;71:245–50.
7. De Dombal FT, Burton I, Goligher JC. Recurrence of Crohn's disease after primary excisional surgery. Gut. 1971;12:519–27.
8. Prantera C, Levenstein S, Capoccia R *et al.* Prediction of surgery for obstruction in Crohn's ileitis. Dig Dis Sci. 1987;32:1363–9.
9. Greenstein AJ, Lachman P, Sachar DB *et al.* Perforating and nonperforating indications for repeated operations in Crohn's disease: evidence for two clinical forms. Gut. 1988;29:588–92.
10. Sachar DB, Subramani K, Mauer K *et al.* Patterns of postoperative recurrence in fistulizing and stenotic Crohn's disease. J Clin Gastroenterol. 1996;22:114–16.
11. Perri F, Annese V, Napolitano G *et al.* Subgroups of patients with Crohn's disease have different clinical outcomes. Inflamm Bowel Dis. 1996;2:1–5.
12. Aeberhard P, Berchtold W, Riedtmann H-J, Stadelmann G. Surgical recurrence of perforating and nonperforating Crohn's disease. Dis Colon Rectum. 1996;39:80–7.
13. Gasche C, Scholmerich J, Brynskov J *et al.* A simple classification of Crohn's disease: report of the Working Party for the World Congresses of Gastroenterology, Vienna 1998. Inflamm Bowel Dis. 2000;6:8–15.
14. Ferguson A, Sedgwick D. Juvenile-onset inflammatory bowel disease: predictors of morbidity and health status in early adult life. J R Coll Phys London. 1994;28:220–7.
15. Wagtmans M, Verspaget H, Lamers C, van Hogezand R. Crohn's disease in the elderly: a comparison with young adults. J Clin Gastroenterol. 1998;27:129–33.
16. Mouzas I, Pallis A, Vlachonikolis G, Manousos O, Bodini P, Fornaciari G. Symptoms at diagnosis and course during the first year in Crohn's disease patients do not differ between the young and the elderly. Gastroenterology. 2001;120 suppl 1:1223(A).
17. Polito II JM, Childs B, Mellits ED, Tokayer AZ, Harris ML, Bayless TM. Crohn's disease: influence of age at diagnosis on site and clinical type of disease. Gastroenterology. 1996;111:580–6.
18. Monsen U, Bernell O, Johansson C, Hellers G. Prevalence of inflammatory bowel disease among relatives of patients with Crohn's disease. Scand J Gastroenterol. 1991;26:302–6.
19. Lee J, Bridger S, Gregor C, Macpherson A, Lennard Jones J. Why children with inflammatory bowel disease are diagnosed at a younger age than their affected parent. Gut. 1994;44:808–11.
20. Borley N, Mortensen N, Jewell D. Preventing postoperative recurrence of Crohn's disease. Br J Surg. 1997;84:1493–502.
21. Cottone M, Rosselli M, Orlando A *et al.* Smoking habits and recurrence in Crohn's disease. Gastroenterology. 1994;106:643–8.
22. Caprilli R, Corrao G, Taddei G, Tonelli F, Torchio P, Viscido A, (GISC). Prognostic factors for postoperative recurrence of Crohn's disease. Dis Colon Rectum. 1996;39:335–41.
23. Lautenbach E, Berlin J, Lichtenstein G. Risk factors for early postoperative recurrence of Crohn's disease. Gastroenterology. 1998;115:259–67.
24. Hanauer SB, Sandborn W and the Practice Parameters Committee of the American College of Physicians. Management of Crohn's disease in adults. Am J Gastroenterol. 2001;96:635–43.
25. Miehsler W, Püspök A, Oberhugen G, Vogelsang H. Impact of different therapeutic regimens on the outcome of patients with Crohn's disease of the upper gastrointestinal tract. Inflamm Bowel Dis. 2001;7:99–105.

13
Early and late inflammatory bowel disease: differential mechanisms

S. KUGATHASAN, D. M. SPENCER, A. D. LEVINE and C. FIOCCHI

INTRODUCTION

Both forms of inflammatory bowel disease (IBD), Crohn's disease (CD) and ulcerative colitis (UC), are chronic conditions that persist during most of the patient's life. After the diagnosis is established, the course of the disease can be extremely diverse, varying from one that only requires sporadic follow-up and occasional treatment, to one where the patient spends a substantial portion of his or her time complaining of symptoms that require frequent visits to the doctor, multiple drug therapy, and eventually a surgical intervention to remove portions of the gastrointestinal tract. Existing knowledge on the causes and mechanisms of IBD is based on two main sources of information: humans with CD or UC, and animals with experimentally induced IBD[1,2]. Investigation performed in humans utilizes cells or tissues primarily from patients who have had IBD for several years and are receiving anti-inflammatory drugs, including immunosuppressive medications or biological immunomodulators, or who have just undergone bowel resection. On the other hand, the majority of studies performed in experimental models are carried out with genetically manipulated animals or animals exposed to pro-inflammatory substances that develop colitis of rapid onset but variable duration[2]. This approach to IBD pathogenesis has created a paradoxical situation where the bulk of knowledge is derived from humans with long-lasting disease or animals with early disease, leaving open a wide gap in our understanding of IBD in humans with early disease and animals with late disease. Some evidence is emerging to indicate that early and late IBD are not only clinically, but also biologically, different, each stage depending on distinct immunological phenomena. Differences in the immune mechanisms of early and late IBD in animals and humans will be presented and their therapeutic implications discussed.

EARLY AND LATE IBD: ANIMAL STUDIES

Animal models of IBD differ in terms of chronicity

Although there are several animal models of IBD, each displays considerable differences in induction and presentation, and much controversy exists as to what is considered an 'acute' or 'chronic' model. There is substantial variation in the time it takes for colitis to occur. Some models are undoubtedly acute, such as those induced by chemical agents that cause damage to the epithelium followed by a superficial mucosal inflammatory response, as in the dextran sulphate sodium (DSS) colitis model[3]. In contrast, other models are proposed to represent more chronic forms of inflammation, such as the colitis induced by the hapten trinitrobenzene sulphonic acid (TNBS) which has been described as chronic because it develops over a 20-day period of time[4]. However, the same TNBS-induced model is described as an acute granulomatous colitis in another report[5]. The SAMP1/Yit mouse model manifests an ileitis histologically similar to human CD and is considered chronic at 30 weeks[6].

One of the most commonly utilized models is the IL-10-deficient mouse colitis, where uncontrolled IL-12 production is implicated in initiation and continuation of chronic colitis at around 3 months of age[7]. However, when we studied mucosal inflammation in this model beyond 3 months into 8 months of duration, we found that inflammation persisted but IL-12 was no longer the responsible mediator[8]. We defined acute and chronic colonic inflammation in the IL-10-deficient mouse based on precise clinical, histological and immunological parameters as they occur in our specific pathogen-free housing facilities: colitis starting at 10 weeks up to 25 weeks is defined as *early* disease, while *late* disease is the inflammation that continues beyond 25 weeks of age. When discussing early and late models of IBD, it is fundamental to remember that, in experimental colitis, inflammation appears at different times, degrees of severity and penetrance vary, and these variables depend not only on the animal's genetic background but also on surrounding environmental factors, among which the microbial ecosystem of the intestinal lumen is fundamental[9].

Clinical features of early and late colitis in IL-10-deficient mice

Various clinical and histological changes occur in the colon of IL-10-deficient mice within the first 25 weeks of age. At the clinical level, there is initially a progressive wasting never observed in wild-type littermates, with a reduced body mass that lasts throughout the life of the animal. Second, stool samples are positive for blood starting at 10 weeks of age and remain so thereafter. Third, serum amyloid A, a classical marker of active inflammation, increases and remains elevated over the course of the disease. Along with these abnormalities, diarrhoea and rectal prolapse are frequently detected beginning at 15 weeks. These clinical manifestations usually start at 10 weeks of age, reach a maximal intensity at around 25 weeks of age, a time when they neither worsen nor resolve, remaining stable for the rest of the animal's survival.

Histologically, inflammation is first detected by 11 weeks of age. Analysis of the colon between 11 and 24 weeks of age reveals mucosal inflammatory infiltrates with skipped lesions, increasing in severity, extent and frequency as the mice age. Beyond 25 weeks no further changes in the degree of inflammation or tissue damage are observed. Early at 12–14 weeks, a few clear sites of inflammation are detected, consisting of both lymphocytic and neutrophilic cell infiltration in the lamina propria. By 14–16 weeks, the size of these infiltrates increases and, at the same time, there is a co-localized loss of goblet cells. The epithelium in the vicinity of inflammation also shows morphological changes, such as regenerative hyperplasia, evidenced by loss of columnar morphology, cell elongation and migration of the nucleus to a more central setting. Epithelial erosions start at 16–18 weeks with occasional ulcerations at around 18–20 weeks. Crypt abscesses are less frequently observed, often surrounded by normal mucosa. Transmural inflammation is only occasionally observed at 20–24 weeks, a time when some mice may also show adenomatous changes and infrequently adenocarcinomas adjacent to active inflammatory sites. When the colitic animals reach 25 weeks of age, these histological features are fully established and persist throughout their life. Interestingly, no noticeable further increase or decrease in the severity, character, or amount of inflammation is noted, and thus histological stability matches that of the clinical parameters. Inflammation of the small intestine is usually minimal and uncommonly detected in either the early or late phase of disease.

Early and late immune responses differ in IL-10-deficient mice

IL-10 is a cytokine with multiple biological properties, among which the most prominent is its ability to inhibit IL-12 production by macrophages and antigen-presenting cells[10]. In the intestine of IL-10-deficient mice, there is excessive synthesis of IL-12, which leads to the subsequent increase in IFN-γ production, and eventually the development of colitis. Before disease onset, colonic lamina propria mononuclear cells (LPMC) from IL-10-deficient mice synthesize low levels of IL-12 but, starting at 10 weeks of age, before the appearance of the first clinical manifestations, production of IL-12 increases dramatically and remains high until 25 weeks of age. Concurrently, IFN-γ synthesis is minimal before disease onset, increasing thereafter in parallel with enhanced IL-12 production. Blocking synthesis of IL-12 *in vivo* with neutralizing antibodies expectedly provides beneficial effects, stimulating weight gain, eliminating blood in the stool, and improving histological inflammation[8]. During treatment, IL-12 is no longer detected in the supernatants of LPMC cultures and IFN-γ levels are comparable to those produced by LPMC isolated from healthy predisease mice. These experiments leave no doubt that IL-12 plays a pivotal role in the early stages of colitis in IL-10-deficient mice.

The clinical and histological steady state observed beyond 25 weeks of age suggests that both IL-12 and IFN-γ synthesis reached a plateau and would remain at the same high level for the duration of the animal survival. To our surprise, however, we discovered otherwise. At around 25 weeks of age, IL-12 and IFN-γ production by LPMC starts to decrease and eventually plummets to the baseline levels found in the predisease state. Since this drop in cytokine production occurs while inflammation persists, we focused our attention on immune events during this late phase of disease. To eliminate the possibility that low undetectable amounts of IL-12 were still playing a role, we blocked its activity

Table 1 Changes in cytokine levels and efficacy of IL-12 blockade in early and late IL-10-deficient mouse colitis

	Predisease	*Early disease*	*Late disease*
IL-12	+	++++	+
IFN-γ	+	++++	+
IL-1β	++	++++	++++
TNF-α	++	+++	+++
IL-18	Not detected	Not detected	Not detected
IL-4	+	+++	+++
IL-13	+	++	+++
IL-12 antibody	Colitis prevention	Colitis reversal	No effect

in vivo with neutralizing antibodies. Even though IL-12 and IFN-γ were no longer detected in LPMC culture supernatants, the clinical or histological manifestations of inflammation were not reversed (Table 1)[8].

A switch in cytokine profile occurs in late disease of IL-10-deficient mice

Since IL-12 and IFN-γ appeared to be no longer required for mediation of active inflammation, other pro-inflammatory cytokines, such as IL-1β, TNF-α, or IL-18, may have assumed the role of maintaining late colitis in the IL-10-deficient mouse. However, there were no significant changes in the production of any of these cytokines by LPMC isolated from colitic mice between the ages of 10 and 35 weeks. This finding indicates that elevated pro-inflammatory cytokine production reflects active inflammation but the immune mechanisms responsible for their induction must vary in the early and late phases of colitis.

One possibility is that the cell composition of the LPMC of IL-10-deficient mice changed over time, somehow resulting in inhibition of macrophage and dendritic cell production of IL-12, as well as of natural killer cell or T-cell production of IFN-γ. To test this possibility, we measured the production of the immunosuppressive cytokines IL-4 and IL-13 by mitogen (concanavalin A)-stimulated LPMC isolated from IL-10-deficient mice between the ages of 7 and 35 weeks. Cells from early and late disease produce significantly greater amounts of both IL-4 and IL-13 compared with LPMC from healthy IL-10-deficient mice at 7 weeks of age. Levels of IL-4 were similar in early and late disease, whereas IL-13 levels significantly increased in late disease (Table 1). It is not clear at this time what role, if any, IL-4 and IL-13 may play in the pathogenesis of late colitis. Future blocking studies should establish whether these cytokines are simple by-products of shifting mucosal T-cell subsets in advanced disease or they actually play a role in perpetuating late disease.

Thus, the evaluation of the mucosal immune response that accompanies the early and late stages of IL-10-deficient murine colitis during a considerable part of the animal's life span leaves no doubt that different biological mechanisms are responsible for the initiation and persistence of intestinal inflammation.

EARLY AND LATE IBD: HUMAN STUDIES

The incidence of IBD is increasing worldwide, and recent epidemiological data show that CD and UC are becoming more frequent in children while the age of onset is decreasing[11]. Since the time between initial symptoms and diagnosis of IBD is usually shorter in children than in adults, investigation of the associated immune abnormalities may provide insight into early mechanisms of IBD before they are modified by drug therapy and disease progression[12]. In addition, as corroborated by the above studies in experimental models of colitis, it is possible that the underlying immune reactivity and cytokine synthesis vary substantially during the evolution of IBD[13]. Since the cytokine milieu at the beginning of the immune response often drives the outcome of the disease, it is important to define at the earliest possible time which mediators are produced in the mucosa affected by early IBD and compare them with those present in the mucosa that has been chronically inflamed.

Since children with IBD do not undergo bowel resection as often as adults, investigation of cytokines can be accomplished using T-cell clones derived from mucosal biopsies of involved tissue. Such clones can be exposed to modulatory agents to gain additional information on whether their reactivity is the same or different in the early and late stages of IBD. Therefore, we measured the production of IFN-γ by *in-vitro* activated T-cells clones and assessed how IFN-γ was modulated by the addition of IL-12 and IL-4, the two key cytokines responsible for inducing Th1 (cell-mediated) and Th2 (antibody-mediated) immune responses[14]. This was accomplished with colonoscopic biopsies from children with typical CD and UC, culture-proven infectious colitis, and control children with radiologically and endoscopically normal colon. Early and late IBD were defined as the first attack of CD or UC, and late CD or UC as disease with at least five years duration from the time of the initial diagnosis and with persistent clinical activity.

T-cell cytokine production and modulation in children with early and late IBD

The capacity to produce IFN-γ varied in T-cells from normal children and children with infectious colitis, early and late CD, as well as early and late UC, but statistically significant differences were not observed among all groups. To determine whether this IFN-γ production was susceptible to regulation, T-cell clones were grown in the presence of IL-12 or IL-4 from the beginning of the culture. When T-cells from normal children were examined, no significant modulatory effect of IL-12 or IL-4 on IFN-γ production was observed. However, T-cells derived from children with infectious colitis showed a marked modulatory effect, with a several-fold increase in IFN-γ production when they were exposed to IL-12 as compared with those grown in the absence of this cytokine[15]. IL-4 had no modulatory effect on T-cell production of IFN-γ. When the modulatory effect of

IL-12 and IL-4 was investigated using T-cells derived from children with early CD or UC, IL-12 also induced a significant increase in IFN-γ production but IL-4 did not, similarly to what was observed in acute infectious colitis. In contrast, when T-cells derived from children with late CD or UC were examined, neither IL-12 nor IL-4 were able to modulate IFN-γ production. Thus, it appears that, during the early stages of IBD, mucosal T-cells mount a typical Th1 response in both CD and UC that resembles an acute infectious process but this response disappears with progression to the late stages of IBD.

Interpreting these observations from a therapeutic standpoint, the greatest opportunity to suppress active IBD should be expected when mucosal T-cells still retain the capacity to be immunologically modulated, as in children with early IBD. At this stage, the promotion of a strong pro-inflammatory Th1 response by high levels of IFN-γ could be blocked by neutralizing IL-12, an approach that should be tested in future clinical trials. Nevertheless, the concept that immunomodulation early in the course of the disease may provide maximal therapeutic efficacy appears correct, as supported by the excellent and lasting beneficial effects seen in children with early CD who are treated with tumour necrosis factor-α antibodies[16].

CONCLUSIONS

Taken together, the results obtained from studies of early and late events in experimental colitis and children with CD or UC indicate that immune phenomena underlying the mucosal inflammation in IBD are not the same throughout the disease, and distinct cellular and molecular responses occur at different times. These responses evolve from an early stage where they are highly susceptible to immunomodulatory agents to later stages when the same agents are less beneficial or their efficacy lasts only for a limited period of time. A better understanding of the key pathophysiological steps responsible for the various stages of IBD immune reactivity should provide a more rational framework for novel time-sensitive therapeutic strategies.

References

1. Fiocchi C. Inflammatory bowel disease: etiology and pathogenesis. Gastroenterology. 1998;115:182–205.
2. Sartor RB. Insights into the pathogenesis of inflammatory bowel diseases provided by new rodent models of spontaneous colitis. Inflamm Bowel Dis. 1995;1:64–75.
3. Cooper HS, Murthy SNS, Shah RS, Sedergran DJ. Clinocopathologic study of dextran sulfate sodium experimental murine colitis. Lab Invest. 1993;69:238–49.
4. Neurath MF, Fuss I, Kelsall BL, Stuber E, Strober W. Antibodies to interleukin 12 abrogate established experimental colitis in mice. J Exp Med. 1995;182:1281–90.
5. Simpson SJ, Shah S, Comiskey M *et al.* T cell-mediated pathology in two models of experimental colitis depends predominantly on the interleukin 12/signal transducer and activator of transcription (stat)-4 pathway, but is not conditional on interferon γ expression by T cells. J Exp Med. 1998;187:1225–34.
6. Kosiewicz MM, Nast CC, Krishnan A *et al.* Th1-type responses mediate spontaneous ileitis in a novel murine model of Crohn's disease. J Clin Invest. 2001;107:695–702.
7. Davidson NJ, Hudak SA, Lesley RE, Menon S, Leach MW, Rennick DM. IL-12, but not IFN-γ, plays a major role in sustaining the chronic phase of colitis in IL-10-deficient mice. J Immunol. 1998;161:3143–9.

8. Spencer DM, Banerjee S, Veldman GM, Levine AD. Anti-IL12 therapy in IL-10-deficient mice prevents the onset of colitis and reverses early disease, but it is ineffective in late disease. Gastroenterology. 1999;116:760(Abstract).
9. Sellon RK, Tonkonogy S, Schultz M *et al.* Resident enteric bacteria are necessary for development of spontaneous colitis and immune system activation in interleukin-10-deficient mice. Infect Immun. 1998;66:5224–31.
10. Fiorentino DF, Zlotnik A, Vieira P *et al.* IL-10 acts on the antigen-presenting cell to inhibit cytokine production by Th1 cells. J Immunol. 1991;146:3444–51.
11. Ekbom A. Epidemiology of inflammatory bowel disease. In: Bistrian BR, Walker-Smith JA, editors. Inflammatory Bowel Diseases. Basel: Karger, 1999:7–21.
12. Cohen MB, Seidman E, Winter H *et al.* Controversies in pediatric inflammatory bowel disease. Inflamm Bowel Dis. 1998;4:203–27.
13. Desreumaux P, Brandt E, Gambiez L *et al.* Distinct cytokine patterns in early and chronic ileal lesions of Crohn's disease. Gastroenterology. 1997;113:118–26.
14. Romagnani S. Th1/Th2 cells. Inflamm Bowel Dis. 1999;5:285–94.
15. Kugathasan S, Binion DG, Itoh J *et al.* Clonal T-cell cytokine secretion is modulated in mucosa of children with recent onset but not chronic inflammatory bowel disease. Gastroenterology. 1997;112:1021(Abstract).
16. Kugathasan S, Werlin SL, Martinez A *et al.* Prolonged duration of response to infliximab in early but not late pediatric Crohn's disease. Am J Gastroenterol. 2000;95:3189–94.

14
Evolution into chronicity

J. C. HOFFMANN and M. ZEITZ

INTRODUCTION

Inflammatory bowel disease (IBD) is generally considered a chronic inflammatory illness of the gastrointestinal tract. To this end, for instance, the German translation for IBD includes the term chronic (chronisch entzündliche Darmerkrankungen). However, IBD occasionally follows a benign course with either long-term remission or even just a single attack[1–3]. Probably, minor forms of bowel inflammation (e.g. ulcerative proctitis) are largely unrecognized because those patients never present to the physician. Little is known about factors which influence the development of chronic inflammation compared with self-limiting acute inflammation. The understanding of these processes seems to be very promising in terms of developing new treatments for those patients who suffer from a chronically active course. Therefore, model systems need to be defined which allow us to investigate and understand the development of chronicity and of protective mechanisms which could counteract IBD. We will describe what is already known from such model systems (particularly animal models and pouchitis), what is not known, and, finally, how we can approach further definition of protective factors in the future. As described below, the genetic background and the environment seem to determine the clinical course of IBD which varies from a single episode to chronic active disease (Figure 1).

LESSONS FROM ANIMAL MODELS

A multitude of IBD animal models has been published over the last two decades, with more than 60 models described so far (Hoffmann *et al.* unpublished database on IBD *in-vivo* models, core facility of the German competence network on IBD; www.kompetenznetz-ced: Forschung: Tiermodelle). Most of these animal models require a certain genetic background which has systematically been investigated for mouse DSS colitis[4]. While C3H/HeJ, C3H/HeJBir, and NOD/LtJ or NOD-scid mice developed colitis after administration of DSS in drinking water for 5 days, other strains (e.g. NON.H2g7 or DBA/2J) do not, or only uncommonly, show colitis after the same treatment. Interestingly, the genetic background even

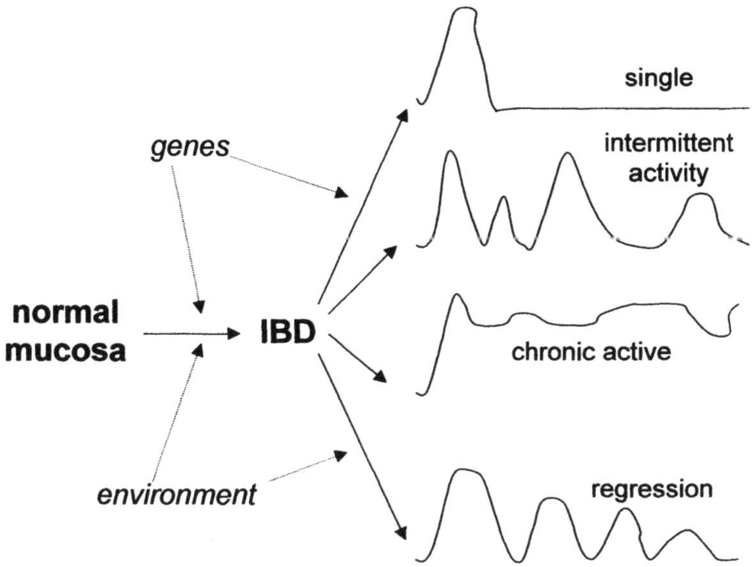

Figure 1 Genes and environment determine the clinical course of IBD

defines the predominant location of inflammation, e.g. inflammation in the caecum but not the remaining colon in 129/SvPas mice and *vice versa* in DBA/2J mice. Also, the genetic background can determine whether chemically induced inflammation becomes chronic or results in resolution of inflammation after a few days. For instance, the hapten TNBS induces an acute but no chronic colitis after weekly intrarectal injections in DBA/2 and C57BL6 mice but a chronic form of colitis in BALB/c and C3H/HeN mice[5]. This phenomenon is not restricted to mice but has also been found in rats (e.g. chronic inflammation in Lewis or Sprague Dawley rats). It is tempting to speculate that genes in man also influence the location of inflammation and the clinical course, i.e. whether chronic inflammation develops.

The flora is certainly important for the development of IBD since most animal models require some kind of flora for the primary inflammation followed by chronicity. Also, the flora can determine whether chronic inflammation or just acute inflammation results after the same single application of the hapten TNBS using BALB/c mice. After a single TNBS injection, chronic inflammation can only be induced in some animal facilities, while in others (even in the same town), only acute inflammation can be observed (unpublished data).

CHRONICITY IN ULCERATIVE COLITIS

As mentioned above, chronicity is often considered to be an essential part of IBD. However, different series have shown that 10–15% of all patients suffering from ulcerative colitis have only a single attack[1,3], while, indeed, at least 85% follow a relapsing course. Further, a subgroup of ulcerative colitis, namely ulcerative proctitis, follows a fairly benign course with more than 40% of patients without further progression[2]. Not uncommonly, extensive disease can regress over long periods of time with a more than 75% cumulative probability for regression both in extensive disease and pancolitis over 25 years[2]. Therefore, there seem to be factors which influence both the extent of disease and the development of chronicity. In general practice, ulcerative colitis is often unrecognized. About 5% of patients presenting with anaemia, constipation, weight loss, abdominal pain, or positive faecal occult blood test had a previously unrecognized ulcerative colitis (Mathysiak-Klose and Braun V, personal communication). It is therefore tempting to speculate that minor forms of ulcerative colitis, particularly proctitis, are either unrecognized or self-limiting. Because of this, large epidemiological studies involving primary care physicians need to be performed in order to determine the 'true' incidence and clinical course of ulcerative proctitis.

LESSONS FROM POUCHITIS: DEVELOPMENT OF CHRONICITY

Proctocolectomy followed by ileopouch–anal anastomosis (IPAA) has become the surgical treatment of choice for patients suffering from severe forms of ulcerative colitis. Over the last decade, it has become clear that inflammation can also develop in the ileal pouch, called pouchitis. This turned out to be a common complication among patients who were operated upon for ulcerative colitis but extremely rare among those patients who had their operation because of familial adenomatous polyposis. In one of the largest cohorts of IPAA (Heidelberg), Heuschen *et al.* described a 10-year cumulative risk of developing pouchitis of 50% among the ulcerative colitis patients[6]. Pouchitis can be divided into primary and secondary, as well as into acute and chronic. Primary pouchitis is defined as inflammation of the pouch without identifiable cause (also known as idiopathic pouchitis). Primary pouchitis shows an acute onset and can often be successfully treated with antibiotics (acute pouchitis). However, more than 10% of these patients follow a chronic course (chronic pouchitis). It is currently unclear what determines how and when pouchitis develops. Furthermore, the factors influencing the occurrence of chronicity are largely unknown. Immunological studies indicate that T helper cells accumulate in the inflamed pouch and secrete T helper 1 cytokines (e.g. interferon γ)[7]. This results in morphological changes in acute pouchitis, particularly crypt hyperplasia and increased villous length[8]. When crypt hyperplasia becomes even more pronounced in chronic pouchitis severe villous atrophy develops (Figure 2). Apart from T helper 1 cytokines, the metalloproteinases 1 and 2 are probably involved in this process[9]. Further studies are required to define the exact series of events looking at immunological, biochemical, and possible microbiological factors in order to determine which patient develops pouchitis, when, and for how long (acute or chronic). Since the earliest point with regard to the initiation of inflammation is known (i.e. the IPAA operation), careful follow-up studies should help us to further understand the evolution of chronicity with regard to pouchitis.

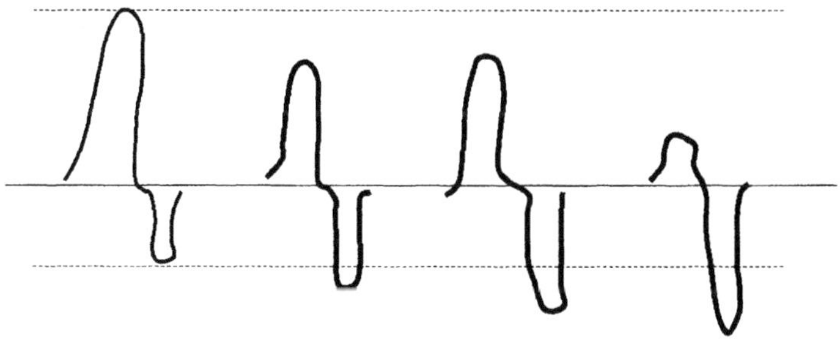

Figure 2 Pattern of mucosal adaptation in ileoanal pouches in relation to disease course (adapted from Reference 8)

PERSPECTIVES WITH REGARD TO UNDERSTANDING EVOLUTION OF CHRONICITY

Two categories of models have been described above, i.e. animal models and pouchitis. Recent studies in animal models have clearly shown that protective mechanism do occur *in vivo*[10–15]. Various cell types can protect or ameliorate bowel inflammation, particularly IL10-secreting CD4 T cells. The phenotype of these cells is characterized by a low expression of CD45RB and an increased expression of CD25. Further, our own studies in the rat also suggest that $\gamma\delta$ T cells might have a protective role in hapten induced colitis[15]. Taken together, genes and flora influence the extent and occurence of inflammation in animal models while protective T cells can either prevent or counteract inflammation. Future studies are needed to further define these protective mechanisms and to transfer these new insights into innovative therapeutic strategies. Looking at human model systems, pouchitis appears to be a perfect model to study both protective mechanisms and the differences between (a) no pouchitis, (b) acute pouchitis, and (c) chronic pouchitis. However, a meticulous follow-up programme is required in order to detect the earliest possible forms of pouchitis. Because of the number of IPAA operations per centre, studies involving several centres hopefully will help to obtain the required samples. Until recently, pouchitis was the only human IBD model since clearly defined genetic markers have been lacking. Lately, three groups have described a genetic marker for Crohn's disease (IBD-1 or NOD2)[16–18]. However, this marker seems to affect only 20% of CD patients. All carriers of a double-mutation in the NOD2 locus investigated so far suffer from Crohn's disease. Single mutations can also occur in the general/healthy population. It is tempting to speculate that such 'healthy' carriers (e.g. relatives of Crohn's disease patients) might develop Crohn's disease in the future. If this turns out to be true, follow-up strategies might help to define early changes and protective factors which determine either an inflammatory or a protected phenotype among these carriers.

Acknowledgement

The authors are supported by the Kompeteurnetzwerk CED of the German Ministry of Research (BNBF).

References

1. Tysk C, Jarnerot G. Ulcerative proctocolitis in Orebro, Sweden. A retrospective epidemiologic study, 1963–1987. Scand J Gastroenterol. 1992;27(11):945–50.
2. Langholz E, Munkholm P, Davidsen M, Nielsen OH, Binder V. Changes in extent of ulcerative colitis: a study on the course and prognostic factors. Scand J Gastroenterol. 1996;31(3):260–6.
3. Langholz E, Munkholm P, Davidsen M, Binder V. Course of ulcerative colitis: analysis of changes in disease activity over years. Gastroenterology. 1994;107(1):3–11.
4. Mahler M, Bristol IJ, Leiter EH *et al.* Differential susceptibility of inbred mouse strains to dextran sulfate sodium-induced colitis. Am J Physiol. 1998;274(3 Pt 1):G544–51.
5. Beagley KW, Black CA, Elson CO. Strain differences in susceptibility to TNBS-induced colitis. Gastroenterology. 1991;100(5):A560.
6. Heuschen UA, Autschbach F, Allemeyer EH *et al.* Long-term follow-up after ileoanal pouch procedure: algorithm for diagnosis, classification, and management of pouchitis. Dis Colon Rectum. 2001;44(4):487–99.
7. Stallmach A, Schafer F, Hoffmann S *et al.* Increased state of activation of CD4 positive T cells and elevated interferon gamma production in pouchitis. Gut. 1998;43(4):499–505.
8. Stallmach A, Moser C, Hero-Gross R *et al.* Pattern of mucosal adaptation in acute and chronic pouchitis. Dis Colon Rectum. 1999;42(10):1311–17.
9. Stallmach A, Chan CC, Ecker KW *et al.* Comparable expression of matrix metalloproteinases 1 and 2 in pouchitis and ulcerative colitis. Gut. 2000;47(3):415–22.
10. Powrie F. T cells in inflammatory bowel disease: protective and pathogenic roles. Immunity. 1995;3(2):171–4.
11. Asseman C, Powrie F. Interleukin 10 is a growth factor for a population of regulatory T cells. Gut. 1998;42(2):157–8.
12. Read S, Malmstrom V, Powrie F. Cytotoxic T lymphocyte-associated antigen 4 plays an essential role in the function of CD25(+) CD4(+) regulatory cells that control intestinal inflammation. J Exp Med. 2000;192(2):295–302.
13. Groux H, O'Garra A, Bigler M *et al.* A CD4+ T-cell subset inhibits antigen-specific T-cell responses and prevents colitis. Nature. 1997;389(6652):737–42.
14. Stallmach A, Wittig B, Giese T *et al.* Protection of trinitrobenzene sulfonic acid-induced colitis by an interleukin 2-IgG2b fusion protein in mice. Gastroenterology. 1999;117(4):866–76.
15. Hoffmann JC, Peters K, Henschke S *et al.* Role of T lymphocytes in rat 2,4,6-trinitrobenzene sulphonic acid (TNBS) induced colitis: increased morality after gammadelta T cell depletion and no effect of alphabeta T cell depletion. Gut. 2001;48(4):489–95.
16. Ogura Y, Bonen DK, Inohara N *et al.* A frameshift mutation in NOD2 associated with susceptibility to Crohn's disease. Nature. 2001;411(6837):603–6.
17. Hugot JP, Chamaillard M, Zouali H *et al.* Association of NOD2 leucine-rich repeat variants with susceptibility to Crohn's disease. Nature. 2001;411(6837):599–603.
18. Hampe J, Cuthbert A, Croucher PJ *et al.* Association between insertion mutation in NOD2 gene and Crohn's disease in German and British populations. Lancet. 2001;357(9272):1925–8.

15
Ulcerative colitis and multiple organ dysfunction syndrome (MODS)

R. CAPRILLI and G. LATELLA

FREQUENCY AND OUTCOME OF MODS IN ULCERATIVE COLITIS

Mortality in acute ulcerative colitis (UC) is commonly attributed to major colonic complications (toxic megacolon, colonic perforation and massive bleeding) or surgical procedures. Early recognition of the severity of colitis ('impending megacolon'), intensive medical treatment and early surgery, have contributed to reduce the mortality rate for severe UC to less than 5% over the last forty years[1,2].

Recently, we observed some fatal cases of severe UC in which death was related to multiple organ dysfunction syndrome (MODS)[3], a condition that occurs in several infectious and non-infectious acute critical diseases[4] but which had never been reported in UC. MODS describes a continuum of abnormalities involving various organs (lung, kidney, heart, nervous system, liver, pancreas, GI tract, and bone marrow) resulting from systemic inflammatory response syndrome (SIRS)[5]. SIRS consists of the massive inflammatory reaction resulting from systemic mediator release[6]. MODS is associated with a very high mortality rate depending on the number of involved organs, duration and degree of organ dysfunction[7,8]. The intestine plays an important role in the development both of SIRS and MODS, being considered in some instances 'the motor' of multiple organ failure[9–11].

In a recent study, we have retrospectively evaluated the frequency and outcome of MODS in a series of 180 consecutive cases of severe UC[12]. All patients were on standard intensive regimen consisting of total parenteral nutrition and hydrocortisone 100 mg qid. Colectomy was performed according to the timing of the Oxford intensive regimen. Of these 180 severe UC patients, 11 (6.1%) experienced clinical and laboratory features of MODS. The lung was involved in 5 patients, the kidney in 3, the liver in 7, the central nervous system in 3, the haematological system in 3 and the pancreas in 1. MODS was preceded by toxic megacolon in 5 patients and by so-called 'impending megacolon' in 4, whereas, in 2 patients, no previous complications of UC were observed. MODS developed during the first attack of colitis in 7 patients, during relapse in 4. The overall mortality rate was 12/180 (6.6%). Note that, of the 12 patients who died, 8 (72.7%) had MODS.

Two main conclusions may be drawn from these data: (1) UC should be included among the causes of MODS, and (2) MODS is responsible for the majority of deaths in acute severe UC.

It appears, therefore, that in the most severe cases of UC, besides a 'colitic' phase, in which inflammation is confined to the intestinal wall, a 'systemic' phase may develop, in which the inflammatory response overflows the intestinal wall. The former is responsible for local complications (toxic megacolon, perforation and massive haemorrhage), the latter for systemic complications (SIRS/MODS) (Figure 1).

Recently, we have confirmed in a prospective study that both intestinal distension and MODS are important clinical features in severe colitis and that they represent powerful prognostic factors. In particular, we evaluated in patients with severe UC the prevalence of gastrointestinal distension and its relationship to clinical outcome, including occurrence of severe complications (TMC and MODS), need for surgery, and mortality[13].

Of 45 patients with severe UC, 24 (53%) had gastrointestinal distension. Three of these had colonic dilatation (TMC) on admission (all underwent surgery and survived), 21 showed increased gastrointestinal gas content (4 developed TMC 1–4 days after the detection of gastrointestinal distension and were operated, 2 developed MODS and died; 8 did not improve, were submitted to surgery and survived). Four of the 21 (19%) patients with increased intestinal gas content had a concomitant abnormal distension of the stomach.

Of the 21 patients with normal gastrointestinal gas content, none had complications; all survived (5 did not improve and required surgery). Thus, only patients with increased gastrointestinal gas content upon admission developed TMC during hospitalization. The need for surgery was higher in patients with

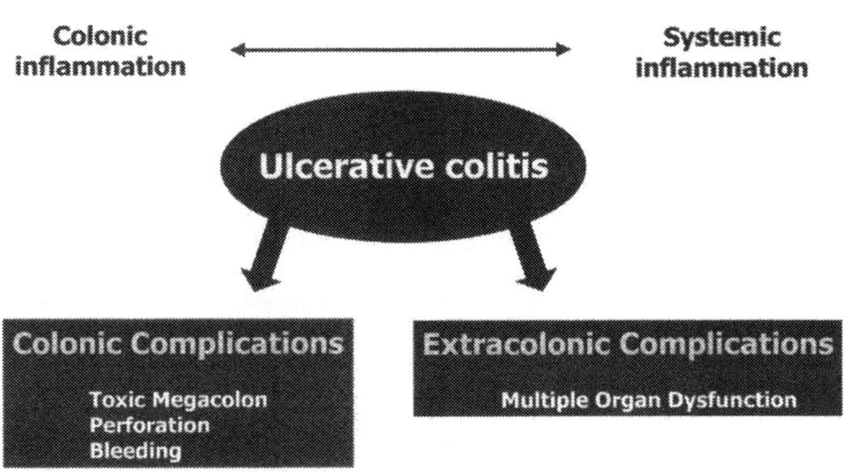

Figure 1 Colonic and extracolonic complications of severe ulcerative colitis

increased gastrointestinal gas (12/21, 57%) compared with those with normal gastrointestinal gas content (5/21, 24%) ($p < 0.05$, OR 4.267, CI 1.134–16.055). The only two deaths observed occurred in patients with MODS, both showing gastrointestinal distension on admission (one 'impending megacolon', one definite toxic megacolon).

The results of this study confirm that, in severe UC, persistent gastrointestinal distension characterizes a subgroup of patients with poor response to medical therapy, at higher risk for TMC and need for surgery. In addition, they show that the development of MODS is the most important predicting factor for fatal outcome.

PATHOGENETIC MECHANISMS

From the presented data it appears that GI distension and MODS are frequently associated. It is therefore possible that they share some pathogenetic mechanisms.

While some data provide possible explanations for the impaired neuromotor function responsible for colonic dilatation in widespread colitis, most of them fail to explain the gaseous distension in the uninflamed small bowel and stomach. Lesions in the myenteric plexus and muscle fibres[14], as well as electrolyte/metabolic imbalance[15], were considered to contribute to the reduction of colonic motor activity[16,17] and the development of TMC. However, electrolyte imbalance is not invariably present, whereas severe anatomical damage can be excluded in those cases in which TMC rapidly subsides.

Today the most convincing explanation for TMC seems to be the excessive local production of nitric oxide (NO) and cytokines, and the activation of viscero-visceral reflexes.

Clinical and experimental data have been reported, suggesting that NO plays a central role in the genesis of colonic distension[18–20]. Increased inducible nitric oxide synthase (iNOS) activity was detected in the inflamed colonic mucosa from patients with UC as compared with controls, with significantly higher levels in TMC than in uncomplicated UC. Similarly, in trinitrobenzenesulphonic acid (TNBS) colitis, an experimental model of acute severe colitis associated with colonic dilatation, a striking increase in the iNOS expression was found, whereas the inhibition of NOS activity by L-NAME, a non-specific NOS inhibitor, prevented colonic dilatation. The observation that some cytokines (IL-1β, TNFα, IFNγ, which are of primary importance in the inflammatory process of severe colitis, as well as free radicals and lipopolysaccharides (LPS) are able to induce iNOS expression in human colonic smooth muscle strips[21,22], further supports the role of iNOS in the genesis of TMC.

The excessive NO generation in the inflamed colon may offer an explanation for distension of the large bowel but not for that of the proximal uninflamed gastrointestinal segments. In fact, NOS activity in the dilated uninflamed colonic segment, in TNBS colitis, was of the same order as that of controls[20]. Furthermore, it is unlikely that NO exerts its inhibitory effect via the blood stream on account of its extremely short half-life[23]. Conversely, this is not the case for cytokines which are present at high concentrations either in the inflamed colonic mucosa or in the serum both of animals with experimental colitis and of patients with severe UC[24]. The cytokines have been demonstrated to suppress neurotransmitter release which may alter neuromuscular function even at the remote site of inflammation[25–27].

An alternative or additional pathogenetic mechanism that might contribute to GI distension in TMC is the activation of intestinal extrinsic inhibitory reflexes[25,28]. Experimental studies have shown that distension or mucosal irritation of one part of the GI tract can inhibit the motor activity of distant segments through the activation of extrinsic neuronal colon–ileal or ileo-colonic inhibitory reflexes[29,30].

Two types of extrinsic reflexes have been identified, namely the 'long reflexes' involving the spinal cord through the dorsal root ganglia and the 'short reflexes' involving only the prevertebral ganglia. The activation of visceral afferent fibres occurs through the stimulation of polymodal (chemical, mechanical etc.) sensory receptors by inflammatory mediators and/or visceral distension[30–32]. The efferent limb, represented by preganglionic and postganglionic sympathetic nerves, innervates mainly the myenteric plexus. Its inhibitory effect on GI tone and motility is primarily mediated by noradrenaline-induced inhibition of acetylcholine and release of tachykinins from post-ganglionic intrinsic cholinergic neurons[33,34].

As far as the development of MODS is concerned, it is directely related to the SIRS which in UC seems to be induced, and then maintained or amplified by colonic inflammation and intestinal bacterial translocation. In severe colitis, ulcerations and extensive mucosal sloughing favour the pathological translocation of bacteria and toxins. At the same time, the exalted immunoinflammatory response of the mucosa induces overproduction of cytokines (IL-1, IL-2, IL-6, IL-8, TNFα, INFγ) and other mediators of the inflammation (eicosanoids, reactive oxygen metabolites)[11,35,36]. Their passage into the systemic circulation, as well as that of bacteria and toxins, activates the circulating immunocompetent cells, especially monocytes and neutrophils, with further production of cytokines and other inflammatory mediators, responsible for systemic haemodynamic and metabolic alterations, which may, in some instances, lead to dysfunction or failure of extraintestinal organs[4,6]. High tissue and plasma levels of cytokines have, indeed, been demonstrated in UC as well as endotoxaemia which was reported in 88% of cases[24,36,37]. Both these findings correlate with the extension and severity of the disease.

In summary, we hypothesized that both GI distension and MODS are strictly related and characterize some of the most severe forms of UC (Figure 2). The increased release of soluble inflammatory mediators (cytokines, reactive oxygen metabolites, eicosanoids, neurotransmitters) in the inflamed colonic mucosa, together with bacterial products, enhance NO generation at muscle level and activate nerve endings of mucosal afferent fibres. NO excess may lead to muscle relaxation and colonic dilatation, whereas the activation of sensory fibres elicits inhibitory reflexes leading to distension of the stomach and small bowel. The distension of small bowel loops might, in turn, aggravate or even trigger the onset of colonic dilatation. On the other hand, the spilling into the systemic blood stream of cytokines and bacterial toxins induces extra-intestinal organ dysfunction (MODS). It may also contribute to the GI distension.

It appears, therefore, that distension of the small bowel and/or of the stomach has the same pathophysiological significance as that of the colon. The finding of

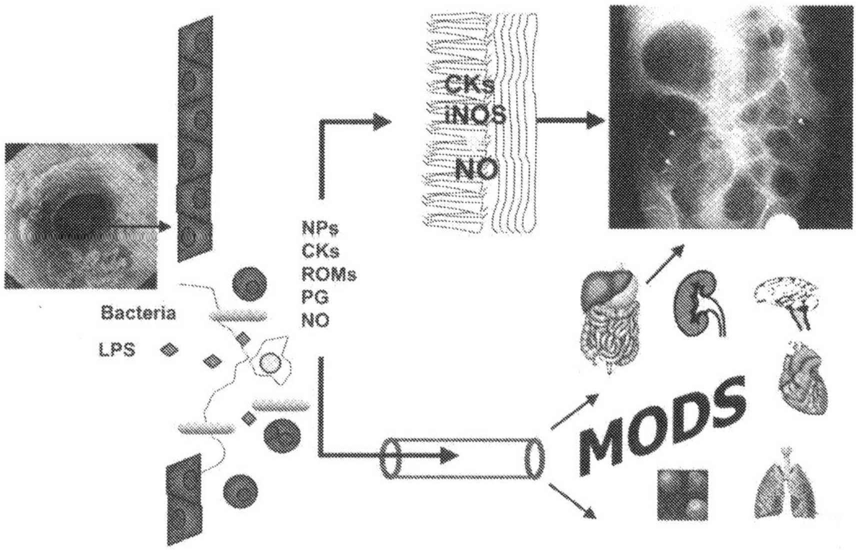

Figure 2 Pathogenetic hypothesis for gastrointestinal distension and MODs in severe ulcerative colitis. LPS = lipopolysaccharides, NPs = neuropeptides, CKs = cytokines, ROMs = reactive oxygen metabolites, PG = prostaglandins, NO = nitric oxide, iNOS = inducible nitric oxide synthase, MODS = multiple organ dysfunction syndrome.

distension in any segment of the GI tract during the clinical course of colitis should, therefore, be considered as an alarm signal for major complications, either local (TMC) or systemic (MODS). Particular attention should be paid to early recognition of the appearance of disproportionate tachycardia, polypnea, hypoxaemia, oliguria, mental confusion and jaundice, that suggest MODS. The detection of one or more of these signs requires an aggressive therapeutic approach. The patient should be moved to an intensive care unit, the main therapeutic goals being maintenance of adequate tissue oxygen supplies and nutritional support (high-calorie/high-protein TPN, supplemented with specific nutrients for the intestinal mucosa) and the minimization of bacterial translocation by means of high doses of antibiotics[4,10,38,39]. Emergency colectomy is the treatment of choice in order to remove, as soon as possible, the main site of intestinal bacteria translocation. Corticosteroids and cyclosporin could prove harmful in MODS as they increase intestinal permeability and reduce both mucosal barrier function and the defensive response of the host[40–43].

References

1. Caprilli R, Vernia P, Latella G, Torsoli A. Early recognition of toxic megacolon. J Clin Gastroenterol. 1987;9:160–4.
2. Hyde GM, Jewell DP. Review article: the management of severe ulcerative colitis. Aliment Pharmacol Ther. 1997;11:419–24.
3. Latella G, Frieri G, Pimpo MT, Caprilli R. Severe ulcerative colitis may induce multiple organ dysfunction. Ital J Gastroenterol. 1996;28(Suppl. 1):A19.

4. Demling R, Lalonde C, Saldinger P, Knox J. Multiple organ dysfunction in the surgical patient: Pathophysiology, prevention and treatment. Curr Prob Surg. 1993;30:347–415.
5. Goris RJA. MODS/SIRS: result of an overwhelming inflammatory response? World J Surg. 1996;20:418–21.
6. Bone RC. Toward a theory regarding the pathogenesis of the systemic inflammatory response syndrome: what we do and do not know about cytokine regulation. Crit Care Med. 1996; 24:163–72.
7. Marshall JC, Cook DJ, Christou NV *et al.* Multiple organ dysfunction score: a reliable descriptor of a complex clinical outcome. Crit Care Med. 1995;23:1638–52.
8. Baue AE, Durham R, Faist E. Systemic inflammatory response syndrome (SIRS), multiple organ dysfunction syndrome (MODS), multiple organ failure (MOD): are we winning the battle? Shock. 1998;10:79–89.
9. Carrico CJ, Meakins JL, Marshall W *et al.* The gastrointestinal tract: the 'motor' of MOF. Arch Surg. 1986;121:196–208.
10. Thompson JS. The intestinal response to critical illness. Am J Gastroenterol. 1995;90:190–200.
11. Marshall JC. Contemporary variations on the ancient theme of the gut in critical illness. Curr Opin Crit Care. 1998;4:101–3.
12. Caprilli R, Latella G, Vernia P, Frieri P. Multiple organ dysfunction in ulcerative colitis. Am J Gastroenterol. 2000;95:1258–62.
13. Latella G, Vernia P, Viscido A *et al.* Gastrointestinal distension in severe ulcerative colitis. Am J Gastroenterol. 2002 (in press).
14. Geboes K, Collins S. Structural abnormalities of the nervous system in Crohn's disease and ulcerative colitis. Neurogastroenterol Motil. 1998;10:189–202.
15. Caprilli R, Vernia P, Colaneri O, Frieri G. Risk factors in toxic megacolon. Dig Dis Sci. 1980;25:817–22.
16. Koch TR, Carney JA, Go VLW, Szurszewski JH. Spontaneous contraction and some electrophysiological properties of circular muscle from normal sigmoid colon and ulcerative colitis. Gastroenterology. 1988;95:77–84.
17. Reddy SN, Bazzochi G, Ghan S *et al.* Colonic motility and transit in health and ulcerative colitis. Gastroenterology. 1991;101:1289–97.
18. Middleton SJ, Shorthouse M, Hunter LO. Increased nitric oxide synthesis in ulcerative colitis. Lancet. 1993;341:465–6.
19. Mourelle M, Casella F, Guarner F *et al.* Induction of nitric oxide synthase in colonic smooth muscle from patients with toxic megacolon. Gastroenterology. 1995;109:1497–502.
20. Mourelle M, Villaseca J, Guarner F *et al.* Toxic dilatation of colon in rat model of colitis is linked to an inducible form of nitric oxide synthase. Am J Physiol. 1996;270:G425–30.
21. Cook HT, Cattel V. Role of nitric oxide in immune-mediated diseases. Clin Sci. 1996;91:375–84.
22. Lundberg JON, Lundberg JM, Alving K, Weitzberg E. Nitric oxide and inflammation: The answer is blowing in the wind. Nature Med. 1997;3:30–1.
23. Moncada S, Palmer RMJ, Higgs EA. Nitric oxide: physiology pathophysiology and pharmacology. Pharmacol Rev. 1991;43:109–42.
24. Fiocchi C. Inflammatory bowel disease. Etiology and pathogenesis. Gastroenterology. 1998;115: 182–205.
25. Caprilli R, Onori L. Pathogenesis of gastrointestinal distension in severe ulcerative colitis: a hypothesis. Gastroenterol Int. 1992;5:268–72.
26. Jackobson K, McHugh K, Collins SM. The mechanism of altered neural function in a rat model of colitis. Gastroenterology. 1997;112:156–62.
27. Sbahidi H, Kilbourn RG. Interleukin-2 therapy in renal cancer induced acute colonic distention. Cancer Metastasis Rev. 1998;17:119–26.
28. Sengupta JN, Gebhart GF. Gastrointestinal afferent fibers and sensation. In: Johnson LR, editor, Physiology of the Gastrointestinal Tract. New York: Raven Press, 1994:483–519.
29. Furness JB, Costa M. Adynamic ileus, its pathogenesis and treatment. Med Biol. 1974;52:82–9.
30. Basilisco G, Phillips SF. Ileal distention relaxes the canine colon: a model of megacolon? Gastroenterology. 1994;106:606–14.
31. Bueno L, Fioramonti J, Delvaux M, Frexinos J. Mediators and pharmacology of visceral sensitivity: from basic to clinical investigations. Gastroenterology. 1997;112:1714–43.
32. Bueno L, Fioramonti J. Effects of inflammatory mediators on gut sensitivity. Can J Gastroenterol. 1999;13(Suppl. A):42A–46A.

33. Reilly WM, Hoyle CHV, Burnstock G. Pre- and postjunctional adrenoceptor types in the circular muscle of the guinea-pig caecum. Naunyn–Schmiedeberg's Arch Pharmacol. 1987;336:37–47.
34. Willis WE. Anatomy and physiology of descending control of nociceptive responses of dorsal horn neurons: a comprehensive review. In: Fields HL, Besson HL, editors, Pain Modulation. Progress in Brain Research. Amsterdam: Elsevier, 1988:1–29.
35. Haglund U. Systemic mediators released from the gut in critical illness. Crit Care Med. 1993;21:S15–S18.
36. Sartor BR. Cytokines in intestinal inflammation. Pathophysiological and clinical considerations. Gastroenterology. 1994;106:533–9.
37. Gardiner KR, Halliday MI, Barclay GR *et al*. Significance of systemic endotoxaemia in inflammatory bowel disease. Gut. 1995;36:897–901.
38. Vincent JL. Prevention and therapy of multiple organ failure. World J Surg. 1996;20:465–70.
39. Wells CL. Editorial response to a decade of experience with selective decontamination of the digestive tract as prophylaxis for infections in patients in the intensive care unit: what have we learned? Clin Infect Dis. 1993;17:1055–7.
40. Spitz JC, Ghandi S, Taveras M *et al*. Characteristics of the intestinal epithelial barrier during dietary manipulation and glucocorticoid stress. Crit Care Med. 1996;24:635–41.
41. Gianotti L, Alexander JW, Fukushima R, Pyles T. Steroid therapy can modulate gut barrier function, host defense, and survival in thermally injured mice. J Surg Res. 1996;62:53–8.
42. Sun S, Greenstein SM, Kim DY *et al*. Nifepidine protects small intestine from cyclosporine-induced hemodynamic and functional impairment. J Surg Res. 1997;69:295–9.
43. Montero EF, Silva RM, Keller R *et al*. Role of cyclosporin A in bacterial translocation. Transplant Proc. 1996;28:2676.

16
Early versus late inflammatory bowel disease: implications for therapy

L. R. SUTHERLAND

INTRODUCTION

This chapter will discuss a variety of possible definitions of 'early vs. late' for Crohn's disease (Table 1). For each definition, the implications of the definition for the management of patients with Crohn's disease will be reviewed.

EARLY INTERVENTION IN THE POPULATION WITH THE GREATEST SUSCEPTIBILITY TO DEVELOP INFLAMMATORY BOWEL DISEASE (PRIMARY PREVENTION)

The best strategy to treat a disease is to prevent it! As we enter the first decade of the 21st century, it is possible to speculate about primary prevention programmes for susceptible populations. Primary prevention of disease is defined by Last as the protection of health by personal and community-wide effects, e.g. preserving good nutritional status, physical fitness and emotional well-being, immunizing against infectious diseases, and making the environment safe[1]. The term is also used to suggest strategies to decrease the incidence of the disease. Most investigators believe that the aetiology of inflammatory bowel disease lies in the interaction between genetic factors, immunological processes and the environment in which we live. As we explore the genome looking for genes associated with Crohn's disease, primary prevention may become a reality.

Table 1 Early interventions in Crohn's disease

Early in the susceptible population
Early onset in life
Early intervention in the course of the disease
Self medication
Early introduction of disease-remitting agents
Early surgery

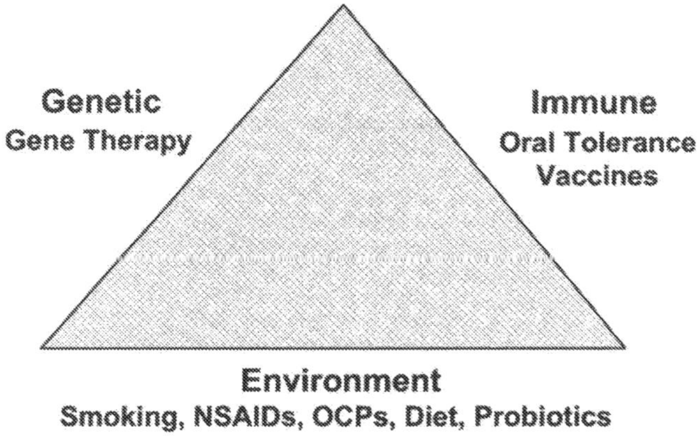

Figure 1 Potential primary prevention strategies for the susceptible population

Figure 1 provides examples of potential modifications that could be introduced to decrease the possibility of developing inflammatory bowel disease. This model might be used for individuals who have a positive family history for Crohn's disease. How would the susceptible population be identified? Siblings of patients with Crohn's disease have an increased risk of developing Crohn's disease compared with the general population. With the ongoing search for genes associated with inflammatory bowel disease, it should be possible in the future to identify the at-risk population more precisely.

Such a programme might, for example, from an environmental perspective provide advice to other family members of patients with Crohn's disease that smoking, non-steroidal anti-inflammatory drugs and perhaps oral contraceptives are risk factors for developing disease. The potential risk from passive smoking might also be included when counselling family members. Perhaps, in the future, gene therapy might be offered to rectify immunological defects in individuals at risk for developing inflammatory bowel disease. If a putative antigen is found, then oral tolerance therapy could be initiated. Conversely, if a microbial factor is important, vaccines might be developed.

EARLY IN THE LIFE OF THE PATIENT

About 20% of patients with Crohn's disease develop their disease in the first two decades of life. Age of onset is one of the three classification variables of the Vienna classification[2]. Paediatric patients are thought to have more severe disease at presentation and to report more extra-colonic manifestations of Crohn's disease than the adult population. Younger patients may be motivated by other factors compared with the adult population. Growth and weight gain as well as completion of puberty are of particular interest to teenagers. Prepubertal teens may be more interested in nutritional approaches to induction of remission given their concerns related to the cosmetic side-effects of corticosteroids.

Various studies have suggested that genetic susceptibility may be more important in familial forms of Crohn's disease than in the sporadic cases which

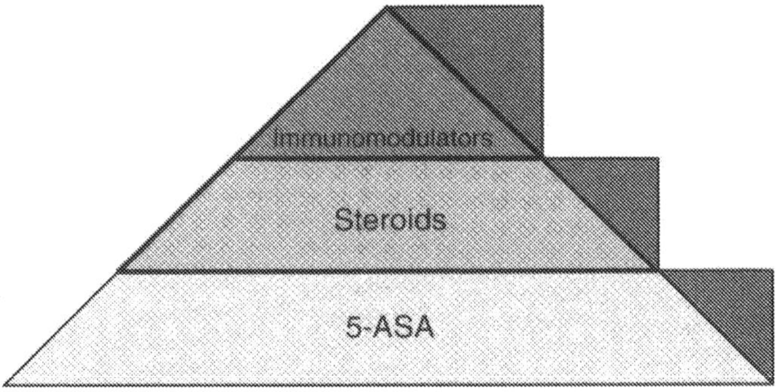

Figure 2 Traditional step-up approach to therapy

develop in the general population. This observation underlies the current search of the genome but might also be expanded to the area of pharmacogenetics. For example, the identification of polymorphisms for anti-TNF-α might be useful in identifying populations that have a greater or lesser chance of responding to the compound.

EARLY AGGRESSIVE INTERVENTION IN THE COURSE OF DISEASE

This definition can be operationalized in a variety of scenarios. First, many patients should be empowered to initiate therapy at the onset of symptoms rather than wait until they are able to see their physician. Early introduction of therapy might abort a flare. There are only a few data which would support this approach. For example, Dickinson and colleagues[3] reported no difference in relapses of patients with ulcerative colitis randomized to sulphasalazine either 2 g bid daily or 3 g initiated at the first onset of flare symptoms. This study suffers from low statistical power and should be repeated.

Recently, there has been interest in moving to the early introduction of more powerful therapy in patients with inflammatory bowel disease. This is driven in part by the approach in rheumatology which emphasizes the use of disease-modifying anti-rheumatic therapy (DMARTs) early in the management of disease. Aggressive therapy has been shown to alter disease progression[4]. Since there are many parallels between inflammatory bowel disease and rheumatoid arthritis (chronic inflammation, early lesions leading to joint and gut damage), it is natural to consider the implications of this approach.

On the negative side, there is the possibility that the subgroup of patients with inflammatory bowel disease who will actually have a more benign course may be unnecessarily exposed to potentially toxic drugs. However, the benefits of a more aggressive approach are demonstrated in a recent report[5]. They reported the results of a follow-up study of patients with early rheumatoid arthritis who had participated in a 9-month placebo-controlled trial assessing the efficacy of hydroxychloroquine therapy. The placebo-treated patients were characterized as the 'late therapy' group and the hydroxychloroquine group were called the 'early therapy' group. After 2 years of follow-up, the early therapy group continued to show ongoing benefits (less pain, improved physical ability, higher physician global assessment scores) compared with the late treatment group.

The management of Crohn's disease for the last two decades has, for the most part, emphasized a 'stepped' approach to therapy with the aminosalicylates followed by corticosteroids as the mainstay of therapy. In most centres across North America, by contrast with Europe, the use of immunosuppressants was restricted to the most challenging of cases. It would not be uncommon for patients to have several relapses and resections before the use of azathioprine, 6-mercaptopurine or more recently methotrexate, would be considered.

In the last few years there has been a change in attitudes to the use of immunomodulators. A recent report summarized the key findings of a survey performed by the International Organization for the Study of Inflammatory Bowel Disease (IOIBD). Six hundred surveys were distributed; 58% were returned. Participants were generally from the academic community. The majority included either azathioprine or 6-MP as part of their therapeutic armenentarium for inflammatory bowel disease[6]. A recent Canadian survey, however, reported that only 7% of patients were taking azathioprine therapy, which suggests that there is room for growth in this area[7].

The paediatric community is providing evidence suggesting that the appropriate strategy in 2001 is to introduce immunomodulators early in the course of the disease. A short course of corticosteroids is provided to induce the remission and immunomodulators maintain the remission. Markowitz and colleages recently reported the final results of their placebo-controlled trial of 6-MP ($1.5\,mg\,kg^{-1}\,day^{-1}$): after 18 months of follow-up, 6-MP-treated patients were twice as likely to remain in remission as the placebo-treated patients (91 vs. 53%, Figure 3)[8]. Discussion of early interventions is particularly appropriate as the new century begins. Although anti-TNF-α is currently only approved for the induction of remission, long-term studies should be initiated to determine if

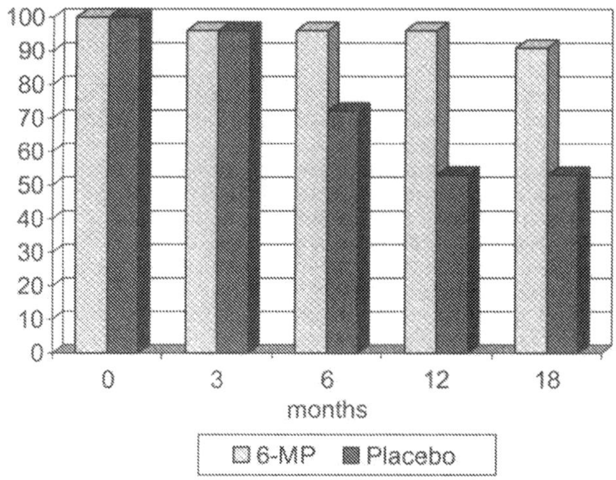

Figure 3 Results of a paediatric trial of 6-MP in maintenance of remission in Crohn's disease

early use of infliximab alters the natural history of disease. Soon DMARTs will give way to biological response modifiers (BRM) offering additional therapeutic options in the treatment of inflammatory bowel disease.

Other early interventions could be non-pharmacological. For example, there is evidence from the management of rheumatic disease that behaviour modification therapy, if introduced early in the management of patients with rheumatic disease, has long-term benefits, including better pain control and less disease-associated depression[9].

Another intervention that should be assessed would be the efficacy of early surgery. Such a trial might compare the long-term outcome, quality of life and economic impact of early surgery compared with a medical model of pharmaco or biological therapy. Such a trial would be difficult. Most of the patients eligible for the trial would be more likely to be seen by community physicians and surgeons and not by trial leaders, who tend to be academic leaders and who see more challenging cases. It might also be difficult to convince patients of the drug-sparing potential benefits of surgery when they have not taken any of the medications up to that time.

In conclusion, we should also realize that we are relatively early in the ultimate journey to determine the cause(s) of inflammatory bowel disease. Once they are identified, a more rational approach to the therapy of these diseases should be possible.

References

1. Last JM. A Dictionary of Epidemiology. 2nd edn. Oxford: Oxford University Press, 1988.
2. Gasche C, Scholmerich J, Brynskov J *et al.* A simple classification of Crohn's disease: Report of the Working Party for the World Congresses of Gastroenterology, Vienna 1998. Inflamm Bowel Dis. 2000;6:8–15.
3. Dickinson RJ, King A, Wight DGD, Hunter JO, Neale G. Is continuous sulfasalazine necessary in the management of patients with ulcerative colitis? Results of a preliminary study. Dis Colon Rectum. 1985;28:929–30.
4. Albers JMC, Palmela L, Kurki P *et al.* Treatment strategy, disease activity, and outcome in four cohorts of patients with early rheumatoid arthritis. Ann Rheum Dis. 2001;60:453–8.
5. Tsakonas E, Fitzgerald AA, Cividino A *et al.* Consequences of delayed therapy with second-line agents in rheumatoid arthritis: A 3 year follow-up on the Hydroxychloroquine in Early Rheumatoid Arthritis (HERA) study. J Rheumatol. 2000;27:623–9.
6. Meuwissen SG, Ewe K, Gassull MA *et al.* IOIBD questionnaire on the clinical use of azathioprine, 6-mercaptopurine, cyclosporin A and methotrexate in the treatment of Crohn's disease. Eur J Gastroenterol Hepatol. 2000;12:13–18.
7. Wallace TM, van Zanten SJO. Frequency of use and standards of care for the use of azathioprine and 6-MP in the treatment of inflammatory bowel disease: A systematic review of the literature and a survery of Canadian gastroenterologists. Can J Gastroenterol. 2001;15:21–8.
8. Markowitz JF, Grancher K, Kohn N, Lesser M, Daum F, The Paediatric 6MP Collaborative Group. A multicenter trial of 6-mercaptopurine and prednisone in children with newly diagnosed Crohn's disease. Gastroenterology. 2000;119:895–902.
9. Sharpe L, Sensky T, Timberlake N, Ryan A, Brewin C, Allard S. A blind, randomized, controlled trial of cognitive-behaviour intervention for patients with recent onset rheumatoid arthritis: preventing psychological and physical morbidity. Pain. 2001;89:275–83.

17
Cells of the intestinal mucosa – from inflammation to fibrosis

G. ROGLER

INTRODUCTION

Fibrosis is a major problem during the course of inflammatory bowel disease. An overzealous repair process leads to the formation of obstruction. About 75% of all patients suffering from Crohn's disease have to undergo surgery at least once during the course of their disease[1,2]. In about 50% of those, the indication for surgery is because of intestinal obstructions and strictures, which means that about one third of all patients with Crohn's disease have to undergo surgery because of intestinal obstructions[1,2]. In a number of patients these obstructions are recurrent[3].

Presently we are just beginning to understand the mechanisms that lead from intestinal inflammation to fibrosis and stenosis of bowel segments during the course of inflammatory bowel disease. Recent data indicate that, in addition to T cells and macrophages, non-classical immune cells, such as epithelial cells and mesenchymal cells, contribute to the initiation and chronic perpetuation of intestinal inflammation. A complex network of signals and mediators between these cells supports cell-to-cell communication. However, it is still unclear which signals can limit an inflammatory response, and whether a lack of such signals may cause chronic or recurrent inflammation. Interestingly, fibrosis is currently not the focus of investigators of inflammatory bowel disease since, at the Digestive Disease Week 2001, only 5–10 out of 4000 abstracts focused on the problem of the pathophysiology of mucosal fibrosis formation despite the severe clinical problems of many of our patients.

In general, fibrosis is thought to be a reactive process. A chronic or recurrent inflammation is regarded to be a necessary condition for the initiation of intestinal fibrosis. According to this view, fibrosis is an overzealous healing response to inflammation-induced injury. It is unclear what triggers increased fibrosis in some patients and not in others. Factors that limit the normal physiological healing response that is essential for the integrity of the intestinal barrier after tissue damage have not been identified.

A number of different cell types play important roles during intestinal inflammation. These cell types interact with each other either directly via intercellular junctions, by surface receptors or by secreted mediators. During inflammation, tissue damage occurs through mediators and enzymes secreted mainly by macrophages and granulocytes. Chronic tissue damage will finally lead to tissue fibrosis.

As fibroblasts and myofibroblasts are the cells finally synthesizing the fibres which are deposited during fibrosis, these cells may be regarded as the central players or as the effectors of intestinal fibrosis. Therefore, after highlighting the mechanisms involved in inflammatory tissue damage, the role of fibroblasts and myofibroblasts in the normal and inflamed mucosa and their interactions with other cell types will be discussed.

TISSUE DAMAGE DURING INTESTINAL INFLAMMATION

Inflammation usually causes damage to the tissue. In the case of the intestinal mucosa, a loss of epithelial cells, ulcerations, submucosal tissue degradation and bleeding occurs. A number of enzymes and other mediators mainly mediated by macrophages and granulocytes is responsible for that tissue damage. There is evidence that these enzymes and mediators have an additive effect.

Oxidative stress

Oxidants like oxygen- or hydroxide-radicals are important contributors to the tissue damage seen in inflammatory bowel disease. In relation to the oxidative stress the colon is subjected to by the production of reactive oxygen species from phagocytic leukocytes during inflammation, the colonic mucosa contains relatively small amounts of antioxidant enzymes[4,5]. During times of active inflammation the colon is overwhelmed with reactive oxygen which can result in intestinal injury.

The production of superoxide and other reactive oxygen intermediates responsible for microbicidal, tumoricidal, and inflammatory activities in phagocytes is mediated by a membrane-associated nicotinamide adenine dinucleotide phosphate (NADPH) oxidase[6,7] (Figure 1). The generation of toxic oxygen species by phagocytes is instrumental for the tissue damage of diverse conditions, including acute or chronic inflammation. The enzyme system responsible for superoxide generation forms a small transmembrane electron transport system that results in the oxidation of NADPH on the cytoplasmic surface and the generation of superoxide on the outer surface of the membrane (Figure 1). The terminal electron donor to oxygen is a flavocytochrome b[8,9] located primarily in the plasma membrane[10]. It is a heterodimer composed of a 91-kDa glycoprotein (termed gp91-phox, for glycoprotein (91 kDa) of phagocyte oxidase) and a 22-kDa polypeptide (p22-phox) (Figure 1)[11]. In addition to the cytochrome b heterodimer, four cytosolic factors (p47-phox, p67-phox, p40-phox and p21 Rac) are required for NADPH oxidase activity[12]. The enzyme is dormant in resting cells and becomes active upon stimulation (Figure 1). PMA initiates translocation of the cytosolic factors to the plasma membrane where they associate with cytochrome b. Superoxide anion is the starting point for the formation of other reactive oxidants, such as hydrogen

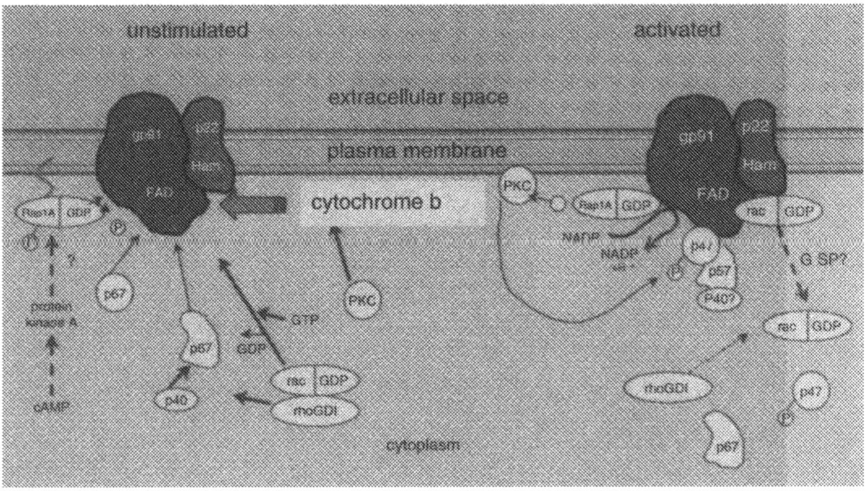

Figure 1 Assembly of the NADPH-oxidase (unstimulated: left, activated: right). During activation, cytosolic components translocate to the plasma membrane. Translocated cytosolic components assemble with the gp91, p22-heterodimer cytochrome b to form the active O_2-generating complex (according to C. Bogdan, 1996, modified)

peroxide, which is further converted by a lysosomal myeloperoxidase to hypochlorous acid. Secretion of these oxidants is definitely associated with inflammatory tissue destruction in ulcerative colitis or Crohn's disease[4,5].

Tissue-degrading enzymes

Besides tissue-degrading radicals during mucosal inflammation, infiltrating and penetrating as well as locally activated immune cells respond to secreted and surface-bound cytokines by secreting extracellular matrix (ECM) modifying and degrading enzymes[13]. This allows the further penetration of invading inflammatory cells into the mucosa (Figure 2). Two major groups of proteinases are secreted: serine proteases and matrix metalloproteinases (MMPs). Tissue degradation is induced by elastase (degrades elastin, fibronectin, laminin, collagen, proteoglycans), heparanase (heparan sulphate), collagenase and other MMPs. Elastase is a serine protease with a broad spectrum of substrates. It also can cleave cell-surface receptors. In contrast to most MMPs, which are secreted as inactive pro-forms (zymogens), elastase can be stored intracellularly in neutrophils and monocytes/macrophages in its active form[13]. The MMP family of enzymes consists of at least 15 distinct members, 9 of which are expressed in leukocytes[13]. All MMPs can degrade ECM components. Their activity is regulated by inhibiting enzymes called tissue inhibitors of metalloproteinases (TIMPs). TIMP-1 and -2 are soluble, whereas TIMP-3 is bound to the ECM. The balance between the tissue-degrading MMPs and their inhibitors may be important for the degree of mucosal damage during mucosal inflammation. Interestingly, in inflammatory bowel disease, an increased expression of MMPs as well as TIMPs has been described. This makes it hard to prove an imbalance of the system.

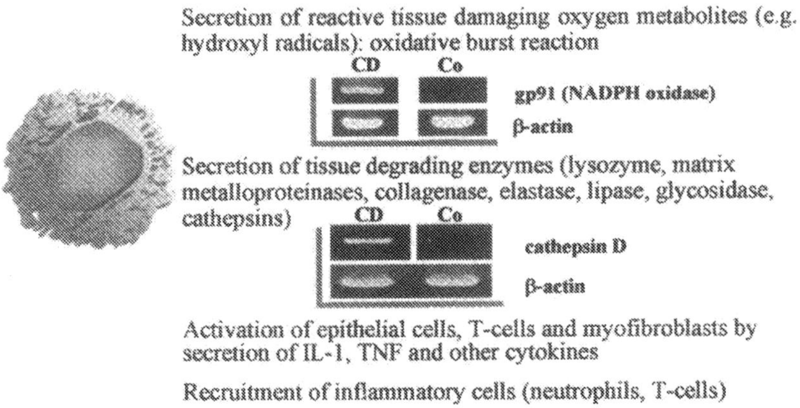

Figure 2 Tissue damage: the role of macrophages. Subtractive hybridizations revealed that, in macrophages isolated from Crohn's disease mucosa, tissue degrading enzymes are dramatically induced, which was confirmed by PCR and Northern blotting. mRNA for gp91 phox, a subunit of the 'oxidative-burst'-inducing NADPH oxidase, is absent in isolated macrophages from control mucosa (Co) but expressed in CD macrophages. The same is true for cathepsin D, which can also contribute to tissue damage and degradation

NF-κB activation

The expression of many of these enzymes is induced by pro-inflammatory mediators, such as TNF and IL-1 during mucosal inflammation. One of the most important mediators of cell activation is the pro-inflammatory transcription factor, nuclear factor-kappaB (NF-κB). Transcription factors of the NF-κB/Rel family form dimeric complexes which control the expression of a variety of inducible genes involved in inflammation and proliferation[14–17]. The prototypic heterodimeric complex NF-κB consists of the subunits p50 and p65 (RelA)[16,18]. The inactive NF-κB dimer is present in the cytosol bound to inhibitory proteins, termed IκB[19,20]. IκBα, IκBβ and IκBε have a similar function in inhibiting the translocation of the NF-κB dimer[21]. The activation of NF-κB by inflammatory cytokines and microorganisms requires the release of IκB from the complex[16,18–20]. The release of IκB is induced by phosphorylation of IκB at two conserved amino-terminal serine residues by a multiprotein IκB–kinase complex containing IκB–kinase alpha (IKK-α), beta (IKK-β) and gamma (IKK-γ)[22–24]. This is followed by a polyubiquination of the IκB proteins by a specialized E3 ubiquitin ligase complex (E3IκB)[25–27] which makes them accessible to proteolytic degradation by the 26S proteasome[21]. The removal of IκB proteins activates respectively exposes nuclear localization signals (NLS) followed by translocation of the activated NF-κB into the nucleus[22]. There, the activated NF-κB dimer interacts with regulatory NF-κB elements in promoters and enhancers.

There is evidence that NF-κB transcription factors might play an important role in the inflammatory process of inflammatory bowel disease. It was shown that the administration of antisense phosphothioate oligonucleotides to the p65 subunit of NF-κB abrogates colitis in IL-10-deficient mice and in the TNBS-colitis model.[28–30] Inhibition of the proteasome complex which is responsible for the rapid degradation of IκB prevented NF-κB activation and attenuated the colonic injury and tissue damage in the PG/PS model[31]. In the DSS model of chronic colitis, the DSS-induced intestinal inflammation was characterized by an increase in NF-κB activity[32]. Blocking NF-κB activation by administering gliotoxin, a fungal product, was accompanied by a significant suppression of intestinal inflammation and mRNA expression of TNF-α and IL-1α *in vivo*[32]. In mucosal biopsies from patients suffering from inflammatory bowel diseases, activation of NF-κB was demonstrated to be mainly localized in two cell types in the intestinal mucosa by double labelling techniques: (1) in lamina propria macrophages, and (2) in epithelial cells[33]. Furthermore, mutations in NOD2, a gene, which is mainly expressed in monocytes/macrophages and activates NF-κB, has been shown to be associated with susceptibility to Crohn's disease[34–36].

A variety of genes induced in the inflamed mucosa have been shown to be regulated by NF-κB, including the genes encoding TNF-α[37] and IL-1β[38]. TNF-α and IL-1 are also able to activate NF-κB, leading to a positive autoregulatory loop[39]. TNF is an important mediator of the mucosal inflammation and is thought to play a key role in the pathophysiology of inflammatory bowel disease[40,41]. The TNF-receptor–IKK–NF-κB cascade is prototypic for a cell-surface-receptor-initiated NF-κB activation. Like TNF, IL-1 is a central regulator of immune functions. It plays a major role in both systemic and local immune responses to bacteria and bacterial wall products such as LPS[42].

Severity of tissue damage: its role for restitution, fibrosis or stenosis

Macrophages and granulocytes are major players in the induction of tissue damage. They secrete tissue-degrading radicals or enzymes that are regulated by pro-inflammatory transcription factors, such as NF-κB. NF-κB itself is activated by cytokines like TNF or IL-1 as well as by oxidative stress or bacterial wall products. This may lead to an auto-inducing loop followed by more and more NF-κB activation and more and more tissue damage. What limits this fatal process? The frustrating answer is: we don't know. During acute inflammation with limited tissue damage, this process obviously comes to an end and is followed by wound healing to a *restitutio ad integrum*. If the basement membrane underlying the injured epithelium is intact, residual epithelial cells at the edge of the wound become motile. They move along the basement membrane until they meet other epithelial cells to form new tight junctions. This process is called restitution[43–45]. Restitution is supported by a number of growth factors secreted by myofibroblasts, such as HGF, KGF, EFG, TGF-β, aFGF and bFGF[43].

If the wound is deep or if there is subepithelial tissue damage, the subepithelial tissue in addition to the epithelial surface must be reconstituted. If the basement membrane has been destroyed, epithelial cells and mesenchymal elements form a new basement membrane[43,46]. Epithelial stem cells undergo mitosis, proliferate and migrate along the newly formed basement membrane[43]. One of the key events in the wound repair process is the contraction of the underlying lamina propria to limit the wound area. Due to their contractile and migratory ability and because of their ability to secrete matrix proteins and growth factors, myofibroblasts play an important role in both the restitution and the repair process.

THE ROLE OF MYOFIBROBLASTS IN WOUND HEALING AND FIBROSIS

Characterization of myofibroblasts

The availability of specific monoclonal antibodies and improved ultrastructural studies has generated evidence that there is a phenotypic heterogeneity among tissue fibroblasts and that some types display features of smooth muscle cell differentiation[47–51]. These cells were termed myofibroblasts[52]. In different tissues, myofibroblasts have similar roles. They play an important role in tissue development and growth[53]. In addition, they are central players during tissue repair that may finally lead to local fibrosis (scars) or generalized fibrosis and stenosis.

Myofibroblasts are thought to be a distinct cell type. However, different authors use different definitions or even completely different terms to describe this cell population, such as 'juxtaparenchymal cells'[43]. Usually they are defined morphologically and immunologically mainly by the expression of cytoskeletal protein[48]. Among these specific features are prominent cytoplasmic actin microfilaments/stress fibres, and the formation of a cell–cell network and intercellular connections via adherens and gap junctions[54–59]. In addition, they show an abundant rough endoplasmic reticulum[60]. The simplest definition used in the literature is by the expression of α-smooth muscle cells actin (α-SMA) (Figure 3). Therefore, they are regarded as an intermediate state between fibroblasts and smooth muscle cells. It is not clear, however, whether they originate from one of those cells types *in vivo*. Other filament proteins are used as well by other authors to define myofibroblasts. Most often used besides α-SMA are vimentin and desmin[43]. Based on the expression of filament protein, a classification of myofibroblasts has been proposed not always involving α-SMA: myofibroblasts only expressing vimentin are called 'V-type' myofibroblasts, those expressing vimentin and desmin 'VD-type', and, when they additionally express α-SMA, they are called 'VAD-type'. In addition, the 'VA-type' (vimentin and α-SMA) and the

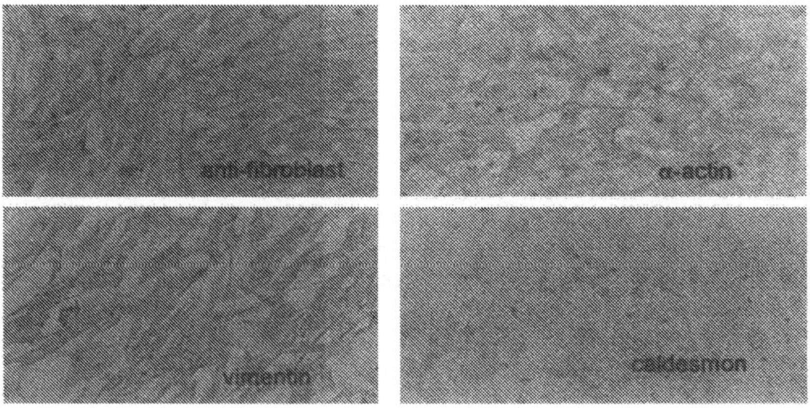

Figure 3 Immunocytochemical characterization of colonic subepithelial myofibroblasts. The cultures show a positive and homogeneous red staining with anti-fibroblast-antibody AsO_2, vimentin and α-actin but not with caldesmon

'VM-type' (vimentin and myosin) have been classified[49,61]. It is unclear whether these phenotypes and their differences in the expression of cytoskeletal proteins are associated with functional differences.

Myofibroblasts in the intestinal mucosa

In the intestinal mucosa, two types of myofibroblasts are found under physiological conditions. Besides the subepithelial myofibroblasts, the interstitial cells of Cajal display a myofibroblast phenotype. The interstitial cells of Cajal are located in the submucosa and muscularis propria in association with the smooth muscle layer of the gut. It is unknown whether subepithelial myofibroblasts and interstitial cells of Cajal like T-cells differentiate from a common precursor (an 'MF_0-cell') or which factors induce this differentiation. Both types of myofibroblasts form a network or syncytium; however, it is unclear whether both networks are interconnected or not[62]. The interstitial cells of Cajal have been proven to be the electrical pacemakers of gastrointestinal motility[62]. The subepithelial myofibroblasts mainly located at the bases of crypts in the lamina propria are morphologically well characterized but their function is less clear[63–68]. They form a three-dimensional network and have contact with each other via gap junctions and adherens junctions, but also with epithelial cells through fenestrations in the basement membrane. In addition, they form contacts with intestinal macrophages. Whereas the interstitial cells of Cajal display the V or VM phenotype, the subepithelial myofibroblasts show the VA-type (vimentin and α-SMA)[43] (Figure 3).

Interestingly, it is still unclear whether intestinal myofibroblasts like other myofibroblasts originate from progenitor stem cells, from the neural crest or simply transdifferentiate from tissue fibroblasts or smooth muscle cells[43] (Figure 4). Platelet-derived growth factor (PDGF) seems to be essential for the differentiation and development of myofibroblasts[43]. Besides PDGF, TGF-β, insulin-like growth factor II (IGF-II) and IL-4 are important factors for the transdifferentiation of fibroblasts to myofibroblasts[43] (Figure 4).

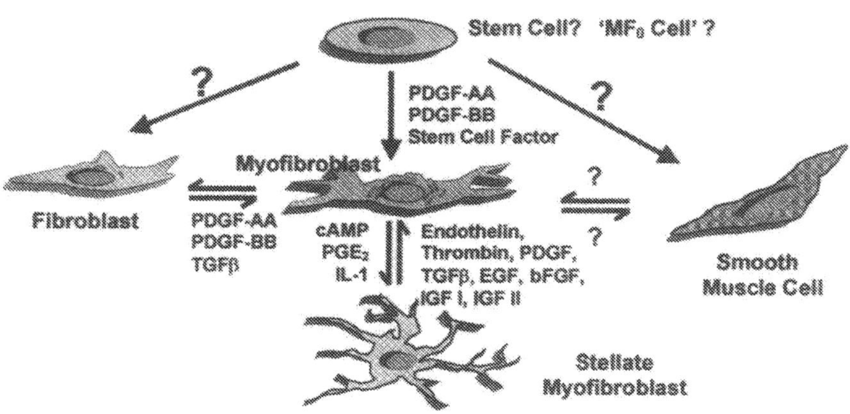

Figure 4 Hypothetical pathways for the transdifferentiation of mesenchymal cells. Modified according to Powel *et al.*[43,62]

It is clear that these subepithelial myofibroblasts have ultrastructural characteristics of activated cells. Recent evidence indicates that subepithelial myofibroblasts are involved in a network of interactions with other cell types. They influence epithelial cell proliferation and differentiation which may become very important during the healing process of mucosal ulcers or in general after mucosal d^mage in inflammatory bowel diseases[69–73]. On the other hand, there is evidence that intestinal epithelial cells may be able to induce a myofibroblast-like phenotype in co-cultured fibroblasts (Dr. Meenhard Herlyn, Philadelphia, personal communication).

Despite these characteristics of 'activated' cells, it must be kept in mind that subepithelial cells display these characteristics physiologically and that usually an activation means a change of function from a resting or inactive state to increased secretion of cellular products. This change does not occur for subepithelial myofibroblasts and it is somewhat a contradiction to talk about 'constitutively activated' cells[74].

Activation of myofibroblasts

Several treatments or pathways lead to an 'activation' of fibroblasts or stellate cells into myofibroblasts. Usually this 'activation' is determined by immunostaining for α-SMC. The appearance of α-SMC staining in fibroblast-like cells is thought to be correlated with cell activation. Among the treatments followed by α-SMC induction is the simple culture of fibroblasts in serum containing growth media. Whereas TGF-β seems to be the most potent and important inductor of α-SMC, other cytokines, such as IL-1, TNF, PDGF, bFGF and IGF, can induce α-SMC expression as well[75]. An important source of TGF-β are epithelial cells hallmarking another cell–cell interaction in intestinal inflammation and fibrosis. The rapid activation of fibroblast or myofibroblasts respectively is supported or made possible by the presence of ECM molecules. In particular, the degradation of fibronectin by MMPS secreted by macrophages allows interaction of fibroblasts/myofibroblasts with the ED-A domain of fibronectin followed by rapid activation of the cells[76]. This ED-A domain of fibronectin increasingly occurring during tissue damage may even be necessary for the TGF-β-triggered expression of α-SMC. After activation of myofibroblasts, PDGF is an important inducer of proliferation or cell migration.

Besides growth factors acting on the MAP-kinase pathways, pro-inflammatory cytokines inducing NF-κB translocation play an important role in the activation of myofibroblasts. IL-1 and TNF secreted by macrophages in the inflamed tissue bind to their specific cell-surface receptors on myofibroblasts, activate NF-κB and have pronounced effects on the synthesis of ECM and cytokine production by myofibroblasts.

The role of subepithelial myofibroblast in intestinal inflammation

Intestinal myofibroblasts are not passive connective tissue cells with only one task, to secrete extracellular matrix, but have been shown to produce a number of important mediators during inflammatory responses[77–81] (see Table 1). A number of these cytokines, chemokines and growth factors have been shown to play an

Table 1 Cytokines, growth factors, chemokines, inflammatory mediators and adhesion molecules secreted or expressed by myofibroblasts (modified according to Reference 43)

Cytokines	*Growth factors*	*Chemokines*	*Inflammatory mediators*	*Adhesion molecules*
IL-1[85–87]	TGF-β[88,89]	IL-8[86,87]	PGE2[98]	ICAM-1[86,87]
IL-6[85–87]	GM-CSF[86]	MCP-1[95]	Prostacyclin	VCAM-1[86,87]
TNF[85,87]	M-CSF[90,91]	GRO-1α[96]	HETEs	NCAM[87]
IL-10[86]	G-CSF[90,91]	MIP-1α[95]	PAF	ACAM[87]
	PDGF-AA[92,93]	RANTES[97]	NO[99]	
	PDGF-AB[92,93]	ENA-78	H_2O_2	
	PDGF-BB[92,93]			
	bFGF			
	IGF-1[93]			
	IGF-II[93]			
	NGF			
	KGF[88]			
	HGF[88]			
	SCF			
	LIF[94]			

important role in the pathogenic process of inflammatory bowel disease[82–84]. Therefore, they are able to modulate the inflammatory response of neighbouring cell types.

LPS stimulation of myofibroblasts was demonstrated to be involved in intestinal fibrosis[100] and disturbance of epithelial cell barrier function[101]. In addition, stimulation with cytokines altered the proliferative response of intestinal myofibroblasts[102], increased prostanoid secretion[98] and altered the overall phenotype[69]. In fetal tissue, secretion of cytokines by myofibroblasts is important for extrathymic T-cell development[103], emphasizing the important role of these cells in the intestinal immune system.

In our own studies, incubation of colonic fibroblasts/myofibroblasts with IL-1, LPS, TNF and PMA induced secretion of IL-6, IL-8, M-CSF and GM-CSF. IL-8 and IL-6 secretion could be stimulated by IL-1α, IL-1β, TNF, PMA and LPS within 6 h of incubation. IL-4 and IL-10 did not change cytokine secretion significantly. TNF and IL-1 induced NF-κB activation. ALLN, a proteasome and NF-κB-activation-inhibitor, reduced TNF-mediated IL-8, GM-CSF and M-CSF induction significantly, whereas induction of IL-6 secretion remained unchanged[104].

The amounts of IL-8 and IL-6 secreted by myofibroblasts after stimulation are comparable to the cytokine secretion of typical immune cells such as, for example, macrophages. These large amounts of IL-8 secretion upon stimulation suggest that colonic fibroblasts/myofibroblasts could play an important role in leukocyte recruitment during mucosal inflammation. Activation of transcription factor NF-κB is involved in the induction of IL-8, GM-CSF and M-CSF secretion in primary human fibroblasts/myofibroblasts by IL-1 and TNF. Activated NF-κB is present in the inflamed intestinal mucosa[33]. In areas of intestinal strictures in Crohn's disease patients, populations of cells showed NF-κB activation that probably represents myofibroblasts.

However, no significant difference in NF-κB activation and induction of cytokine secretion between fibroblasts/myofibroblasts from normal or IBD mucosa could be detected. On the basis of this observation, it is likely that activation *in vivo* is a transient property caused by interaction with surrounding cells and not a different stage of differentiation. A terminal differentiation caused by acute or chronic mucosal inflammation would affect the response to stimulation of isolated myofibroblast even under *in-vitro* conditions.

IFN-γ can induce the expression of CD40 on primary human colonic myofibroblasts. Ligation of CD40 on these cells by CD40L induces NF-κB activation and subsequent secretion of NF-κB-dependent cytokines. Not only is soluble CD40L able to induce cytokine secretion by myofibroblasts but also interaction of CD4+ T cells expressing CD40L with human colonic myofibroblasts can induce cytokine secretion from these cells. This is a new mechanism of cell–cell interaction that may be responsible for the induction of cytokine secretion during mucosal inflammation. During inflammatory bowel disease, colonic myofibroblasts display CD40 *in vivo*, indicating that this mechanism could be of pathophysiological importance.

Recently, Liu and co-workers showed that CD40L is expressed on freshly isolated T cells of patients with inflammatory bowel disease[105]. CD40L expression on these T cells induced IL-12 and TNF production by normal monocytes. In immunohistochemical studies, the authors showed that the number of CD40- and CD40L-positive cells was significantly increased in inflamed mucosa. These data support the concept that CD40–CD40L interaction could be relevant during mucosal inflammation. Non-classical immune cells, such as myofibroblasts, can play an important role in cell–cell interactions during inflammation. CD40L-positive T cells activate cytokine secretion not only in macrophages but also in primary myofibroblasts. Among the molecules induced by CD40 ligation on colonic myofibroblasts are: IL-8, which can attract neutrophils; MCP-1, which attracts monocytes/macrophages; and ICAM-1. It has been shown previously that activation of intestinal fibroblasts induces ICAM-1 surface expression and mRNA as well as adhesiveness for T cells[106]. ICAM-1 may be essential for intestinal fibroblast binding of T cells. Musso and co-workers concluded from their data that intestinal fibroblasts may have a crucial regulatory role in mucosal immunity and they may be potential targets for therapeutic intervention in intestinal inflammation[106]. The interaction of CD40- with CD40L-displaying T cells may induce ICAM-1 expression or be associated with ICAM-1 expression which then increases T cell adhesiveness and further improves the ability of fibroblasts to interact with T cells. Other chemokines relevant for the pathophysiology of the mucosal inflammation may be induced by CD40 ligation as well, as suggested by studies on fibroblasts from other origins.

Migration of intestinal myofibroblasts as a prerequisite for repair functions

As mentioned, intestinal subepithelial fibroblasts form a network of cells located beneath the basement membrane stretching from the oesophagus to the anus[62]. They have contact with intestinal epithelial cells via fenestrations of the basement membrane[62]. During tissue injury, these subepithelial myofibroblasts migrate to the site of tissue damage and contract the surrounding tissue. Subepithelial myofibroblasts express smooth muscle myosin and actin, which is necessary for this contractile function. Migration of fibroblasts into and through the extracellular matrix during the initial phase of wound healing appears to be a fundamental component of wound contraction. After the wound has been repopulated and the chemotactic gradient that was established by inflammatory cells is decreased, fibroblast migration will cease[107]. Subepithelial myofibroblasts can stimulate their own migration by autocrine and paracrine factors. However, the migratory response of subepithelial myofibroblasts isolated from Crohn's disease mucosa was found to be significantly reduced when compared with cells isolated from control cells. In myofibroblasts from normal mucosa, a similar persistent reduction of migration can be induced by incubation with TNF or IFN-γ. How this reduced migratory potential contributes to fibrosis in inflammatory bowel disease is still unclear.

SUMMARY

During intestinal inflammation, interactions between a number of different cell populations in the mucosa take place (Figure 5). Activation of NF-κB in leukocytes induces the secretion of pro-inflammatory cytokines, which further activate these leukocytes in an autocrine loop, as well as neighbouring cells such as epithelial cells or myofibroblasts. Macrophages and granulocytes induce tissue damage by secreting reactive oxygen radicals. The same cells, as well as lymphocytes, myofibroblasts and epithelial cells, secrete metalloproteinases followed by a degradation of extracellular matrix. This is followed by increased levels of pro-inflammatory cytokines previously bound to the matrix as well as chemotactic and cell-activating effects of matrix degradation products (peptides).

If the tissue damage is severe and no simple wound healing with complete restitution can be achieved, myofibroblasts migrate to the sites of tissue defects.

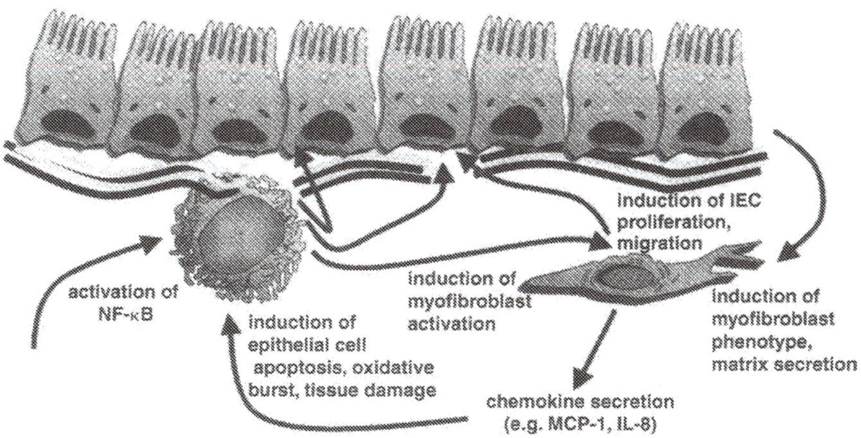

Figure 5 Schematic representation of cell–cell interactions during the inflammation–fibrosis transition

They display an activated phenotype and contract the tissue. In addition, they secrete extracellular matrix compounds to allow a 'defect healing' and repair of the tissue.

Two hypotheses for the development of strictures in inflammatory bowel disease have been described. On one hand, an ongoing activation of the collagen producing myofibroblasts has been postulated. If this is true, our efforts should focus on the mechanisms of how these cells are activated and how those activated mechanisms could be terminated. On the other hand, there is some evidence that signals that physiologically limit the repair process are not recognized or sent during stricture formation in Crohn's disease. If this is the case, our investigations should concentrate on the mechanisms of limitation of myofibroblast activation to be finally able to use these mechanisms in the patients applying pharmaceutically generated 'limiting-signals'.

Another approach for the future is the investigation of mechanisms to limit tissue damage during intestinal inflammation. It seems that the amount of tissue degradation varies dramatically in individual patients and that sometimes control of the inflammation itself is just not enough. In selected patients, inhibition of NADPH oxidase or of certain metalloproteinases could be of great benefit.

In general, research on the pathophysiology of stricture formation in inflammatory bowel disease should be encouraged. As about 50% of all our patients have to undergo surgery during the course of Crohn's disease because of obstruction, more effort to elucidate the pathways from inflammation to fibrosis is well worth while.

References

1. Farmer RG, Whelan G, Fazio VW. Long-term follow-up of patients with Crohn's disease. Relationship between the clinical pattern and prognosis. Gastroenterology. 1985;88:1818–25.
2. Andres PG, Friedman LS. Epidemiology and the natural course of inflammatory bowel disease. Gastroenterol Clin N Am. 1999;28:255–81,vii.
3. Whelan G, Farmer RG, Fazio VW, Goormastic M. Recurrence after surgery in Crohn's disease. Relationship to location of disease (clinical pattern) and surgical indication. Gastroenterology. 1985;88:1826–33.
4. Allgayer H. Clinical relevance of oxygen radicals in inflammatory bowel disease – facts and fashion. Klin Wochenschr. 1991;69:1001–3.
5. Yamada T, Grisham MB. Role of neutrophil-derived oxidants in the pathogenesis of intestinal inflammation. Klin Wochenschr. 1991;69:988–94.
6. Chanock SJ, el Benna J, Smith RM, Babior BM. The respiratory burst oxidase. J Biol Chem. 1994;269:24519–22.
7. Henderson LM, Chappel JB. NADPH oxidase of neutrophils. Biochim Biophys Acta. 1996;1273:87–107.
8. Segal AW, Jones OT, Webster D, Allison AC. Absence of a newly described cytochrome b from neutrophils of patients with chronic granulomatous disease. Lancet. 1978;2:446–9.
9. Segal AW, Abo A. The biochemical basis of the NADPH oxidase of phagocytes. Trends Biochem Sci. 1993;18:43–7.
10. Jesaitis AJ, Buescher ES, Harrison D. Ultrastructural localization of cytochrome b in the membranes of resting and phagocytosing human granulocytes. J Clin Invest. 1990;85:821–35.
11. Parkos CA, Allen RA, Cochrane CG, Jesaitis AJ. Purified cytochrome b from human granulocyte plasma membrane is comprised of two polypeptides with relative molecular weights of 91,000 and 22,000. J Clin Invest. 1987;80:732–42.
12. Bastian NR. Assembly and regulation of NADPH oxidase and nitric oxide synthase. Curr Opin Immunol. 1994;6:131–9.

13. Vaday GG, Lider O. Extracellular matrix moieties, cytokines, and enzymes: dynamic effects on immune cell behavior and inflammation. J Leukoc Biol. 2000;67:149–59.
14. Lenardo MJ, Baltimore D. NF-kappa B: a pleiotropic mediator of inducible and tissue-specific gene control. Cell. 1989;58:227–9.
15. Baeuerle PA. The inducible transcription activator NF-kappa B: regulation by distinct protein subunits. Biochim Biophys Acta. 1991;1072:63–80.
16. Baeuerle PA, Henkel T. Function and activation of NF-kappa B in the immune system. Annu Rev Immunol. 1994;12:141–79.
17. Baeuerle PA, Baltimore D. NF-kappa B: ten years after. Cell. 1996;87:13–20.
18. Grilli M, Chiu JJ, Lenardo MJ. NF-kappa B and Rel: participants in a multiform transcriptional regulatory system. Int Rev Cytol. 1993;143:1–62.
19. Baeuerle PA, Baltimore D. I kappa B: a specific inhibitor of the NF-kappa B transcription factor. Science. 1988;242:540–6.
20. Cheng Q, Cant CA, Moll T *et al.* NK-kappa B subunit-specific regulation of the I kappa B alpha promoter. J Biol Chem. 1994;269:13551–7.
21. Huxford T, Malek S, Ghosh G. Structure and mechanism in NF-kappa B/I kappa B signaling. Cold Spring Harb Symp Quant Biol. 1999;64:533–40.
22. Maniatis T. Catalysis by a multiprotein IkappaB kinase complex. Science. 1997;278:818–19.
23. Mercurio F, Zhu H, Murray BW *et al.* IKK-1 and IKK-2: cytokine-activated IkappaB kinases essential for NF-kappaB activation. Science. 1997;278:860–6.
24. Woronicz JD, Gao X, Cao Z, Rothe M, Goeddel DV. IkappaB kinase-beta: NF-kappaB activation and complex formation with IkappaB kinase-alpha and NIK. Science. 1997;278:866–9.
25. Karin M. How NF-kappaB is activated: the role of the IkappaB kinase (IKK) complex. Oncogene. 1999;18:6867–74.
26. Karin M. The beginning of the end: IkappaB kinase (IKK) and NF-kappaB activation. J Biol Chem. 1999;274:27339–42.
27. Karin M, Delhase M. The I kappa B kinase (IKK) and NF-kappa B: key elements of proinflammatory signalling. Semin Immunol. 2000;12:85–98.
28. Neurath MF, Pettersson S. Predominant role of NF-kappa B p65 in the pathogenesis of chronic intestinal inflammation. Immunobiology. 1997;198:91–8.
29. Neurath MF, Pettersson S, Meyer zum Buschenfelde KH, Strober W. Local administration of antisense phosphorothioate oligonucleotides to the p65 subunit of NF-kappa B abrogates established experimental colitis in mice. Nat Med. 1996;2:998–1004.
30. Neurath MF, Becker C, Barbulescu K. Role of NF-kappaB in immune and inflammatory responses in the gut. Gut. 1998;43:856–60.
31. Conner EM, Brand S, Davis JM *et al.* Proteasome inhibition attenuates nitric oxide synthase expression, VCAM-1 transcription and the development of chronic colitis. J Pharmacol Exp Ther. 1997;282:1615–22.
32. Herfarth H, Brand K, Rath HC *et al.* Nuclear factor-kappa B activity and intestinal inflammation in dextran sulphate sodium (DSS)-induced colitis in mice is suppressed by gliotoxin. Clin Exp Immunol. 2000;120:59–65.
33. Rogler G, Brand K, Vogl D *et al.* Nuclear factor kappaB is activated in macrophages and epithelial cells of inflamed intestinal mucosa [see comments]. Gastroenterology. 1998;115:357–69.
34. Hugot JP, Chamaillard M, Zouali H *et al.* Association of NOD2 leucine-rich repeat variants with susceptibility to Crohn's disease. Nature. 2001;411:599–603.
35. Ogura Y, Bonen DK, Inohara N *et al.* A frameshift mutation in NOD2 associated with susceptibility to Crohn's disease. Nature. 2001;411:603–6.
36. Ogura Y, Inohara N, Benito A *et al.* Nod2, a Nod1/Apaf-1 family member that is restricted to monocytes and activates NF-kappa B. J Biol Chem. 2001;276: 4812–18.
37. Muller JM, Ziegler-Heitbrock HW, Baeuerle PA. Nuclear factor kappa B, a mediator of lipopolysaccharide effects. Immunobiology. 1993;187:233–56.
38. Pullman WE, Elsbury S, Kobayashi M, Hapel AJ, Doe WF. Enhanced mucosal cytokine production in inflammatory bowel disease. Gastroenterology. 1992;102:529–37.
39. Hiscott J, Marois J, Garoufalis J *et al.* Characterization of a functional NF-kappa B site in the human interleukin 1 beta promoter: evidence for a positive autoregulatory loop. Mol Cell Biol. 1993;13:6231–40.
40. Targan SR, Kagnoff MF, Brogan MD, Shanahan F. Immunologic mechanisms in intestinal diseases. Ann Intern Med. 1987;106:853–70.

41. Targan SR. Biology of inflammation in Crohn's disease: mechanisms of action of anti-TNF-a therapy. Can J Gastroenterol. 2000;14(Suppl. C):13C–16C.
42. Cao Z, Tanaka M, Regnier C *et al.* NF-kappa B activation by tumor necrosis factor and interleukin-1. Cold Spring Harb Symp Quant Biol. 1999;64:473–83.
43. Powell DW, Mifflin RC, Valentich JD *et al.* Myofibroblasts. I. Paracrine cells important in health and disease. Am J Physiol. 1999;277:C1–C19.
44. Podolsky DK. Healing the epithelium: solving the problem from two sides. J Gastroenterol. 1997;32:122–6.
45. Silen W, Ito S. Mechanisms for rapid re-epithelialization of the gastric mucosal surface. Annu Rev Physiol. 1985;47:217–29.
46. Wallace JL, Granger DN. The cellular and molecular basis of gastric mucosal defense. FASEB J. 1996;10:731–40.
47. Komuro T. Re-evaluation of fibroblasts and fibroblast-like cells. Anat Embryol. 1990;182:103–12.
48. Sappino AP, Schurch W, Gabbiani G. Differentiation repertoire of fibroblastic cells: expression of cytoskeletal proteins as marker of phenotypic modulation. Lab Invest. 1990;63:144–61.
49. Schmitt-Graff A, Desmouliere A, Gabbiani G. Heterogeneity of myofibroblast phenotypic features: an example of fibroblastic cell plasticity. Virchows Arch. 1994;425:3–24.
50. Skalli O, Schurch W, Seemayer T *et al.* Myofibroblasts from diverse pathologic settings are heterogeneous in their content of actin isoforms and intermediate filament proteins. Lab Invest. 1989;60:275–85.
51. Fries KM, Blieden TM, Looney RJ *et al.* Evidence of fibroblast heterogeneity and the role of fibroblast subpopulations in fibrosis. Clin Immunol Immunopathol. 1994;72:283–92.
52. Gabbiani G, Ryan GB, Majne G. Presence of modified fibroblasts in granulation tissue and their possible role in wound contraction. Experientia. 1971;27:549–50.
53. Simon-Assmann P, Kedinger M, De Arcangelis A, Rousseau V, Simo P. Extracelluair matrix components in intestinal development. Experientia. 1995;51:883–900.
54. Spanakis SG, Petridou S, Masur SK. Functional gap junctions in corneal fibroblasts and myofibroblasts. Invest Ophthalmol Vis Sci. 1998;39:1320–8.
55. Jamieson S, Going JJ, D'Arcy R, George WD. Expression of gap junction proteins connexin 26 and connexin 43 in normal human breast and in breast tumours. J Pathol. 1998;184:37–43.
56. Petridou S, Masur SK. Immunodetection of connexins and cadherins in corneal fibroblasts and myofibroblasts. Invest Ophthalmol Vis Sci. 1996;37:1740–8.
57. Sims DE. Orientation of adhering junctions between bovine pulmonary fibroblasts. Acta Anat. 1991;140:245–9.
58. Neumuller J, Tohidast-Akrad M, Ammer K *et al.* Ultrastructural and autoradiographic investigations of cell cultures derived from tendons or ligamentous material from patients with fibromatous disorders. Exp Cell Biol. 1988;56:113–30.
59. Gabbiani G, Chaponnier C, Huttner I. Cytoplasmic filaments and gap junctions in epithelial cells and myofibroblasts during wound healing. J Cell Biol. 1978;76:561–8.
60. Eyden B. The myofibroblast: an assessment of controversial issues and a definition useful in diagnosis and research. Ultrastruct Pathol. 2001;25:39–50.
61. Schmitt-Graff A, Kruger S, Bochard F, Gabbiani G, Denk H. Modulation of alpha smooth muscle actin and desmin expression in perisinusoidal cells of normal and diseased human livers. Am J Pathol. 1991;138:1233–42.
62. Powell DW, Mifflin RC, Valentich JD *et al.* Myofibroblasts. II. Intestinal subepithelial myofibroblasts. Am J Physiol. 1999;277:C183–201.
63. Guldner FH, Wolff JR, Keyserlingk DG. Fibroblasts as a part of the contractile system in duodenal villi of rat. Z Zellforsch Mikrosk Anat. 1972;135:349–60.
64. Joyce NC, Haire MF, Palade GE. Morphologic and biochemical evidence for a contractile cell network within the rat intestinal mucosa. Gastroenterology. 1987;92:68–81.
65. Kaye GI, Pascal RR, Lane N. The colonic pericryptal fibroblast sheath: replication, migration, and cytodifferentiation of a mesenchymal cell system in adult tissue. 3. Replication and differentiation in human hyperplastic and adenomatous polyps. Gastroenterology. 1971;60:515–36.
66. Kaye GI, Lane N, Pascal RR. Colonic pericryptal fibroblast sheath: replication, migration, and cytodifferentiation of a mesenchymal cell system in adult tissue. II. Fine structural aspects of normal rabbit and human colon. Gastroenterology. 1968;54:852–65.
67. Komuro T. Comparative morphology of interstitial cells of Cajal: ultrastructural characterization. Microsc Res Tech. 1999;47:267–85.

68. Pascal RR, Kaye GI, Lane N. Colonic pericryptal fibroblast sheath: replication, migration, and cytodifferentiation of a mesenchymal cell system in adult tissue. I. Autoradiographic studies of normal rabbit colon. Gastroenterology. 1968;54:835–51.
69. Fritsch C, Simon-Assmann P, Kedinger M, Evans GS. Cytokines modulate fibroblast phenotype and epithelial–stroma interactions in rat intestine. Gastroenterology. 1997;112:826–38.
70. Fritsch C, Orian-Rousseaul V, Lefebvre O *et al.* Characterization of human intestinal stromal cell lines: response to cytokines and interactions with epithelial cells. Exp Cell Res. 1999;248:391–406.
71. Kedinger M, Duluc I, Fritsch C, Lorentz O, Plateroti M, Freund JN. Intestinal epithelial–mesenchymal cell interactions. Ann NY Acad Sci. 1998;859:1–17.
72. Duluc I, Lorentz O, Fritsch C *et al.* Changing intestinal connective tissue interactions alters homeobox gene expression in epithelial cells. J Cell Sci. 1997;110:1317–24.
73. Halttunen T, Marttinen A, Rantala I, Kainulainen H, Maki M. Fibroblasts and transforming growth factor beta induce organization and differentiation of T84 human epithelial cells. Gastroenterology. 1996;111:1252–62.
74. Pucilowska JB, Williams KL, Lund PK. Fibrogenesis. IV. Fibrosis and inflammatory bowel disease: cellular mediators and animal models. Am J Physiol Gastrointest Liver Physiol. 2000;279:G653–9.
75. Kovacs EJ, DiPietro LA. Fibrogenic cytokines and connective tissue production. FASEB J. 1994;8:854–61.
76. Jarnagin WR, Rockey DC, Koteliansky VE, Wang SS, Bissell DM. Expression of variant fibronectins in wound healing: cellular source and biological activity of the EIIIA segment in rat hepatic fibrogenesis. J Cell Biol. 1994;127:2037–48.
77. Smith RE, Hogaboam CM, Strieter RM, Lukacs NW, Kunkel SL. Cell-to-cell and cell-to-matrix interactions mediate chemokine expression: an important component of the inflammatory lesion. J Leukoc Biol. 1997;62:612–19.
78. Schor SL, Grey AM, Ellis I *et al.* Fetal-like fibroblasts: their production of migration-stimulating factor and role in tumor progression. Cancer Treat Res. 1994;71:277–98.
79. Smith RS, Smith TJ, Blieden TM, Phipps RP. Fibroblasts as sentinel cells. Synthesis of chemokines and regulation of inflammation. Am J Pathol. 1997;151:317–22.
80. Murakami S, Okada H. Lymphocyte-fibroblast interactions. Crit Rev Oral Biol Med. 1997;8:40–50.
81. Low RB. Modulation of myofibroblast and smooth-muscle phenotypes in the lung. Curr Top Pathol. 1999;93:19–26.
82. Rogler G, Andus T. Cytokines in inflammatory bowel disease. World J Surg. 1998;22:382–9.
83. Fiocchi C. Intestinal inflammation: a complex interplay of immune and nonimmune cell interactions. Am J Physiol. 1997;273:G769–75.
84. Dammeier J, Brauchle M, Falk W, Grotendorst GR, Werner S. Connective tissue growth factor: a novel regulator of mucosal repair and fibrosis in inflammatory bowel disease? Int J Biochem Cell Biol. 1998;30:909–22.
85. Strong SA, Pizarro TT, Klein JS, Cominelli F, Fiocchi C. Proinflammatory cytokines differentially modulate their own expression in human intestinal mucosal mesenchymal cells. Gastroenterology. 1998;114:1244–56.
86. Pang G, Couch L, Batey R, Clancy R, Cripps A. GM-CSF, IL-1 alpha, IL-1 beta, IL-6, IL-8, IL-10, ICAM-1 and VCAM-1 gene expression and cytokine production in human duodenal fibroblasts stimulated with lipopolysaccharide, IL-1 alpha and TNF-alpha. Clin Exp Immunol. 1994;96:437–43.
87. Chakravortty D, Kumar KS. Interaction of lipopolysaccharide with human small intestinal lamina propria fibroblasts favors neutrophil migration and peripheral blood mononuclear cell adhesion by the production of proinflammatory mediators and adhesion molecules. Biochim Biophys Acta. 1999;1453:261–72.
88. Maas-Szabowski N, Fusenig NE. Interleukin-1-induced growth factor expression in postmitotic and resting fibroblasts. J Invest Dermatol. 1996;107:849–55.
89. Beltinger J, McKaig BC, Makh S, Stack WA, Hawkey CJ, Mahida YR. Human colonic subepithelial myofibroblasts modulate transepithelial resistance and secretory response. Am J Physiol. 1999;277:C271–9.
90. Fibbe WE, Van Damme J, Billiau A *et al.* Human fibroblasts produce granulocyte-CSF, macrophage-CSF, and granulocyte-macrophage-CSF following stimulation by interleukin-1 and poly(rI).poly(rC). Blood. 1988;72:860–6.

91. Hamilton JA, Piccoli DS, Cebon J *et al.* Cytokine regulation of colony-stimulating factor (CSF) production in cultured human synovial fibroblasts. II. Similarities and differences in the control of interleukin-1 induction of granulocyte-macrophage CSF and granulocyte-CSF production. Blood. 1992;79:1413–19.
92. Palman C, Bowen-Pope DF, Brooks JJ. Platelet-derived growth factor receptor (beta-subunit) immunoreactivity in soft tissue tumors. Lab Invest. 1992;66:108–15.
93. Homma S, Nagaoka I, Abe H *et al.* Localization of platelet-derived growth factor and insulin-like growth factor I in the fibrotic lung. Am J Respir Crit Care Med. 1995;152:2084–9.
94. Knight DA, Lydell CP, Zhou D, Weir TD, Robert Schellenberg R, Bai TR. Leukemia inhibitory factor (LIF) and LIF receptor in human lung. Distribution and regulation of LIF release. Am J Respir Cell Mol Biol. 1999;20:834–41.
95. Hogaboam CM, Steinhauser ML, Chensue SW, Kunkel SL. Novel roles for chemokines and fibroblasts in interstitial fibrosis. Kidney Int. 1998;54:2152–9.
96. Cuenca RE, Azizkhan RG, Haskill S. Characterization of GRO alpha, beta and gamma expression in human colonic tumours: potential significance of cytokine involvement [published erratum appears in Surg Oncol 1992 Dec;1(6):417]. Surg Oncol. 1992;1:323–9.
97. Maune S, Werner JA, Sticherling M, Schroder JM. Fibroblasts obtained from human nasal, laryngeal and tracheal mucosa produce the chemokine RANTES. Otolaryngol Pol. 1997;51:3–10.
98. Kim EC, Zhu Y, Andersen V *et al.* Cytokine-mediated PGE2 expression in human colonic fibroblasts. Am J Physiol. 1998;275:C988–94.
99. Chakravortty D, Kumar KS. Induction of cell proliferation and collagen synthesis in human small intestinal lamina propria fibroblasts by lipopolysaccharide: possible involvement of nitric oxide. Biochem Biophys Res Commun. 1997;240:458–63.
100. van Tol EA, Holt L, Li FL *et al.* Bacterial cell wall polymers promote intestinal fibrosis by direct stimulation of myofibroblasts. Am J Physiol. 1999;277:G245–55.
101. Chakravortty D, Kumar KS. Modulation of barrier function of small intestinal epithelial cells by lamina propria fibroblasts in response to lipopolysaccharide: possible role in TNFalpha in inducing barrier dysfunction. Microbiol Immunol. 1999;43:527–33.
102. Jobson TM, Billington CK, Hall IP. Regulation of proliferation of human colonic subepithelial myofibroblasts by mediators important in intestinal inflammation. J Clin Invest. 1998;101: 2650–7.
103. Murray AM, Simm B, Beagley KW. Cytokine gene expression in murine fetal intestine: potential for extrathymic T cell development. Cytokine. 1998;10:337–45.
104. Rogler G, Gelbmann CM, Vogl D *et al.* Differential activation of cytokine secretion in primary human colonic fibroblast/myofibroblast cultures. Scand J Gastroenterol. 2001;36:389–98.
105. Liu Z, Colpaert S, D'Haens GR *et al.* Hyperexpression of CD40 ligand (CD154) in inflammatory bowel disease and its contribution to pathogenic cytokine production. J Immunol. 1999;163:4049–57.
106. Musso A, Condon TP, West GA *et al.* Regulation of ICAM-1-mediated fibroblast-T cell reciprocal interaction: implications for modulation of gut inflammation. Gastroenterology. 1999; 117:546–56.
107. Nedelec B, Ghahary A, Scott PG, Tredget EE. Control of wound contraction. Basic and clinical features. Hand Clin. 2000;16:289–302.

Section IV
Bacteria and gut inflammation

18
Bacteria and gut inflammation: a case report

G. ZOLI, D. ORSI and S. PARRO

INTRODUCTION

Ulcerative colitis represents a clinical entity characterized by spontaneous relapses due to immunity disregulation versus inflammatory stimuli. The gut mucosa, with its absorbent function, plays an important role as a selective barrier between the internal (microcirculation, lymphoid tissue) and the external (intestinal lumen) environment.

In an individual with genetic susceptibility, an intercurrent event may lead to a perturbation in the gut ecosystem equilibrium, causing a breakdown of mucosal tolerance by immune sensibilization. Once this occurs, the integrity of the barrier and its functions become compromised, leaving mucosal injury and increased intestinal permeability[1].

The present report describes how alteration of the gut microflora induced by an intestinal infection could act as a promotor for the onset of ulcerative colitis in a genetically predisposed individual.

CASE REPORT

A young couple, a 37-year-old male manager and a 35-year-old female working as a customer assistant, travelled to Mexico for their honeymoon. After a few days, they both developed acute diarrhoea. They both took rifaximine; the man promptly improved and the diarrhoea disappeared. The lady, however, did not improve and she needed hospitalization because of dehydration. In the hospital, therapy with rifaximine was continued and she received liquids, improving in a few days; a stool examination for possible intestinal infection was not performed.

Back home, the young woman continued with intermittent but increasingly persistent symptoms of diarrhoea and abdominal pains; a stool test did not reveal growth of pathological bacteria.

In the past, the lady had always had regular bowel movements or intermittent diarrhoea, and had been diagnosed with irritable bowel syndrome.

This time, after 2 weeks of antibiotics, the diarrhoea improved and she became better but the diarrhoea did not disappear completely.

After 1 month, she again had abdominal pain with diarrhoea, mucus and blood, and was losing weight (4 kg in 1 month). The General Practitioner initially diagnosed irritable bowel syndrome with haemorrhoids but, when fever appeared, he ordered blood tests, that showed anaemia, a high erythrocyte sedimentation rate and positive C-reactive protein. He finally ordered a sigmoidoscopy with biopsies; leading to a diagnosis of ulcerative colitis.

Treatment with mesalazine was started, both orally and topically, and she improved after 2 weeks of treatment.

DISCUSSION

The colon and the distal small intestine have the highest bacterial concentration and it is not surprising, therefore, that the gut forms the largest immune tissue of the human body.

Infectious aetiology for ulcerative colitis has long been sought because of features similar to those of infectious enteritis, including response to antibiotics. Great efforts are now being made to isolate and identify the millions of species normally present in the gut ecosystem[2–4].

Studies on mice with immunogenetic alteration growing in germ-free conditions have shown that bacteria are necessary for the onset of colitis and also that enterocolitis is milder when the mice are kept in a restricted microbial environment[5,6].

It is known that abnormal bacteria can cause inflammation through the impairment of epithelial cell metabolism. Colonic anaerobic bacteria able to interfere in the energetic metabolism of the colonocytes may lead to the onset of disease. Also, an excess of sulphate-reducing bacteria is responsible for the onset of a chronic colitis in guinea pigs[7,8].

In our report, the first step to take is the differential diagnosis between acute infectious-type colitis (AIC) and ulcerative colitis. Presentation of AIC is characterized by the rapid onset of diarrhoea usually accompanied by fever and abdominal pain, while UC normally has an insidious onset and is dominated by phases of remission and relapse. The two diseases frequently overlap, delaying diagnosis. AIC may have a prolonged course (lasting even for several months) with bloody diarrhoea; equally, UC may have an abrupt onset and even the endoscopic and histological specimens can resemble one another in the initial phase; however, clinical presentation and histological findings could be helpful in cases of doubt.

Attention must be paid to anamnesis, particularly with regard to the diagnosis; as in our case report, a symptomatic infectious colitis could unmask or precipitate a chronic inflammatory disease with a pathogenetic model described in our introduction. It has been reported that 60% of IBD patients with acute or subacute onset had gastroenteritis, were on antibiotics therapy or travelled abroad immediately before the onset.

Development of irritable bowel syndrome after a gastroenteric infectious disease has been described. One hypothesis could be that our laboratory methods were not sensitive enough to detect a persistent pathogen or toxins in this patient.

Several studies are underway to clarify the beneficial effects of probiotics in the treatment of IBD patients in order to assess new therapeutic strategies.

The use of probiotics without proinflammatory activity has shown a favourable effect on the gut mucosa, participating in the composition of the intestinal environment, and promoting immune modulation and epithelial regeneration[9].

The role of probiotics, once the disease is manifest, is probably to restore the initial ecosystem and to diminish contact with antigens by normalization of increased intestinal permeability[10]. Probiotics are also protective against colon cancer and can prevent atopic disease[11,12].

In addition, the beneficial effect of antibiotics on relapse of the disease is probably due to a reduction of bacteria quantity and composition.

In conclusion, the hypothesis of a trigger event, a possible transient infection in predisposed individuals, as in this case report, could promote the rupture of the gut barrier which leads to reduced mucosal tolerance to normal microflora or their products, resulting in a chronic stimulation of the immune system. This confirms epidemiological data that support the interaction between genetic factors and gut environmental ecosystem.

Whether chronic recurring inflammation is triggered by infection of a specific pathogen, by exaggerated absorption of resident normal luminal bacteria products, by dietary antigens or by other environmental factors is still unclear.

References

1. Garcia-Lafuente A, Antolin M, Guarner F *et al.* Modulation of colonic barrier function by the composition of the commensal flora in rat. Gut. 2001;48(4):449.
2. Campieri M, Giochetti P. Bacteria as the cause of ulcerative colitis. Gut. 2001;48:132–5.
3. Sanderson JD, Moss MT, Tizard ML *et al. Mycobacteria paratuberculosis* found in Crohn's disease DNA in Crohn's disease tissue. Gut. 1992;33:890–6.
4. Derfeuille-Michaud A, Neut C, Barnich N *et al.* Presence of adherent *Escherichia coli* strain in ileal mucosa of patient with Crohn's disease. Gastroenterology. 1998;115:1405–13.
5. Sadlack B, Merz H, Schorle H, Scimpi A, Feller AC, Horak I. Ulcerative colitis-like disease in mice with a disruptive interleukin-2 gene. Cell. 1993;75:253–61.
6. Kuhn R, Lohler J, Rennick D, Rajeski K, Mullere W. IL-10 deficient mice develop chronic enterocolitis. Cell. 1993;75:263–74.
7. Roedingen WEW. The colonic epithelium in chronic ulcerative colitis: an energy deficiency disease? Lancet. 1980;2:712–15.
8. Pitcher MCL, Cummings JH. Hydrogen sulphide: a bacterial toxin in ulcerative colitis? Gut. 1996;39:1–4.
9. Shanahan F. Probiotics in inflamatory bowel disease. Gut. 2001;48(5):609.
10. Isolauri E, Sutas Y, Kankaanpaa P, Arvilommi H, Salminen S. Probiotics: effects on immunity. Am J Clin Nutr. 2001;73(2 Suppl):444S–50S.
11. Dugas B, Mercenier A, Lenoir-Wijnkoop I *et al.* Immunity and probiotics. Immunol Today. 1999;20:387–90.
12. Kalliomaki M, Salminen S, Arvilommi H *et al.* Probiotics in primary prevention of atopic disease: a randomised placebo-controlled trial. Lancet. 2001;357(9262):1057–9.

19
Bacteria and gut inflammation

R. N. FEDORAK

BACKGROUND

Inflammatory bowel disease (IBD) is the result of an unchecked intestinal inflammatory response. While the exact aetiology and pathogenesis of IBD remain unclear, initiation of the inflammatory response is probably caused by luminal environmental factors, very likely bacteria or bacterial products, serving as activating antigens. By sieving through a permeable epithelial barrier, this initiating factor leads to an increased exposure of the mucosal immune system to luminal antigens and toxins. In the genetically susceptible individual, this process results in an inappropriate and unrestrained mucosal immune response and ensuing tissue injury.

THE ROLE MICROBES PLAY IN INFLAMMATORY BOWEL DISEASE: EVIDENCE FROM ANIMAL STUDIES

The role of resident bacteria in initiating and perpetuating IBD

The individual aspects of immune, genetic and environmental elements that ultimately result in human IBD have been investigated through studies on various animal models. These studies have identified the ways in which multiple gastrointestinal physiological and morphological alterations lead to inflammation. These alterations include imbalances in cytokines[1,2], loss of specific cell populations and their regulatory functions[3,4], abrogation of oral tolerance[5], and alterations in epithelial barrier integrity[6–8].

A common element seen in each of these experimental animal models is an association with luminal bacteria. Indeed, to date, all IBD models that develop intestinal inflammation when housed under conventional environmental conditions (i.e. in the presence of luminally normal enteric flora) have remained histologically disease free when raised in a germ-free (i.e. luminally sterile) environment[2,9,10]. Conversely, when these germ-free animals are exposed to and colonized by normal enteric flora, they develop an intestinal inflammation similar to that found in conventionally raised animals[10,11]. Furthermore, while antibiotic treatment does not completely prevent or abolish colitis, it does reduce the inflammation and delay onset[12,13]. Again, these findings imply that bacteria play a central role in the pathogenesis of IBD.

It is important to note, however, that the host's genetic background and the age at which bacterial colonization occurs determines the immune response to these bacterial antigenic stimuli. For instance, while HLAB27 transgenic rats develop colitis when exposed to *Bacteroides vulgatus*, interleukin-10-gene-deficient mice develop little, if any, intestinal inflammation when exposed to this luminal microbe.

Collectively, these investigations provide strong support for the contention that indigenous intestinal flora play a role in the initiation and perpetuation of intestinal mucosal inflammation in genetically susceptible hosts.

The role of live bacteria and bacterial products

It is not yet known whether live bacteria are necessary to the initiation or perpetuation of IBD, or whether certain bacterial antigens will cause these effects. In experiments in which bacterial antigens have been used to stimulate T-cell activity in inflamed and uninflamed tissue, T cells and T-cell clones isolated from the intestinal mucosa of control subjects responded *in vitro* to non-living bacterial sonicates prepared from the intestinal flora of different subjects (heterologous antigens) but not to sonicates prepared from a subject's own flora (autologous antigens)[14]. Nonetheless, T cells derived from IBD patients[15], and from IBD animal models[16], are reactive to their own (autologous) bacterial antigens, raising the possibility that, once activated, lymphocytes may respond to non-bacterial autologous antigens. This possibility implies that an autoimmune process may perpetuate the disease, even after an initiating event has been concluded or an initiating element has been removed.

This research suggests that, under normal conditions, the animal model shows tolerance towards resident bacterial antigens but that this tolerance is broken down under inflammatory conditions. However, the tolerance has not been investigated in terms of individual bacteria.

The role of the mucosal immune system in bacterially initiated inflammatory processes

CD4+ T cells play a central role in the immune perturbation of IBD. In many rodent models of IBD, mucosal inflammation can be transferred through injecting immune-deficient mice with CD4+ cells derived from either the spleen or mucosa of diseased animals[17–20]. Similarly, the transfer of lamina propria lymphocytes from IL-10-deficient mice, to syngeneic SCID mice causes a fatal inflammation in the colon of the recipients. Additionally, $CD45Rb^{hi}$ transfer animal model studies show that transferred CD4+ cells have to be reactivated in the host to be able to travel to the intestine and cause disease[21]. Reactivation appears to be antigen dependent and class-II restricted[21]. One possibility is that a bacterial antigen might provide the necessary stimuli for the activation of these transferred T cells. Whether bacterial antigens on their own, or live bacteria alone, will allow for the transferred cells to be reactivated is unknown. It is possible that pathogenic T cells may not require bacteria or bacterial antigens at all; they may be restimulated by their own proteins in an autoimmune fashion.

The role of beneficial bacteria

Certain bacterial species, such as *Lactobacillus* spp. and *Bifidobacterium*, collectively termed probiotics, have been shown to play a protective role in animal models that develop bacteria-induced intestinal inflammation[22]. Probiotic bacteria are living microorganisms which, upon ingestion in certain numbers, exert beneficial effects beyond those of basic nutrition. Mechanisms by which probiotics may exert their beneficial activity include: (1) competitive exclusion of bacterial adherence and/or translocation, (2) stimulation of both a cellular and a humoral immune response, (3) antimicrobial activity, and (4) enhancement of barrier integrity. Indeed, *Lactobacillus* spp. treatment reverses the changes associated with colonic mucosal adherence by injurious bacterial strains in IL-10 gene-deficient mice; the treatment thereby prevents the development of colitis[23].

Taken together, IBD animal model results indicate that bacterial flora in genetically susceptible hosts may stimulate a pathogenic cellular immune response consequent upon defective immunological tolerances and the lack of appropriate mucosal defences.

THE ROLE OF MICROBES IN INFLAMMATORY BOWEL DISEASES: EVIDENCE FROM HUMAN STUDIES

The alteration of resident bacteria

Despite many years of extensive research, scientists do not fully understand the pathogenesis of inflammatory bowel diseases. Genetic factors as well as environmental triggers seem to play substantial roles. In the case of environmental triggers, bacterial and viral organisms are among the best studied[24].

Although studies of experimental IBD models indicate that the normal resident luminal bacteria are significantly involved in the onset and chronicity of inflammation, a fundamental question of aetiology remains: Is the disease caused by aberrant intestinal flora, or does disease result from an overly aggressive immune response to normal resident flora?

IBD occurs in sites with the highest concentration of luminal bacteria, such as the colon and terminal ileum[25]. Diversion of the faecal stream away from the site of IBD often results in improvement, not only of symptoms, but also of the mucosal injury profile.

Giaffer *et al.* have shown that the intestinal flora of patients with active Crohn's disease and ulcerative colitis is considerably different than that seen in patients with quiescent disease, ulcerative colitis, or normal controls[24]. In the case of active IBD, aerobic bacteria concentrations were elevated, especially *Escherichia coli*; among the anaerobic bacteria, *Bacteroides fragilis* and *Bacteroides vulgatus* were increased. Additionally, for all patients with IBD, levels of *Bifidobacteria* were decreased. Similar reductions in luminal and mucosal adherent levels of *Bifidobacterium* and lactobacillus in humans with active IBD have been described by Favier *et al.*[26] and Fabia *et al.*[27], respectively.

Thus, it is very plausible that the elimination of the subset of aggressive luminal bacteria along with a repopulation by beneficial (probiotic) bacteria will lead to a blockade of pro-inflammatory cytokines and TH1 lymphocytes, while providing a simultaneous enhancement of anti-inflammatory and protective immune responses.

References

1. Kuhn R, Lohler J, Rennick D, Rajewsky K, Muller W. Interleukin-10-deficient mice develop chronic enterocolitis [see comments]. Cell. 1993;75:263–74.
2. Sadlack, B, Merz H, Schorle H, Schimpl A, Feller AC, Horak I. Ulcerative colitis-like disease in mice with a disrupted interleukin-2 gene [see comments]. Cell. 1993;75:253–61.
3. Hollander GA, Simpson SJ, Mizoguchi E *et al.* Severe colitis in mice with aberrant thymic selection. Immunity. 1995;3:27–38.
4. Mowat AM, Lamont AG, Strobel S, Mackenzie S. The role of antigen processing and suppressor T cells in immune responses to dietary proteins in mice. Adv Exp Med Biol. 1987;216A:709–20.
5. Gardiner KR, Anderson NH, Rowlands BJ, Barbul A. Colitis and colonic mucosal barrier dysfunction. Gut. 1995;37:530–5.
6. Hermiston ML, Gordon JI. Inflammatory bowel disease and adenomas in mice expressing a dominant negative N-cadherin. Science. 1995;270:1203–7.
7. Panwala CM, Jones JC, Viney JL. A novel model of inflammatory bowel disease: mice deficient for the multiple drug resistance gene, mdr1a, spontaneously develop colitis. J Immunol. 1998;161:5733–44.
8. Onderdonk AB, Franklin ML, Cisneros RL. Production of experimental ulcerative colitis in gnotobiotic guinea pigs with simplified microflora. Infect Immun. 1981;32:225–31.
9. Madsen KL, Malfair D, Gray D, Doyle JS, Jewell LD, Fedorak RN. Interleukin-10 gene-deficient mice develop a primary intestinal permeability defect in response to enteric microflora. Inflamm Bowel Dis. 1999;5:262–70.
10. Sellon RK, Tonkonogy S, Schultz M *et al.* Resident enteric bacteria are necessary for development of spontaneous colitis and immune system activation in interleukin-10-deficient mice. Infect Immun. 1998;66:5224–31.
11. Rath HC, Herfarth HH, Ikeda JS *et al.* Normal luminal bacteria, especially Bacteroides species, mediate chronic colitis, gastritis, and arthritis in HLA-B27/human beta2 microglobulin transgenic rats. J Clin Invest. 1996;98:945–53.
12. Onderdonk AB, Hermos JA, Dzink JL, Bartlett JG. Protective effect of metronidazole in experimental ulcerative colitis. Gastroenterology. 1978;74:521–6.
13. Madsen KL, Doyle JS, Tavernini MM, Jewell LD, Rennie RP, Fedorak RN. Antibiotic therapy attenuates colitis in interleukin 10 gene-deficient mice. Gastroenterology. 2000;118:1094–105.
14. Duchmann R, Kaiser I, Hermann E, Mayet W, Ewe K, Meyer zum Buschenfelde KH. Tolerance exists towards resident intestinal flora but is broken in active inflammatory bowel disease (IBD) [see comments]. Clin Exp Immunol. 1995:102:448–55.
15. Duchmann R, May E, Heike M, Knolle P, Neurath M, Meyer zum Buschenfelde KH. T cell specificity and cross reactivity towards enterobacteria, bacteroides, bifidobacterium, and antigens from resident intestinal flora in humans [see comments]. Gut. 1999;44:812–18.
16. Duchmann R, Schmitt E, Knolle P, Meyer zum Buschenfelde KH, Neurath M. Tolerance towards resident intestinal flora in mice is abrogated in experimental colitis and restored by treatment with interleukin-10 or antibodies to interleukin-12. Eur J Immunol. 1996;26:934–8.
17. Aranda R, Sydora BC, McAllister PL *et al.* Analysis of intestinal lymphocytes in mouse colitis mediated by transfer of CD4+, CD45Rbhigh T cells to SCID recipients. J Immunol. 1997;158:3464–73.
18. Rennick DM, Fort MM, Davidson NJ. Studies with IL-10-/- mice: an overview. J Leuk Biol. 1997;61:389–96.
19. Morrissey PJ, Charrier K, Braddy S, Liggitt D, Watson JD. CD4+ T cells that express high levels of CD45RB induce wasting disease when transferred into congenic severe combined immunodeficient mice. Disease development is prevented by cotransfer of purified CD4+ T cells. J Exp Med. 1993;178:237–44.
20. Matsuda JL, Gapin L, Sydora BC *et al.* Systemic activation and antigen-driven oligoclonal expansion of T cells in a mouse model of colitis. J Immunol. 2000;164:2797–806.

21. Schultz M, Sartor RB. Aberrant host immune responses to luminal bacteria in the pathogenesis of chronic inflammatory bowel disease. In: Ernst PB, Michetti P, Smith PD, editors, The Immunobiology of H. pylori: From Pathogenesis to Prevention. Philadelphia: Lippincott-Raven Publishers, 1997:67–182.
22. Bengmark S. Probiotics and prebiotics in prevention and treatment of gastrointestinal diseases. Gastroenterol Int. 1998;11(Suppl. 1):4–7.
23. Madsen KL, Doyle JS, Jewell LD, Tavernini MM, Fedorak RN. Lactobacillus species prevents colitis in interleukin-10 gene-deficient mice. Gastroenterology. 1999;116:1107–14.
24. Giaffer MH, Holdsworth CD, Duerden BI. The assessment of faecal flora in patients with inflammatory bowel disease by a simplified bacteriological technique. J Med Microbiol. 1991;35A:238–43.
25. Lashner BA. Clinical features, laboratory findings, and course of Crohn's disease. In: Kirshner JB, editor, Inflammatory Bowel Disease. Philadelphia: W.B. Saunders, 2000:305–15.
26. Favier C, Neut C, Mizon C, Cortol A, Colombel JF, Mizon J. Fecal beta-D-galactosidase production and Bifidobacteria are decreased in Crohn's disease. Dig Dis Sci. 1997;42:817–22.
27. Fabia R, Ar'Rajab A, Johansson ML *et al.* Impairment of bacterial flora in human ulcerative colitis and experimental colitis in rat. Digestion. 1993;54:248–55.

20
Dietary components as antigens, haptens and mitogens in the pathogenesis of inflammatory bowel disease

J. M. RHODES

FOOD ANTIGENS IN ULCERATIVE COLITIS

In this condition food antigens probably play relatively little part. Several well-conducted trials[1] have shown no benefit in severe colitis from bowel rest by either intravenous or enteral feeding or by surgical exclusion. A study by Wright and Truelove over thirty years ago did, however, show that about one in five patients with ulcerative colitis benefits from exclusion of dairy products (unrelated to the hypolactasia that often accompanies a severe attack)[2]. Their study has never been refuted.

FOOD ANTIGENS IN CROHN'S DISEASE

Lipids, detergents and emulsifiers

The case for a role of food antigens in the pathogenesis of Crohn's disease is much stronger. There is evidence that components in the faecal stream are responsible for maintaining disease activity[3] and a major component may be vegetable fibre which many patients find provokes symptoms and which has been shown in provocation studies to induce biochemical as well as symptomatic relapse (Figure 1). Remission, associated with healing of ileal ulceration, can be induced with either intravenous feeding or enteral feeding. Initial success was obtained using amino-acid-based feeds[4]. Results with polymeric feeds have ranged from excellent[5] to poor and it has been pointed out that there is a good inverse correlation between the long-chain fat content of the feed and the therapeutic response, feeds with a low fat content producing a better response[6]. In a recent study, in conjunction with the group in Cambridge, we have, however,

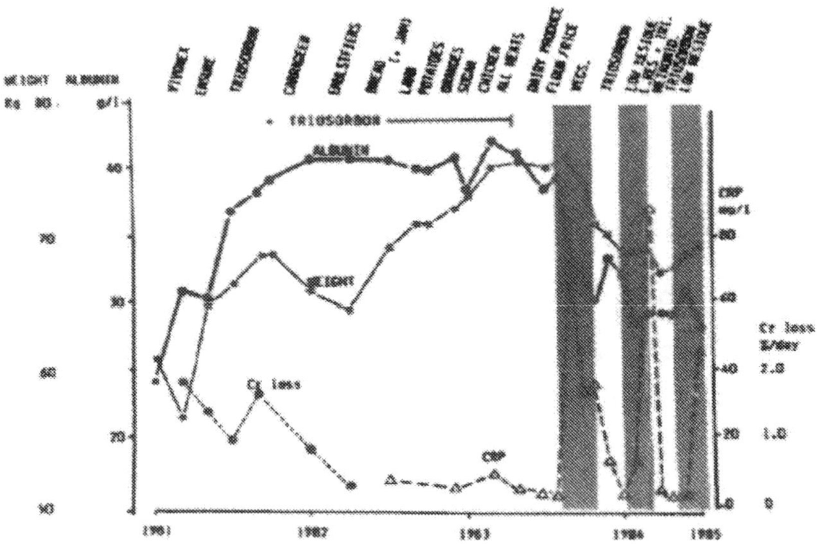

Figure 1 An extended study of dietary challenge in a patient with multiple small bowel strictures due to Crohn's disease. Remission was induced with enteral feeding and a series of dietary challenges was carried out over a three-year period. It can be seen: (1) that vegetable fibre eaten in late 1983 caused not only symptomatic relapse but also a rapid rise in serum C reactive protein, (2) that the changes in CRP/disease activity are too rapid to be accounted for by changes in nutritional status, (3) that, after the first relapse, the patient was no longer able to tolerate the low-residue diet he had been managing without problems before the relapse. This suggests that, when the intestine is ulcerated, the patient may become intolerant of a range of foods that he/she might be able to tolerate when fully in remission with a healed mucosa. Taken from Reference 5

found no difference in efficacy between a high-fat and a low-fat feed[7]. We can only speculate that there may be some other component of the less successful polymeric feeds that was reducing their efficacy. One possibility might be an increased content of emulsifiers which are in effect detergents and which would be expected to increase intestinal permeability.

Nanoparticles as haptens – the titanium dioxide story

One fascinating story that is under investigation in London is the possibility that Crohn's disease may be at least in part due to the presence in the diet of nanoparticles. These are insoluble particles which have a diameter in the order of nanometres. By virtue of their very high ratio of surface area to mass, they act as biological catalysts. The nanoparticle which is probably most prevalent in the modern diet is titanium dioxide, a white pigment that has been extensively used in the food industry for about one hundred years. The group at St Thomas' Hospital in London have shown that the presence of titanium oxide increases about one hundred fold the lymphocyte response to bacterial lipopolysaccharide[8] and have reported remarkably good results in a small controlled trial comparing a particle-free with a standard diet[9] (Figure 2).

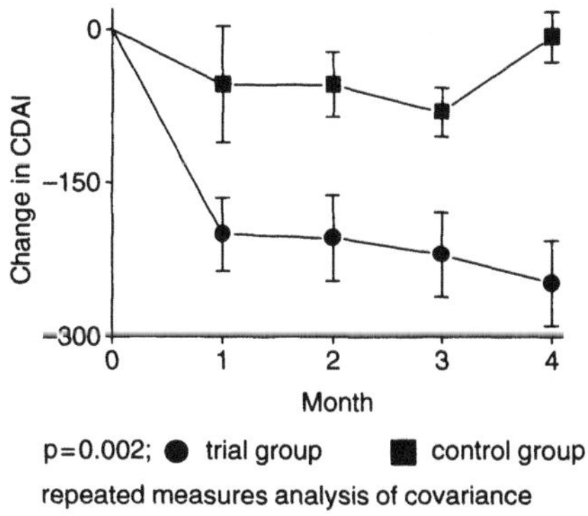

Figure 2 Double-blind study of low microparticle and sham manipulated diet in active Crohn's disease (n=10 for each group). This shows a remarkable response to avoidance of microparticles (including but not exclusively titanium dioxide). Taken from Reference 9

Microbial cell wall oligomannan, the epitope for the anti-*Saccharomyces cerevisiae* antibody (ASCA), has the potential to induce a localized mucosal defect in phagocytic cell function

It has recently been shown that about two thirds of Crohn's disease patients have circulating antibodies (ASCA) to baker's yeast (*Saccharomyces cerevisiae*)[10]. The epitope for this antibody is a polysaccharide: oligomannan, with specific alpha 1–3 linkages between the mannose residues[11]. It is likely that this is present on a range of bacterial cell walls as well as on the cell walls of baker's yeast and the presence of ASCA probably reflects penetration of the mucosa by a range of different microbes rather than a food allergy. A study published nearly twenty years ago showed that the presence of oligomannan markedly suppressed the release of myeloperoxidase from neutrophil polymorphs[12], thus inducing a very similar defect to that seen in the hereditary condition, chronic granulomatous disease, where the bowel becomes affected by a condition that closely mimics Crohn's disease[13]. We have therefore speculated that the granulomatous reaction of Crohn's disease may be a consequence of a mucosal defect in phagocytic cell function that is the result of mucosal bacterial invasion and shedding of bacterial cell wall oligomannan[14] (Figure 3).

Microbial and dietary lectins and their interactions with dietary fibre and with the mucosa

Mucosal glycosylation changes are common in both ulcerative colitis and Crohn's disease and closely mimic those seen in colorectal cancer and adenoma. They include shortening of O-linked oligosaccharide chain length, reduced sulphation, increased sialylation and increased expression of oncofetal antigens such as the galactose-terminated Thomsen-Friedenreich blood group antigen (galactose β1,3 *N*-acetylgalactosamine α)[15]. These changes affect both secreted mucins[16] and cell-surface glycoproteins, such as CD44[17]. We have speculated that this may allow recruitment of microbial and/or dietary lectins which would otherwise pass by in the colon lumen without interaction[18]. Since lectins often

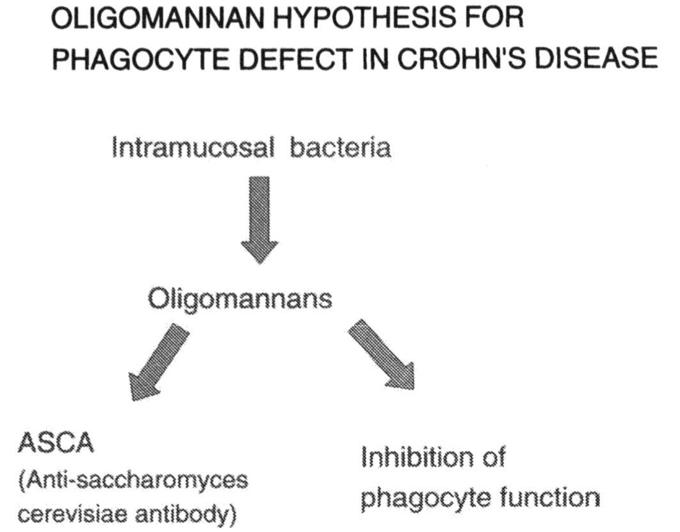

Figure 3 About two thirds of patients with Crohn's disease have circulating antibodies to Baker's yeast (*Saccharomyces cerevisiae*). The epitope for this antibody is oligomannan with an alpha 1–3 linkage between its mannose residues. This is not specific to baker's yeast and is likely to be present on a range of bacterial cell walls. The hypothesis is proposed that intramucosal shedding of bacterial cell wall oligomannan may interact with phagocytic cells, inducing a local defect in phagocytic cell function within the mucosa, analogous to that seen in chronic granulomatous disease. This is supported by the study of Wright *et al.* who showed that oligomannan inhibits the release of myeloperoxidase from neutrophils[12].

have a mitogenic effect on cells to which they bind, we have speculated that this may have a cancer-promoting effect. As proof of the concept of this hypothesis, we have shown that individuals with a histologically normal colon but with increased expression of Thomsen-Friedenreich antigen in their colonic mucosa have a 40% increase in rectal mucosal proliferation following one week of dietary supplementation with peanuts, which are a potent source of a Thomsen-Friedenreich-binding lectin[19]. We have also shown, in a case-control study of diet and sporadic colon cancer, that, whereas total dietary fibre intake had a neutral effect on colon cancer risk, a high intake of fibres containing galactose (which are almost exclusively fruit and vegetable fibres rather than cereal fibres) had a significant protective effect against colon cancer[20].

Work is ongoing in our laboratory to explore further the hypothesis that the mucosal-associated flora that are found in Crohn's disease may have been attracted there by virtue of lectin/carbohydrate interactions specifically directed against the oncofetal carbohydrate structures that are so markedly up-regulated in the inflammatory bowel disease mucosa. If this hypothesis is correct, then high-galactose fibres may also have the potential to act as 'negative prebiotics' by competitively inhibiting the mucosal attraction of potentially harmful bacteria.

Dietary therapy, along with azathioprine and infliximab, are the only therapies so far shown to heal the ileal ulcers of Crohn's disease. It seems highly likely that a better understanding of the relationship between Crohn's disease and diet may lead to effective methods of prevention.

References

1. Dickinson RJ, Ashton MG, Axon AT, Smith RC, Yeung CK, Hill GL. Controlled trial of intravenous hyperalimentation and total bowel rest as an adjunct to the routine therapy of acute colitis. Gastroenterology. 1980;79:1199–204.
2. Wright R, Truelove SC. A controlled therapeutic trial of various diets in ulcerative colitis. Br Med J. 1965;2:138–41.
3. Harper PH, Lee EC, Kettlewell MG, Bennett MK, Jewell DP. Role of the faecal stream in the maintenance of Crohn's colitis. Gut. 1985;26:279–84.
4. O'Morain C, Segal AW, Levi AJ. Elemental diets in treatment of acute Crohn's disease. Br Med J. 1980;281:1173–5.
5. Raouf AH, Hildrey V, Daniel J, Walker RJ, Krasner N, Elias E, Rhodes JM. Enteral feeding as sole therapy for Crohn's disease: A controlled trial of whole protein versus amino-acid based feed and a case study of dietary challenge. Gut. 1991;32:702–7.
6. Fernandez-Banares F, Cabré E, Gonzalez-Huix F, Gassull MA. Enteral nutrition as primary therapy in Crohn's disease. Gut. 1994;35(Suppl. 1):S55–9.
7. Leiper K, Woolner J, Mullan MMC, Parker T, van der Vliet M, Fear S, Rhodes JM, Hunter JO. A randomised controlled trial of high versus low long chain triglyceride whole protein feed in active Crohn's disease. Gut. 2001;49:790–4.
8. Powell JJ, Harvey RS, Ashwood P, Wolstencroft R, Gershwin ME, Thompson RP. Immune potentiation of ultrafine dietary particles in normal subjects and patients with inflammatory bowel disease. J Autoimmun. 2000;14:99–105.
9. Lomer MC, Harvey RS, Evans SM, Thompson RP, Powell JJ. Efficacy and tolerability of a low microparticle diet in a double blind, randomized, pilot study in Crohn's disease. Eur J Gastroenterol Hepatol. 2001;13:101–6.
10. Sendid B, Colombel JF, Jacquinot PM, Faille C, Fruit J, Cortot A, Lucidarme D, Camus D, Poulain D. Specific antibody response to oligomannosidic epitopes in Crohn's disease. Clin Diagn Lab Immunol. 1996;3:219–26.
11. Young M, Davies MJ, Bailey D *et al.* Characterization of oligosaccharides from an antigenic mannan of Saccharomyces cerevisiae. Glycoconj J. 1998;15:815–22.
12. Wright CD, Bowie JU, Nelson RD. Influence of yeast mannan on release of myeloperoxidase by human neutrophils: determination of structural features of mannan required for formation of myeloperoxidase–mannan–neutrophil complexes. Infect Immun. 1984;43:467–71.
13. Ament ME, Ochs HD. Gastrointestinal manifestations of chronic granulomatous disease. N Engl J Med. 1973;288:382–7.
14. Rhodes JM. Lectins, colitis and colon cancer. J R Coll Phys. 2000;34:191–6.
15. Rhodes JM. Mucins and inflammatory bowel disease. Q J Med. 1997;90:79–82.
16. Campbell BJ, Hounsell E, Finnie IA, Rhodes JM. Direct demonstration of increased expression of Thomsen-Friedenreich antigen (Galβ1–3GalNAc) by mucus in colon cancer and inflammatory bowel disease. J Clin Invest. 1995;95:571–6.
17. Singh R, Campbell BJ, Yu L-G, Fernig DG, Milton JD, Goodlad RA, FitzGerald AJ, Rhodes JM. Cell surface-expressed Thomsen-Friedenreich antigen in colon cancer is predominantly carried on high molecular weight splice variants of CD44. Glycobiology. 2001;11:587–92.
18. Rhodes JM. Unifying hypothesis for inflammatory bowel disease and related colon cancer: sticking the pieces together with sugar. Lancet. 1996;347:40–4.
19. Ryder SD, Jacyna MR, Levi AJ, Rizzi PM, Rhodes JM. Eating peanuts increases rectal proliferation in individuals with mucosal expression of peanut lectin receptor. Gastroenterology. 1998;114:44–9.
20. Evans RC, Ashby D, Hackett A, Williams E, Rhodes JM. Consumption of peanuts, which contain a galactose-binding lectin, associates with increased risk for colorectal cancer whereas high non-starch polysaccharide galactose intake associates with reduced risk. Gut. 1997;41(Suppl. 3):A124.

21 Use of antibiotics and probiotics in Crohn's disease

C. PRANTERA, M. L. SCRIBANO and R. MANGIAROTTI

Crohn's disease (CD) is a chronic inflammatory bowel disease of uncertain origin. The hypothesis that intestinal bacteria play a role in the pathogenesis of CD lesions is supported by many experimental and clinical data[1–3]. Bacteria live predominantly in the sites which are commonly affected by CD lesions and are the cause of animal and human intestinal diseases similar to CD. Spontaneous colitis that develops in genetically engineered rodent models does not occur when the animals are raised in germ-free conditions[4]. The luminal content is necessary for causing the intestinal lesions, and some studies have shown that, when it was diverted from the gut, inflammatory lesions of CD did not appear[5]. Moreover, when the effluent of ileostomy was reintroduced into the intestine, it caused inflammatory changes and triggered postoperative recurrence of the disease[6]. The ultrafiltrated effluent was without effect.

On the basis of these and other observations, antibiotics are often employed in the treatment of CD as an alternative to, or in combination with, corticosteroids in spite of few studies supporting their efficacy in this disease.

METRONIDAZOLE

Among the various antibiotics, metronidazole, active against some parasites and most anaerobic bacteria, is now the most widely employed. This imidazole compound was first reported to be effective in CD in an open study in 1975[7]. It is widely used in treating perianal CD and open studies have shown its efficacy in closing fistula and healing perianal abscesses, even if these lesions do often reappear when the therapy is discontinued[8–10]. Randomized controlled trials of metronidazole therapy in active CD have demonstrated that this antibiotic is efficacious in Crohn's colitis or ileocolitis but not in small bowel location (Table 1). The positive results obtained with metronidazole when only the colon is involved might be due to the higher concentration of anaerobic bacteria in

Table 1 Randomized controlled trials on efficacy of metronidazole in active Crohn's disease

Reference	*Study duration (months)*	*Patients (n)*	*Dose (mg/day)*	*Control*	*Remission (%)*	
					Treatment	*Control*
Blichfeldt *et al.**[11] (1978)	4	40	1000	Placebo	NS	
Ursing *et al.**[12] (1982)	4	78	800	SASP	NS	
Ambrose *et al.*[13] (1985)	1	72	800	Placebo	Improvement 44 M 57 M + C 62 C	 41
Sutherland *et al.*[14] (1991)	4	99	20/kg 10/kg	Placebo	27 36	25

SASP, sulphasalazine; NS, not significant; M, metronidazole; C, cotrimoxazole; M + C, metronidazole plus cotrimoxazole; *crossover study.

colitis, and the efficacy of this antibiotic seems to be correlated with luminal *Bacteroides* concentration. A trial of metronidazole in recurrence prevention of Crohn's ileitis after intestinal resection seems to confirm this explanation[15]. The study showed that the antibiotic, used for a 3-month period, significantly decreased the severity of early endoscopic recurrence in the neoterminal ileum, in comparison to placebo, and also seemed to delay the symptomatic recurrence at 1 year. More recently, the same authors have demonstrated that ornidazole, given for 1 year after surgery, is efficacious in preventing severe endoscopic recurrence of CD[16]. Preliminary results of the trial have shown the presence of severe endoscopic lesions after 12 months in 94% of the placebo patients compared with 62% of the ornidazole patients.

Metronidazole is generally well tolerated, and its side-effects vary between 10% and 20% depending on the dosage and the length of treatment. The most frequent are gastrointestinal intolerance, neurotoxicity and metallic taste. Peripheral neuropathy occurs in 50–85% of long-term metronidazole use[9].

CIPROFLOXACIN

Another antibiotic used in CD is ciprofloxacin, a quinolone derivative with a selective suppressive effect on the intestinal microflora. *Escherichia coli* and Enterobacteriacae are especially sensitive to this antibiotic, which, by contrast, does not particularly affect anaerobic bacteria.

Ciprofloxacin has been anecdotally reported to be effective in the long-term treatment of 10 patients with active perianal CD[17], in 4 cases of Crohn's ileitis[18] and, associated with metronidazole, in an uncontrolled series of 31 patients with active CD[19]. Five randomized controlled trials have employed ciprofloxacin in the treatment of acute phases of CD, reporting interesting results (Table 2).

Table 2 Randomized controlled trials on efficacy of ciprofloxacin in active Crohn's disease

Reference	*Study duration (weeks)*	*Patients (n)*	*Dose (mg/day)*	*Control*	*Remission (%)*	
					Treatment	*Control*
Turunen *et al.*[20] (1995)	26	89	1000–1500 + metronidazole steroid	Placebo + metronidazole steroid	NS	
Prantera *et al.*[21] (1996)	12	41	1000 + 1000 metronidazole	Steroid	45.5	63
Colombel *et al.*[22] (1999)	6	40	1000	Mesalamine	56	55
Arnold *et al.*[23] (1999)	26	36	1000	Placebo	$p < 0.001$	
Steinhart *et al.*[24] (2001)	130	8	1000+1000 metronidazole + budesonide	Placebo + budesonide	33	38

NS, not significant.

The efficacy of a therapy with ciprofloxacin, alone or associated with metronidazole, in active CD has been confirmed in a retrospective analysis on 233 patients seen at our Inflammatory Bowel Disease Clinic during the period 1984–1996[25]. Similar rates of success, defined as remission [Simple Index (SI) ≤2] or improvement (SI ≤50% of basal value), were achieved with the three schemes of treatment: 70.6% with the antibiotic combination, 69% with ciprofloxacin and 72.8% with metronidazole. Considering that the patients treated with only one antibiotic had a milder form of disease or received, at the same time, immunosuppressive drugs, the efficacy of metronidazole and ciprofloxacin in combination was the most impressive. All the diseased locations responded to the treatment, although there was reduced efficacy of ciprofloxacin in colitis. The poor efficacy of this antibiotic against anaerobic bacteria could be the cause. Recurrent ileitis responded better than primary ileitis to the antibiotics alone or in association. When the ileocaecal valve is resected, the concentration of anaerobes in the ileum is similar to the concentration in the colon, and the small bowel overgrowth can become more relevant in causing symptoms such as abdominal pain and diarrhoea. As expected, a higher percentage of side effects responsible for interruption of therapy was reported with the antibiotic association (21.8%). The most common were epigastric pain, nausea and vomiting.

The percentage of side effects reported in the studies on ciprofloxacin depends on the dosage and the length of treatment. The most frequent are of gastrointestinal origin but skin reactions and increase in transaminase level have been described.

In conclusion, metronidazole and ciprofloxacin have shown themselves to be an effective alternative to steroids in the treatment of acute flares of CD, particularly in patients with abscesses, fever, pus in the stools and toxic signs, all of which suggest a bacterial participation in the inflammatory process.

PROBIOTICS

Manipulation of enteric flora with probiotic compounds is conceptually more appealing than the suppression of bacteria with antibiotics. Administration of probiotics may counterbalance the harmful intestinal flora with a beneficial flora, and therefore might be of therapeutic advantage in patients with CD. At the present time, few data are available on the role of probiotics in CD[26,27] and very few clinical trials have investigated the effectiveness of probiotic agents on CD.

The non-pathogenic *Escherichia coli* strain Nissle 1917 has been used as maintenance therapy in patients with CD[28]. Twenty-eight patients with active colonic disease were treated over 1 year with prednisolone together with the non-pathogenic *Escherichia coli* or placebo. All patients randomized to receive the probiotic were able to stop taking the steroids within 6 months, whereas a few patients on placebo could not completely stop taking the prednisolone. Moreover, a relapse rate of 33.3% in the *Escherichia coli* group compared with 63.6% in the control group was observed. However, these interesting results are hampered by the interference of a contemporaneous long-term treatment with corticosteroids.

Clinical and experimental observations have suggested that the intestinal flora may play a role in post-surgical recurrence of CD. Consequently, the operated patients offer the best *in-vivo* opportunity for studying the influence of endoluminal bacteria on the recurrent lesions.

In a recent study on the prevention of post-surgical recurrence of CD, forty patients were treated either with an antibiotic, rifaximin 1.8 g/day, for 3 months followed by a probiotic, VSL#3, for 9 months, or with mesalazine 4 g/day for 12 months[29]. After 1 year, 20% of patients in the antibiotic/probiotic group had a severe endoscopic recurrence, compared with 40% on mesalazine.

We have conducted a randomized controlled trial with a probiotic, *Lactobacillus rhamnosus* strain GG (LGG), in the prevention of post-operative recurrence of CD[30]. The first aim of our study has been to evaluate the efficacy of this probiotic in preventing the appearance of recurrent lesions or in reducing their severity at 1 year after the surgery. Forty-five patients have been randomized to receive for 12 months LGG or placebo, given immediately after the operation, when all the diseased gut was removed. Preliminary results on 26 of the 45 patients have

Table 3 Preliminary results of LGG in the prevention of post-operative recurrence of Crohn's disease

	LGG (n = 14)	*Placebo (n = 12)*
Non-compliance (%)	2 (14.2)	1 (8.3)
Protocol violation (%)	3 (21.4)	1 (8.3)
Clinical remission* (%)	7 (77.7)	8 (80.0)
Endoscopic remission† (%)	4 (57.1)	5 (62.5)
Endoscopic recurrence† (%)	3 (42.9)	3 (37.5)

*CDAI ≤ 150 after 52 weeks of therapy; †Rutgeerts scoring system: 0–1 = remission; 2–4 = recurrence.

shown no differences in endoscopic and clinical remission between the two groups (Table 3), suggesting that LGG offers no benefit with respect to placebo in prevention of recurrence after surgery.

Preliminary results of probiotic treatment in patients with CD are encouraging, but more information on mechanisms by which probiotics confer their therapeutic effect is needed and, above all, more controlled studies are required to evaluate the real efficacy of these compounds in managing CD.

References

1. Prantera C, Scribano ML, Berto E, Zannoni F. Antibiotic use in Crohn's disease. Why and how? BioDrugs. 1997;8:293–306.
2. Prantera C, Scribano ML. Crohn's disease: the case for bacteria. Ital J Gastroenterol Hepatol. 1999;31:244–6.
3. Sartor RB. Enteric microflora in IBD: pathogens or commensals? Inflamm Bowel Dis. 1997;3:230–5.
4. Sartor RB. Insights into the pathogenesis of inflammatory bowel disease provided by new rodent models of spontaneous colitis. Inflamm Bowel Dis. 1995;1:64–75.
5. Rutgeerts P, Goboes K, Peeters M *et al.* Effect of faecal stream diversion on recurrence of Crohn's disease in the neoterminal ileum. Lancet. 1991;338:771–4.
6. D'Haens GR, Geboes K, Peeters M *et al.* Early lesions of recurrent Crohn's disease caused by infusion of intestinal contents in excluded ileum. Gastroenterology. 1998;114:262–7.
7. Ursing B, Kamme C. Metronidazole for Crohn's disease. Lancet. 1975;1:775.
8. Bernstein LH, Frank MS, Brandt LJ *et al.* Healing of perianal Crohn's disease with metronidazole. Gastroenterology. 1980;79:357–65.
9. Brandt LJ, Bernstein LH, Boley SS *et al.* Metronidazole therapy for perianal Crohn's disease: a follow-up study. Gastroenterology. 1982;83:383–7.
10. Jacobovitis J, Shuster M. Metronidazole therapy for Crohn's disease and associated fistulae. Am J Gastroenterol. 1984;79:533–40.
11. Blichfeldt P, Blomhoff JP, Myhre E *et al.* Metronidazole in Crohn's disease: a double-blind cross-over clinical trial. Scand J Gastroenterol. 1978;13:123–7.
12. Ursing B, Alm T, Barany F *et al.* A comparative study of metronidazole and sulfasalazine for active Crohn's disease: the Cooperative Crohn's Disease Study in Sweden: II. Result. Gastroenterology. 1982;83:550–62.
13. Ambrose NS, Allan RN, Keighley MRB *et al.* Antibiotic therapy for treatment in relapse of intestinal Crohn's disease: a prospective randomized study. Dis Colon Rectum. 1985;28:81–5.
14. Sutherland L, Singleton J, Sessions J *et al.* Double-blind, placebo controlled trial of metronidazole in Crohn's disease. Gut. 1991;32:1071–5.
15. Rutgeerts P, Hiele M, Geboes K *et al.* Controlled trial of metronidazole treatment for prevention of Crohn's recurrence after ileal resection. Gastroenterology. 1995;108:1617–21.
16. Rutgeerts PJ, D'Haens G, Baert F *et al.* Nitroimidazol antibiotics are efficacious for prophylaxis of postoperative recurrence of Crohn's disease: a placebo controlled trial. Gastroenterology. 1999;116:A808.
17. Turunen U, Farkkila M, Valtonen V *et al.* Long-term outcome of ciprofloxacin treatment in severe perianal or fistulous Crohn's disease. Gastroenterology. 1993;104:A793.
18. Peppercorn MA. Is there a role for antibiotics as primary therapy in Crohn's ileitis? J Clin Gastroenterol. 1993;17:235–7.
19. Prantera C, Kohn A, Zannoni F *et al.* Metronidazole plus ciprofloxacin in the treatment of active, refractory Crohn's disease: results of an open study. J Clin Gastroenterol. 1994;19:79–88.
20. Turunen U, Farkkila M, Hakala K *et al.* Ciprofloxacin treatment combined with conventional therapy in Crohn's disease: a prospective, double blind, placebo controlled study. Gut. 1995;37:A193.
21. Prantera C, Zannoni F, Scribano ML *et al.* An antibiotic regimen for the treatment of active Crohn's disease: a randomized, controlled clinical trial of metronidazole plus ciprofloxacin. Am J Gastroenterol. 1996;91:328–32.
22. Colombel JF, Lemann M, Cassagnou M *et al.* A controlled trial comparing ciprofloxacin with mesalazine for the treatment of active Crohn's disease. Am J Gastroenterol. 1999;94:674–8.

23. Arnold GL, Patel H, Beaves M, Boyd H. Ciprofloxacin in active Crohn's disease: preliminary report of a 6 month randomized placebo controlled study. Gastroenterology. 1999;116:A664.
24. Steinhart AH, Feagan BG, Greenberg GR *et al.* Combined budesonide and antibiotic therapy for active Crohn's disease: a randomized controlled trial. Gastroenterology. 2001;102:A126.
25. Prantera C, Berto E, Scribano ML, Falasco G. Use of antibiotics in the treatment of active Crohn's disease: experience with metronidazole and ciprofloxacin. Ital J Gastroenterol Hepatol. 1998;30:602–6.
26. Malin M, Suomalainen H, Saxelin M, Isolauri E. Promotion of IgA immune response in patients with Crohn's disease by oral bacteriotherapy with Lactobacillus GG. Ann Nutr Metab. 1996;40: 137–45.
27. Favier C, Neut C, Mizon C *et al.* Fecal β-galactosidase production and bifidobacteria are decreased in Crohn's disease. Dig Dis Sci. 1997;42:817–22.
28. Malchow HA. Crohn's disease and *Escherichia coli.* A new approach in therapy to maintain remission of colonic Crohn's disease? J Clin Gastroenterol. 1997;25:653–8.
29. Campieri M, Rizzello F, Venturi A *et al.* Combination of antibiotic and probiotic treatment is efficacious in prophylaxis of post-operative recurrence of Crohn's disease: a randomized controlled study vs mesalamine. Gastroenterology. 2000;118:A781.
30. Scribano ML, Falasco G, Prantera C. Lactobacillus GG in the prevention of postoperative recurrence of Crohn's disease: preliminary results of a 12 months randomized, double-blind, placebo controlled clinical trial. Digest Liver Dis. 2000;32(2):A60.

22
Probiotics in IBD

P. GIONCHETTI, F. RIZZELLO, C. AMADINI, A. VENTURI, V. PALMONARI, R. ROMAGNOLI, C. MORSELLI, D. MATTEUZZI, P. BRIGIDI and M. CAMPIERI

PROBIOTICS

The use of lactic acid bacteria in foods has a long history; in fact, fermented milk products with live bacteria have been consumed for centuries.

However, the first to propose the use of probiotics for the purpose of health maintenance and disease prevention was Elie Metchnikoff, the Russian Nobel Prize winner who, at the beginning of the 20th century, suggested that a high concentration of lactobacilli in the intestinal flora was important for health and longevity in humans[1]. At the same time, Tissier showed that bifidobacteria were the predominant intestinal microbial flora in breast-fed infants; and it was speculated that infant diarrhoea could be treated by the administration of large doses of bifidobacteria[2]. The term 'probiotic' was first introduced in 1965 by Lilly and Stillwell: they used it to describe any substance or organism that contributes to intestinal microbial balance[3]. This definition was subsequently modified by Fuller, who stressed the importance of a live microbial feed supplement to beneficially affect the host by improving the intestinal microbial balance[4]. More recently, probiotics have been defined as 'living organisms, which upon ingestion in certain numbers, exert health benefits beyond inherent basic nutrition'[5], emphasizing the importance of maintaining a sufficient population of live micro-organisms in the gut, and further implying that benefits, such as improvement in microbial balance, may be associated with other effects, such as immunomodulation.

Bacteria associated with probiotic activity are most commonly lactobacilli, bifidobacteria and streptococci but other non-pathogenic bacteria, such as some strains of *Escherichia coli*, and non-bacterial organisms, such as the yeast *Saccharomyces boulardii*, have been used.

Probiotic strains must possess some necessary characteristics. They must be normal inhabitants of the intestinal tract and of human origin, because some health-promoting effects may be species specific. They also need to be able to survive the acid of the stomach, the digestive enzymes and bile salts. They must have the ability to be metabolically active within the luminal flora, where, ideally, they should survive, but not persist in the long term. They should be antagonistic against pathogenic bacteria and, obviously, they must be safe for human use and should maintain their viability and beneficial properties during manufacturing processes[6].

The 'probiotic concept' is still rather controversial because the beneficial effects of probiotics have been demonstrated almost exclusively under experimental conditions, and because the precise mechanisms by which probiotic micro-organisms exert their effect on the host *in vivo* are not yet well defined.

Several mechanisms have been proposed to account for probiotic action; these include antagonistic activity against pathogenic bacteria either by inhibition of adherence and translocation or by production of antibacterial substances, such as antimicrobial peptides (bacteriocins) and hydrogen peroxide. Probiotics also stimulate mucosal defence, both at the level of immune and epithelial function, with increase of sIgA production, blockade of proinflammatory cytokines, enhancement of anti-inflammatory cytokines levels, stimulation of intestinal mucin expression and improvement of gut permeability. Finally, they are able to produce nutrients of special importance to the intestine, such as short-chain fatty acids and vitamins.

PROBIOTICS AND IBD

The rationale for using probiotics in IBD (inflammatory bowel disease) is based on convincing evidence implicating intestinal bacteria in the pathogenesis of IBD.

The distal ileum and the colon are the areas with the highest bacterial concentrations and represent the sites of inflammation in IBD[7]; similarly, pouchitis, the non-specific inflammation of the ileal reservoir after ileo–anal anastomosis, appears to be associated with bacterial overgrowth and dysbiosis. Enteric bacteria or their products have been found within the inflamed mucosa of patients with Crohn's disease (CD).

There is evidence of a loss of immunological tolerance to the enteric flora in IBD[8,9]. Decreasing bacterial concentration with antibiotics or faecal stream diversion decrease activity in CD, with disease recurrence occurring after restoration of faecal stream[10]. Patients with pouchitis may also be effectively treated with antibiotics. Additionally, recent studies have shown the ability of luminal contents, presumably dominated by bacteria or their products, to trigger post-operative recurrence of CD in the neoterminal ileum within a few days[11]. But the most compelling evidence is derived from animal models; despite great diversity in genetic defects and immunopathology, a consistent feature of many transgenic and knockout mutant murine models of colitis is dependency on the presence of normal enteric flora for full expression of inflammation[12].

All these observations have suggested that it may be possible to prevent or treat IBD by manipulating intestinal microflora, and increasing evidence supports a potential therapeutic role of probiotics in IBD[13].

Encouraging results have been obtained with probiotic therapy in experimental colitis. Administration of *Lactobacillus reuteri* was shown to significantly reduce inflammation in acetic acid- and methotrexate-induced colitis in rats[14,15]. More recently, *Lactobacillus* spp. were shown to be able to prevent the development of spontaneous colitis in interleukin-10- (IL-10) deficient mice[16], and continuous feeding with *Lactobacillus plantarum* could attenuate an established colitis in the same knockout model[17]. A strain of *Lactobacillus salivarius* (subsp. *salivarius*) reduced the rate of progression from inflammation through dysplasia and colonic cancer in IL-10-deficient mice[18], and a novel strain of bifidobacterium, (*B. longum*) was able to attenuate inflammation in a lymphocyte transfer model in severe combined immunodeficient mice[19].

Coming to human data, the efficacy of a non-pathogenic strain of *Escherichia coli* (Nissle 1917) in the treatment of IBD has been tested in four recent trials. In the first pilot study, treatment with capsules containing *E. coli* Nissle 1917 was compared with the administration of placebo in maintenance of steroid-induced remission of colonic CD. Twelve patients were treated with *E. coli* Nissle 1917 and 11 with placebo; at the end of the treatment period (12 weeks), relapse rates were 33% in the *E. coli* group and 63% in the placebo group, but, unfortunately, because of the very small number of patients treated, this difference did not reach statistical significance[20]. In the other three controlled studies, *E. coli* Nissle 1917 has been found to exhibit efficacy similar to that of mesalazine in the maintenance treatment of ulcerative colitis (UC). But the short follow-up period of only 3 months and the low dose of mesalazine used in the first study, the heterogeneous group of patients, the low dose of mesalazine in the prevention of relapse part of the study and the high relapse rate in both groups (about 70%) in the second study, and the low dose of mesalazine used in the third study, limit, at least partially, the findings of these studies[21–23].

In a small comparative controlled trial, Guslandi *et al.* have evaluated the efficacy of *Saccharomyces boulardii* in maintenance treatment of CD[24]. Thirty-two patients with CD in remission were randomized to receive either mesalazine (3 g/day) or the association of mesalazine (2 g/day) and *Saccharomyces boulardii* (1 g/day). After a period of 6 months, 37% of patients receiving mesalazine alone and 6.2% of patients treated with the combined treatment had relapsed[24].

We have recently explored another strategy using a probiotic preparation (VSL#3) characterized by a very high bacterial concentration and the presence of a cocktail of eight different bacterial species. This product contains 300 billions/g of viable lyophilized bacteria of four strains of lactobacilli (*L. casei*, *L. plantarum*, *L. acidophilus*, *L. delbrueckii* subsp. *bulgaricus*), three strains of bifidobacteria (*B. longum*, *B. breve*, *B. infantis*) and one strain of *Streptococcus salivarius* subsp. *thermophilus*. Every strain of probiotic bacteria has different and specialized metabolic activities and, in theory, a composite mixture of a large number of different strains, with potential synergistic relationships, could represent the ideal treatment.

Firstly, we carried out a pilot study using VSL#3 as maintenance treatment in patients with UC in remission, allergic or intolerant to sulphasalazine and mesalazine to verify the impact of this preparation on the faecal flora. Twenty patients received 6 g/day of VSL#3 for 12 months and were assessed clinically and endoscopically at baseline and at 6 and 12 months or if relapse occurred. Stool culture and determination of faecal pH were also performed at different intervals. Microbiological determination showed a significant increase in concentration of lactobacilli, bifidobacteria and *Streptococcus thermophilus*, which was evident already after 20 days and persisted through the treatment period with a return to basal levels within 15 days after stopping treatment, with no modification of faecal concentration of *Bacteroides*, enterococci, coliforms, *Clostridia* or total anaerobes and aerobes. Faecal pH was significantly reduced by the treatment and 15 of the 20 patients (75%) remained in remission[25].

This preparation has also been tested in experimental models of colitis. In collaboration with Rachmilewitz and colleagues, we have shown a significant attenuation of inflammation with a decrease of MPO (myeloperoxidase) and NOS (nitric oxide synthase) activity in iodoacetamide-induced colitis in rats[26], while Madsen and colleagues have reported a significant improvement in inflammation together with a reduction in mucosal levels of proinflammatory cytokines and a normalization of colonic barrier integrity in IL-10 KO mice[27].

In a double-blind study we have, subsequently, compared the efficacy of this probiotic preparation with placebo in the maintenance treatment of chronic pouchitis. Forty patients who obtained clinical and endoscopic remission after 1 month of combined antibiotic treatment were randomized to receive VSL#3 6 g daily or an identical-appearing placebo for 9 months. Clinical assessment was made every month; endoscopic and histological assessment were performed at entry and every 2 months. Stool culture was done before and after antibiotic treatment and subsequently every month during maintenance treatment. Relapse was defined as an increase of at least 2 points in the clinical portion of pouchitis activity index and should be confirmed endoscopically and histologically. All 20 patients treated with placebo had a relapse during the follow-up period; in contrast, 17 of the 20 patients treated with VSL#3 were still in remission after 9 months. Interestingly, all these 17 patients had a relapse within 4 months after suspension of the active treatment. Faecal concentrations of lactobacilli, bifidobacteria and *Streptococcus salivarius* subsp. *thermophilus* were significantly increased within 1 month after starting VSL#3 treatment and remained stable throughout the study but this increase did not affect the concentration of the other bacterial groups, suggesting that the effect was not mediated by suppression of endogenous luminal bacteria[28].

With regard to the mechanisms of action, in these patients, we found that continuous administration of VSL#3 determined a significant increase in IL-10 tissue levels together with a significant decrease in tissue levels of proinflammatory cytokines, TNF-α, IL-1 and IFN-γ, and a decrease in matrix metalloproteinase activity[29].

We have also carried out a double-blind placebo-controlled trial to evaluate the efficacy of VSL#3 in the prevention of pouchitis onset in patients operated for ileal pouch–anal anastomosis (IPAA) for UC. Forty patients, within 1 week after ileostomy closure, were randomized to receive VSL#3 3 g/day or an identical placebo for 12 months; patients were assessed clinically, endoscopically and histologically at 1, 3, 6, 9 and 12 months according to PDAI.

Patients treated with VSL#3 had a significantly lower incidence of acute pouchitis compared with those treated with placebo during the first year after ileostomy closure (10% vs. 40%; $p < 0.05$)[30].

Finally, we carried out a single-blind study to compare a combined antibiotic–probiotic treatment with mesalazine in the prevention of postoperative recurrence of CD; 40 patients, within 1 week after curative surgery, were randomized to receive a high dose of rifaximin, a non-absorbable wide-spectrum antibiotic, for 3 months, followed by VSL#3, 6 g/day for 9 months, or mesalazine, 4 g/day for 12 months. Patients were assessed clinically and endoscopically at 3 and 12 months; the combined antibiotic–probiotic treatment resulted in a significantly lower incidence of severe endoscopic recurrence both at 3 and 12 months (respectively 10% and 20% vs. 40% and 40%; $p < 0.01$)[31].

CONCLUSIONS

Many clinical and experimental observations do suggest an involvement of the intestinal microflora in the pathogenesis and the perpetuation of IBD.

Probiotics may provide a simple and attractive way to treat IBD, and patients find the probiotic concept appealing. Highly concentrated probiotics are a valid approach for prevention of pouchitis onset and relapse. The encouraging results obtained in ulcerative colitis and Crohn's disease need to be assessed further in large double-blind trials.

It is, however, important to select a well-characterized probiotic preparation; in fact, the viability and survival of many available preparations are unproven.

Future research on probiotic bacteria needs to be focused on a better understanding of the composition of enteric flora or 'the neglected organ', and of the intestinal physiology and its relationship with the luminal ecosystem. This information will allow the fulfilment of the therapeutic potential of probiotics.

References

1. Metchnikoff E. The Prolongation of Life: Optimistic Studies: Mitchell C, ed. London: William Heinemann, 1907:161–83.
2. Tissier H. Traitement des infections intestinales par la méthode de la flore bactérienne de l'intestin. CR Soc Biol. 1906;60:359–61.
3. Lilly DM, Stillwell RH. Probiotics: growth promoting factors produced by microorganisms. Science. 1965;47:747–8.
4. Fuller R. Probiotics in human medicine. Gut. 1991;32:439–42.
5. Schaafsma G. State of the art concerning probiotic strains in milk products. IDF Nutr Newslett. 1996;5:23–4.
6. Lee YK, Salminen S. The coming age of probiotics. Trends Food Sci Technol. 1995;6:241–5.
7. Sartor RB. Enteric microflora in IBD: pathogens or commensals? Inflamm Bowel Dis. 1997;3:230–5.
8. Duchmann R, Kaiser I, Hermann E, Mayet W, Ewe K, Meyer zum Buschenfelde K-H. Tolerance exists towards resident intestinal flora but is broken in active inflammatory bowel disease (IBD). Clin Exp Immunol. 1995;102:104–8.
9. MacPherson A, Khoo UY, Forgacs I, Philpott-Howard J, Bjarnason I. Mucosal antibodies in inflammatory bowel disease are directed against intestinal bacteria. Gut. 1996;38:365–75.
10. Janowitz HD, Croen EC, Sachar DB. The role of the faecal stream in Crohn's disease: an historical and analytic perspective. Inflamm Bowel Dis. 1998;4:29–39.
11. D'Haens GR, Geboes K, Peeters M, Penninckx F, Rutgeers SP. Early lesions of recurrent Crohn's disease caused by infusion of intestinal contents in excluded ileum. Gastroenterology. 1998;114:771–4.
12. Sartor RB. Insights into the pathogenesis of inflammatory bowel disease provided by new rodent models of spontaneous colitis. Inflamm Bowel Dis. 1995;1:64–75.
13. Campieri M, Gionchetti P. Probiotics in inflammatory bowel disease: New insight to pathogenesis or a possible therapeutic alternative? Gastroenterology. 1999;116:1246–9.
14. Fabia R, Ar'rajab A, Johansson M-L *et al*. The effect of exogenous administration of *Lactobacillus reuterii* R2LC and oat fiber on acetic acid-induced colitis in the rat. Scand J Gastroenterol. 1993;28:155–62.

15. Mao Y, Nobaek S, Kasravi B *et al.* The effects of *Lactobacillus* strains and oat fibre on methotrexate-induced enterocolitis in rats. Gastroenterology. 1996;111:334–44.
16. Madsen KL, Tavernini MM, Doyle JSG, Fedorak RN. *Lactobacillus* sp prevents development of enterocolitis in interleukin-10 gene-deficient mice. Gastroenterology. 1999;116:1107–14.
17. Schultz M, Veltkamp C, Dieleman LA, Wyrick PB, Tonkonogy SL, Sartor RB. Continuous feeding of *Lactobacillus plantarum* attenuates established colitis in interleukin-10 deficient mice. Gastroenterology. 1998;114:A1081.
18. Collins JK, Murphy L, O'Mahony L, Dunne C, O'Sullivan GC, Shanahan F. A controlled trial of probiotic treatment of IL-10 knockout mice (abstr.). Gastroenterology. 1999;116:G2981.
19. Murphy L, Byrne F, Collins JK, Shanahan F, O'Sullivan GC, Aranda R. Evaluation and characterisation of probiotic therapy in the CD45RBhi transfer model of colitis. Gastroenterology. 1999;20:387–90.
20. Malchow HA. Crohn's disease and Escherichia coli. A new approach in therapy to maintain remission of colonic Crohn's disease? J Clin Gastroenterol. 1997;25:653–8.
21. Kruis W, Schuts E, Fric P, Fixa B, Judmaier G, Stolte M. Double-blind comparison of an oral Escherichia coli preparation and mesalazine in maintaining remission of ulcerative colitis. Aliment Pharmacol Ther. 1997;11:853–8.
22. Rembacken BJ, Snelling AM, Hawkey P, Chalmers DM, Axon TR. Non pathogenic Escherichia coli vs mesalazine for the treatment of ulcerative colitis: a randomised trial. Lancet. 1999;354: 635–9.
23. Kruis W, Fric P, Stolte M. Maintenance of remission in ulcerative colitis is equally effective with *Escherichia Coli Nissle 1917* and with standard mesalamine. Gastroenterology. 2001; 120 suppl:A127.
24. Guslandi M, Mezzi G, Sorghi M *et al.* *Saccharomyces boulardii* in maintenance treatment of Crohn's disease. Dig Dis Sci. 2000;45:1462–4.
25. Venturi A, Gionchetti P, Rizzello F *et al.* Impact on the faecal flora composition of a new probiotic preparation. Preliminary data on maintenance treatment of patients with ulcerative colitis (UC) intolerant or allergic to 5-aminosalicylic acid (5 ASA). Aliment Pharmacol Ther. 1999;13: 1103–8.
26. Shibolet O, Karmeli F, Eliakim R *et al.* Probiotics ameliorate iodoacetamide-induced colitis. Gastroenterology. 1999;116:A818.
27. Madsen K, Cornish A, Soper P *et al.* Probiotic bacteria enhance murine and human intestinal epithelial barrier function. Gastroenterology. 2001;121:580–91.
28. Gionchetti P, Rizzello F, Venturi A *et al.* Oral bacteriotherapy as maintenance treatment in patients with chronic pouchitis: a double-blind, placebo-controlled trial. Gastroenterology. 2000;119:305–9.
29. Ulisse S, Gionchetti P, D'Alò S *et al.* Increased expression of cytokines, inducible nitric oxide synthase and matrix metalloproteinases in pouchitis: effects of probiotic treatment (VSL#3). Gastroenterology. 2001;120 suppl:A281.
30. Gionchetti P, Rizzello F, Venturi A *et al.* Prophylaxis of pouchitis onset with probiotic therapy: a double blind, placebo controlled trial. (Abstr.) Gastroenterology. 2000;118:A190.
31. Campieri M, Rizzello F, Venturi A *et al.* Combination of antibiotic and probiotic treatment is efficacious in prophylaxis of post-operative recurrence of Crohn's disease: a randomised controlled study vs mesalazine. Gastroenterology. 2000;118:A781.

Section V
Refractory CD

23
Prevention and management of postoperative recurrence in Crohn's disease

G. D'HAENS

INTRODUCTION

The incidence of Crohn's disease recurrence following 'curative' resection is high. The disease almost invariably recurs on the ileal side of the ileocolonic anastomosis, although rectal and colonic recurrence have also been reported. The clinical picture of recurrent disease resembles that of the preoperative disease. We will review medical therapies tested to prevent postoperative recurrence and/or reoperation. Many clinical trials have shown that the benefit from mesalamine therapy is rather limited. Immunosuppressives, such as 6-mercaptopurine or azathioprine, seem to be more promising. Nitro-imidazole antibiotics reduce the severity of endoscopic and clinical relapse. The answer to the question if all patients operated on for Crohn's disease need prophylactic treatment depends on a number of variables and strategies which will be discussed in the last part of this chapter.

DIAGNOSIS OF EARLY CROHN'S DISEASE RECURRENCE

Postoperative recurrence of Crohn's disease can be defined as clinical, endoscopic or radiological recurrence. The incidence of clinical recurrence of Crohn's disease averages about 10% of all operated patients per year postoperatively[1,2], although Olaison and colleagues reported clinical recurrence in up to one third of their patients as early as 3 months following surgery[3]. The use of clinical parameters to diagnose recurrence, however, has serious shortcomings, for certain symptoms (e.g. diarrhoea) can be a consequence of the surgical resection itself, and the variability in individual perception and interpretation of symptoms can be significant. The need for repeated surgery ('surgical recurrence') is, fortunately, much lower, varying between 16% and 65% at 10 years after the first resection[4,5]. Undoubtedly, endoscopic examination has been the most sensitive method to document significant recurrence. Signs of early recurrent Crohn's disease have been observed in 73% to 93% of all patients at 1 year, and in 85% of all patients at 3 years, postoperatively[3,6]. The ensuing clinical disease course correlates well with the endoscopic appearance of the neoterminal ileum 1 year after surgery[6]. Because of this correlation, ileocolonoscopy has become the gold standard to document recurrence and to assess its severity. The majority of recent pharmaceutical recurrence prevention trials has indeed used endoscopic parameters as an endpoint. Endoscopic recurrence can be classified as mild or severe, but a more detailed score developed by Rutgeerts *et al.* allows a more precise classification. A score of 'i0' ('i' stands for 'ileal') means absence of any lesion, 'i1' fewer than 5 aphthous ulcers (<5 mm), 'i2' more than 5 aphthous ulcers with normal mucosa between the lesions OR lesions confined to the ileocolonic anastomosis (<1 cm), 'i3' diffuse aphthous ileitis with diffusely inflamed mucosa and 'i4' diffuse ileitis with larger ulcers, nodularity and/or narrowing[6].

The ultimate goal of recurrence prevention consists of a reduction in clinical recurrence and reoperation and an improvement in quality of life when compared with untreated patients. The main problem when studying this phenomenon is the sometimes long delay between surgery and clinical recurrence. For this reason, a reduction in endoscopic lesions in the first 1 or 2 years following surgery has been considered a valuable aim, which probably predicts a more benign clinical course. This concept which is based on the Leuven studies has recently been questioned and merits further confirmation[7].

RISK FACTORS FOR RECURRENCE

The risk profile of the individual patient should play an important part in the decisions whether or not and how to treat Crohn's disease patients prophylactically. Recurrence rates are higher, for instance, in patients operated at a younger age than in those undergoing a resection at an older age[8]. Patients with a preoperative disease history of more than 10 years at the time of surgical intervention do better than those with a shorter disease history[9]. Smoking is also associated with higher recurrence rates, particularly in female patients[10,11]. Patients with combined ileocolonic disease suffer higher recurrence rates than those with predominantly ileal disease[12] or with isolated colonic disease[13]. Finally, the behaviour of Crohn's disease appears to be a determining risk factor for recurrence. The time to reoperation ('surgical recurrence') is significantly shorter in patients operated on for perforating as opposed to non-perforating disease[14].

MEDICAL PROPHYLAXIS OF CROHN'S DISEASE RECURRENCE

Since many indicators point towards the persistence of minimal disease in the macroscopically 'healthy' residual gut, medical strategies should be targeted at the suppression of this minimal inflammation and the prevention of macroscopic lesions which lead to symptoms. Although the mechanisms involved in 'established disease' may be different from those in early recurrent disease[15], the drugs used to prevent recurrence are the same as the ones used to maintain remission in full-blown Crohn's disease. Nonetheless, one of the most potent acute anti-inflammatory therapies for Crohn's disease, namely corticosteroids, has been ineffective to prevent postoperative recurrence. In a randomized placebo-controlled and double-blind study with budesonide vs. placebo, recurrence rates were not lower in the budesonide group, except when patients operated on for 'active disease' were analysed separately[16]. Similarly, in a placebo-controlled trial with IL-10 given subcutaneously for the first 3 months following surgery, no difference between IL-10 treatment and placebo was observed. The latter study, however, had a limited follow-up of only 3 months and comprised a large subgroup of patients operated on for inactive obstructive disease, which is a situation in which recurrence appears later anyway[17]. Significant reduction in recurrence rates has been observed with aminosalicylates, antibiotics and the immunosuppressive drugs like 6-mercaptopurine.

Sulphasalazine and 5-aminosalicylates

By far the largest number of recurrence prevention trials has been performed with mesalamine (5-ASA). This medication is considered safe and well-tolerated but is rather expensive when used chronically in appropriate doses and its benefit as a maintenance agent for full-blown Crohn's disease is questionable[18–20]. Post-operative prevention studies with 5-ASA have produced varying results, possibly because of different pharmacological preparations, different doses and time points for the start of the postoperative treatment (from less than 10 days to 8 weeks following surgery). In addition, endpoints of the studies differed in that they used endoscopic, clinical and/or radiological endpoints as primary criteria (Table 1).

Ewe and colleagues showed that the parent drug of mesalamine, sulphasalazine, was significantly more effective than placebo in the first 2 years of therapy for maintaining clinical remission of Crohn's disease after resection[21]. Surprisingly, their recurrence rates were higher in the group of patients treated with radical resection than in those with more limited resections. Both strategies were additive: non-radical operation and sulphasalazine had the best prognosis[21].

Table 1 Prevention of postoperative recurrence with 5-ASA

Reference	*Product*	*Dose*	*Start*	*Endpoint*	*Result*
Florent *et al.*[26]	Claversal	3 g/d	<15 days	Endo 12 weeks	50% vs. 63% (NS)
Fiasse *et al.*[27]	Eudragit 5-ASA	3 g/d	3 mo	RX 12 mo Clin 12 mo	NS NS
Caprilli *et al.*[22]	Asacol	2.4 g/d	<15 days	Endo 6, 12, 24 mo	24 mo: 52% vs. 85% ($p < 0.002$)
				Clin 6, 12, 24 mo	24 mo:18% vs. 41% ($p = 0.006$)
Brignola *et al.*[24]	Pentasa	3 g/d	<30 days	Endo 12 mo	Severe 24% vs. 56% ($p < 0.008$)
McLeod *et al.*[23]	Salofalk	3 g/d	<8 weeks	Endo+clin+RX	Clin 3 years 27% vs. 47%
Lochs *et al.*[25]	Pentasa	4 g/d	<10 days	Clin 18 mo	NS except for small bowel alone

clin = clinical criteria; endo = endoscopic criteria; RX = radiological criteria; mo = months.

Caprilli and colleagues demonstrated a preventive effect of 2.4 g/d Asacol, with a significant reduction in the 2-year endoscopic and clinical recurrence rate[22]. The authors observed a 39% prevention of all recurrences and 55% prevention of severe recurrences. This study, however, was not placebo-controlled and the recurrence rates in the no-treatment group were rather low[22]. A large Canadian multicentre trial with an appropriate placebo group confirmed these results to a certain extent: the overall 3-year symptomatic recurrence was 27% on 1.5 g mesalamine (Salofalk) twice daily started within 8 weeks after curative resection as compared with 47% on placebo. The most important limitation of this study was the time point at which therapy was initiated. Eight weeks after surgery, some patients undoubtedly already had microscopic (and endoscopic) signs of Crohn's recurrence. Based on the placebo results in this study, one could argue that 53% of the patients received unnecessary treatment for 3 years[23].

Mesalamine in a slow-release formulation (Pentasa) was compared with placebo in a double-blind Italian multicentre trial and more recently in the German–Austrian ECCDS IV study. In the Italian study with 3 g/d Pentasa, severe endoscopic recurrence was documented in 56% of the placebo patients versus in 24% of the Pentasa patients ($p < 0.004$) after 12 months, although the clinical relapse rate was not significantly reduced[24]. In the ECCDS trial with 4 g/d Pentasa, only clinical parameters (CDAI) were used to determine recurrence and all types of resections for CD were included. After 18 months, clinical relapse rates were not significantly lower in Pentasa- than in placebo-treated patients. Subgroup analysis, however, did show a significant effect on patients operated on for small bowel disease alone[25].

Another trial used Claversal (Eudragit-coated 5-ASA) at a dose of 3 g/d for 12 weeks following surgery. There was a slight, though insignificant, trend toward greater benefit with Claversal (50% vs. 63% endoscopic signs of recurrence, $p=0.16$)[26]. The same drug at a dose of 1.5 g/d, started as late as 3 months after resection, was studied by Fiasse *et al.* There was no significant difference in clinical or radiological recurrence rates in the patients who completed the trial[27]. In a meta-analysis adjusted for confounding variables, the advantage of taking mesalamine in the postoperative setting of Crohn's disease was estimated to offer a reduction in recurrence rates of approximately 13%[20].

Nitroimidazole antibiotics

Metronidazole is effective to control active Crohn's disease[28,29]. It has also been shown that high concentrations of anaerobic bacteria are present in the terminal ileum in Crohn's disease after ileal resection, and that bacterial antigens may possibly play a role in the induction of Crohn's inflammation[30,31]. For these reasons, Rutgeerts and colleagues performed a controlled trial with metronidazole, 20 mg kg^{-1} d^{-1}, or placebo started within a week after resection and continued for 3 months[32]. At 12 weeks, 75% of patients had recurrent lesions in the neoterminal ileum in the placebo group vs. 52% in the metronidazole group. Interestingly, metronidazole reduced the clinical recurrence rates at 1 year (4% vs. 25%), but not at 2 and 3 years. Unfortunately, the rate of adverse events in the metronidazole-treated patients was considerable[32]. A comparable beneficial effect of nitroimidazole antibiotics on endoscopic recurrence was recently demonstrated in the preliminary results of a trial with ornidazole (Roche, Tiberal) 500 mg bid given for a full year after surgery. At 3 months, 74% of placebo-treated patients had severe endoscopic recurrence (i2–i4) versus 41% of ornidazole-treated patients ($p = 0.02$). At 1 year, 94% of the placebo patients had i2–i4 vs. 62% of the ornidazole patients[33]. Given the toxicity of nitroimidazole antibiotics when given for a long time and/or in high doses, they can probably only be used as initial short-term prevention therapy.

Immunosuppressives: 6-mercaptopurine

Immunomodulators like azathioprine and 6-mercaptopurine are the most potent agents in the maintenance treatment of Crohn's disease[18,34,35]. It was therefore logical that the benefit of these agents to prevent postsurgical recurrence was tested. One hundred and eighteen patients were enrolled in a North American–European multicentre trial with randomization to 50 mg 6-mercaptopurine/d, 3 g Pentasa (12 × 250 mg tablets)/d or placebo in a double-blind, double-dummy fashion. Follow-up lasted 2 years with clinical check-ups and ileocolonoscopies 6, 12 and 24 months after surgery. During the trial, a considerable number of patients dropped out of the study because of adverse events or lack of compliance (16 in the Pentasa group, 16 in the 6-MP group and 11 in the placebo group). Intent-to-treat analysis showed absence of endoscopic relapse in 32% of the patients on 6-MP (p=0.04), in 20% on Pentasa (NS) and in 10% on placebo at 2 years. Severe endoscopic relapse at 2 years (score >i2) was more frequently observed with placebo and Pentasa than with 6-MP (p=0.01 vs. placebo and 0.07 vs. Pentasa). The clinical relapse rate was reduced by both Pentasa and 6-MP but statistical significance was only achieved with 6-MP (p=0.04). The authors concluded that 6-MP is the strongest recurrence prevention therapy up to date and that higher doses may lead to even lower recurrence rates[36].

Besides their efficacy to prevent severe recurrence, immunosuppressives have also been useful in the treatment of *established* recurrent ileitis, not only to control symptoms but also to induce mucosal healing[37]. Patients who undergo balloon dilation of an anastomotic stenosis have longer remissions if they are treated with a short course of budesonide CIR and further azathioprine maintenance than if they remain untreated[38].

SURGICAL PROPHYLAXIS OF CROHN'S DISEASE RECURRENCE

Surgeons have looked at various strategies to decrease the risk of postsurgical recurrence. A recent clinical trial where patients were randomized to 2- or 10-cm margins performed at the Cleveland clinic detected no difference in recurrence rates[39]. The type of anastomosis (end-to-end vs. end-to-side ileocolonic anastomosis) also has no effect on the rate of recurrence[40]. In some centres, an end-to-end ileocolonic anastomosis is preferred because anastomotic strictures can be treated endoscopically more easily with this construction. Finally, the presence of microscopic signs of inflammation at the resection margin does not affect recurrence either[41]. Given these findings, resections should be as limited as possible and surgically safe.

A STRATEGY FOR THE PREVENTION AND THE TREATMENT OF ILEAL RECURRENCE OF CROHN'S DISEASE

Based on all the available evidence, we do not think it is necessary to treat every patient operated on for Crohn's disease prophylactically. Patients should be stratified according to their risk profile for recurrence. Those with a low risk profile for recurrence (non-smokers, first resection, fibrostenotic disease) do not receive treatment at our centre but are advised to undergo an ileocolonoscopy 6–12 months after surgery. In cases with no or mild endoscopic lesions, patients are reassured about the unlikelihood of serious future problems and remain untreated. If more severe endoscopic lesions are present and the patient is free of symptoms, we institute treatment with a 5-ASA preparation at a dose of 3–4 g/d. In patients with both severe endoscopic lesions (i3 or i4) and symptoms, we immediately start with a 3-month course of budesonide CIR and azathioprine 2–2.5 mg kg^{-1} day^{-1}. The same strategy is followed in patients undergoing balloon dilatation of the ileocolonic anastomosis in the presence of severe ileitis.

Patients with a high risk of early recurrence are approached differently. If they undergo a second, third or fourth resection, or if they undergo surgery for medically intractable disease, they will immediately be started on azathioprine, often accompanied by metronidazole 250 mg tid in the first 3 months. Patients already taking azathioprine will be kept on it (Figure 1).

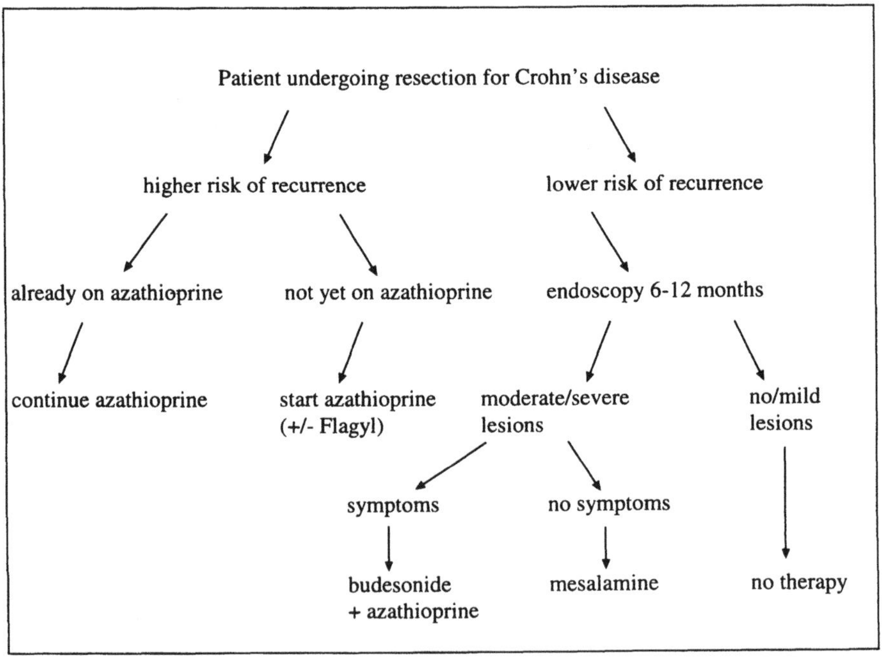

Figure 1 Algorithm for an approach to patients operated on for Crohn's disease

CONCLUSION

The large number of studies looking at risk factors for postoperative recurrence of Crohn's disease allows us to estimate the individual risk and to stratify patients with regard to the need for prophylactic treatment. The findings at an early ileocolonoscopy provide relevant information about the further clinical course. In patients with a low risk, recurrence prevention is not always necessary, although maintenance therapy with mesalamine may be of benefit. High-risk patients or early relapsers are preferably treated with immunomodulators, such as azathioprine or 6-MP, initially in combination with metronidazole (immediately after surgery) or with budesonide (in the presence of symptoms).

References

1. Kyle J. Prognosis after ileal resection for Crohn's disease. Br J Surg. 1971;58:735–7.
2. Lennard-Jones JE, Stalder GA. Prognosis after resection of chronic regional enteritis. Gut. 1967;8:332–6.
3. Olaison G, Smedh K. Sjödahl R. Natural course of Crohn's disease after ileocolic resection: endoscopically visualized ileal ulcers preceding symptoms. Gut. 1992;33:331–5.
4. Greenstein AJ, Sachar DB, Pasternack BS, Janowitz HD. Reoperation and recurrence in Crohn's colitis and ileocolitis. N Engl J Med. 1975;293:685–90.
5. Whelan G, Farmer RG, Fazio VW, Goormastic M. Recurrence after surgery in Crohn's disease. Gastroenterology. 1985;88:1826–33.
6. Rutgeerts P, Geboes K, Vantrappen G *et al.* Predictability of the postoperative course of Crohn's disease. Gastroenterology. 1990;99:956–63.
7. McLeod RS, Wolff B, Steinhart H *et al.* Risk and significance of endoscopic/radiological evidence of recurrent Crohn's disease. Gastroenterology. 1997;113:1823–7.
8. Hellers G. Crohn's disease in Stockholm Country 1955–1974. A study of epidemiology, results of surgical treatment and long-term prognosis. Acta Chir Scand. 1979;490(suppl.):5–81.
9. Baker WNW. The results of ileorectal anastomosis at St. Mark's Hospital from 1953 to 1968. Gut. 1970;11:235–9.
10. Sutherland LR, Ramcharan S, Bryant H *et al.* Effect of cigarette smoking on recurrence of Crohn's disease. Gastroenterology. 1990;98:1123–8.
11. Cottone M, Rosselli M, Orlando A *et al.* Smoking habits and recurrence in Crohn's disease. Gastroenterology. 1994;106:643–8.
12. Griffiths AM, Wesson DE, Shandling B *et al.* Factors influencing postoperative recurrence of Crohn's disease in childhood. Gut. 1991;32:491–5.
13. Caprilli R, Corroa G, Taddei G *et al.* Prognostic factors for postoperative recurrence of Crohn's disease. Dis Col Rect. 1996;39:335–41.
14. Aeberhard P, Berchtold W, Riedtmann HJ *et al.* Surgical recurrence of perforating and nonperforating Crohn's disease. Dis Col Rect. 1996;39:80–7.
15. Desreumaux P, Brandt E, Gambiez L *et al.* Distinct cytokine patterns in early and chronic ileal lesions of Crohn's disease. Gastroenterology. 1997;113:118–26.
16. Hellers G, Cortot A, Jewell D *et al.* Oral budesonide for prevention of postsurgical recurrence in Crohn's disease. Gastroenterology. 1999;116:294–300.
17. Colombel JF, Rutgeerts P, Malchow H *et al.* Safety and tolerance of subcutaneous recombinant human interleukin-10 in subjects with Crohn's disease after first ileal or ileocolonic resection. Gut. 2001;49:42–6.
18. D'Haens G, Rutgeerts P. Maintenance and prophylactic therapy for Crohn's disease. Curr Opin Gastroenterol. 1997;13:312–16.
19. Sutherland LR, Martin F, Bailey RJ *et al.* and the Canadian Mesalamine for Remission Study Group. A randomized, placebo-controlled, double-blind trial of mesalamine in the maintenance of remission of Crohn's disease. Gastroenterology. 1997;112:1069–77.
20. Camma C, Giunta M, Roselli M, Cottone M. Mesalamine in the maintenance treatment of Crohn's disease: a meta-analysis adjusted for confounding variables. Gastroenterology. 1997; 113:1465–73.

21. Ewe K, Herfarth C, Malchow H *et al.* Postoperative recurrence of Crohn's disease in relation to radicality of operation and sulfasalazine prophylaxis: a multicenter trial. Digestion. 1989;42: 224–32.
22. Caprilli R, Andreoli A, Capurso L *et al.* Oral mesalazine (Asacol) for the prevention of postoperative recurrence of Crohn's disease. Eur J Gastroenterol Hepatol. 1994;8:35–43.
23. McLeod RS, Wolff BG, Steinhart AH *et al.* Prophylactic mesalamine treatment decreases postoperative recurrence of Crohn's disease. Gastroenterology. 1995;109:404–13.
24. Brignola C, Cottone M, Pera A *et al.* Mesalamine in the prevention of endoscopic recurrence after intestinal resection for Crohn's disease. Gastroenterology. 1995;108:345–9.
25. Lochs H, Mayer M, Fleig WE *et al.* Prophylaxis of postoperative relapse in Crohn's disease with mesalazine (Pentasa) in comparison to placebo. Gastroenterology. 2000;118:264–73.
26. Florent C, Cortot A, Quandale P *et al.* Placebo-controlled clinical trial of mesalazine in the prevention of early endoscopic recurrences after resection for Crohn's disease. Eur J Gastroenterol Hepatol. 1996;8:229–33.
27. Fiasse R, Fontaine F, Vanheuverzwyn R. Prevention of Crohn's disease recurrences after intestinal resection with Eudragit-L-coated 5-ASA. Gastroenterology. 1991;100:A208.
28. Ursing B, Kamme G. Metronidazole for Crohn's disease. Lancet. 1975;1:775–7.
29. Blichfeldt P, Blomhoff JP, Myhre E, Gjone E. Metronidazole in Crohn's disease. Scand J Gastroenterol. 1978;13:123–7.
30. Rath HC, Herfarth HH, Ikeda JS *et al.* Normal luminal bacteria, especially Bacteroides species, mediate chronic colitis, gastritis and arthritis in HLA-B27/β2 microglobulin transgenic rats. J Clin Invest. 1996;98:945–53.
31. Gorbach SL, Tabaqchali S. Bacteria, bile and the small bowel. Gut. 1969;10:963–71.
32. Rutgeerts P, Peeters M, Hiele M *et al.* A placebo controlled trial of metronidazole for recurrence prevention of Crohn's disease after resection of the terminal ileum. Gastroenterology. 1995;108:1617–21.
33. Rutgeerts P, D'Haens G, Baert F *et al.* Nitroimidazol antibiotics are efficacious for prophylaxis of postoperative recurrence of Crohn's disease: a placebo controlled trial. Gastroenterology. 1999;116:A808.
34. Willoughby JM, Beckett J, Kumar PJ, Dawson AM. Controlled trial of azathioprine in Crohn's disease. Lancet. 1971;2:944–7.
35. Present DH, Korelitz BI, Wisch N *et al.* Treatment of Crohn's disease with 6-mercaptopurine. A long-term randomized double-blind study. N Engl J Med. 1980;302:981–7.
36. Korelitz B, Hanauer S, Rutgeerts P *et al.* Postoperative prophylaxis with 6-MP, 5-ASA or placebo in Crohn's disease: a two year multicenter trial. Gastroenterology. 1998;114:A1011.
37. D'Haens G, Geboes K, Ponette E *et al.* Healing of severe recurrent ileitis with azathioprine therapy in patients with Crohn's disease. Gastroenterology. 1997;112:1475–81.
38. Raedler A, Peters I, Screiber S. Treatment with azathioprine and budesonide prevents reoccurence of ileocolonic stenosis after endoscopic dilatation in Crohn's disease. Gastroenterology. 1997;112:A1067.
39. McLeod RS. Is it possible to prevent recurrent Crohn's disease with medical or surgical interventions? Neth J Med. 1996;48:68–70.
40. Cameron JL, Hamilton SR, Coleman J *et al.* Patterns of ileal recurrence in Crohn's disease. Ann Surg. 1992;215:546–51.
41. Kotanagi HH, Kramer K, Fazio VW, Petras RE. Do microscopic abnormalities at resection margins correlate with increased anastomotic recurrence in Crohn's disease? Retrospective analysis of 100 cases. Dis Colon Rectum. 1991;34:909–16.

24
Refractory Crohn's disease – discussion of the case

M. VECCHI, S. SAIBENI, C. ABBIATI and R. DE FRANCHIS

GENERAL COMMENTS

The course of the disease observed in this lady has been very unfortunate, as is pointed out in her history. First of all, she has been suffering, at different times of her disease, from a pan-enteritis with inflammatory involvement from the duodenum to the entire colon. Although we all know that Crohn's disease may involve the whole GI system, such extensive involvement is rare and duodenal Crohn's disease is observed in less than 10% of patients. Such diffuse involvement in turn reduces the therapeutic options and surgery cannot easily be proposed. Indeed, she has experienced several failures of usually effective therapies, such as methotrexate, infliximab and thalidomide, as well as several rather rare side-effects from other potentially effective drugs leading to treatment discontinuation.

DISEASE REFRACTORINESS

No matter how refractoriness in Crohn's disease is defined there is no doubt that this patient can be considered to have refractory Crohn's disease. In general, when we are confronted by refractory disease, a re-evaluation of the diagnosis should be carefully considered and this should also be performed in this lady.

DIAGNOSTIC CONSIDERATIONS

Although it is extremely improbable that intestinal tuberculosis might persist for so many years and after so many immunomodulating treatments without being complicated by overt infection and miliary diffusion, an extensive search for mycobacterial agents should be performed in this lady by means of cultural and molecular methods, both on ileal effluents and on intestinal biopsies. Indeed, this patient appeared to have poor therapeutic response to usually highly effective treatments; many treatments have been detrimental to her disease. In addition, tubercular infection has shown a sharp increase in incidence in the last 20 years in western countries, due both to the migration of populations from countries where endemic infection exists and to the diffusion of acquired immunodeficiency[1]. One should also bear in mind that around 80% of intestinal tubercular infections occur without any evidence of current or past pulmonary infection. Other, even less probable diagnostic possibilities that need to be ruled out in this case include ischaemic enteritis and mesenteric vasculitides.

THERAPEUTIC CONSIDERATIONS

As previously stated, many forms of therapy have been ineffective in the treatment of this lady. Other drugs have caused severe side-effects, leading to treatment discontinuation. The results of the drugs utilized in this case are summarized in Table 1. The only drugs that appear to have given some response in this patient are corticosteroids and IL-10. The latter, however, was used in the course of a clinical trial and, despite a partial (and most probably temporary) clinical improvement, the patient had a caecal perforation at the colonoscopy performed at the end of treatment. Corticosteroids, on the other hand, may have been effective during the early stages of the disease, but, most probably, the patient was addressed to azathioprine due to steroid dependency or steroid resistance.

Thus, should the patient be treated again with steroids, she would most probably become steroid dependent or resistant; in this 65-year-old lady, the chronic use of steroids might be very harmful due to its role in diabetes, osteoporosis and eye cataract. Low-bioavailability steroids are characterized by a fairly good safety profile, with a prevalence of side-effects similar to those reported for placebo, both in short- and long-term treatment. However, a recent meta-analysis[2] has shown that budesonide, the most extensively studied of these molecules, is significantly less effective than traditional steroids in active phases and has no therapeutic advantage over placebo in maintenance treatment.

Thus, a non-steroidal drug effective in the treatment of acute phases should be considered in order to avoid steroids; the possible long-term use of the same drug or of an alternative drug should also be considered for the purpose of maintenance therapy. In general, infliximab would be the drug of choice in this setting, on the basis of its effectiveness in acute phases and the possibility of repeated long-term infusions[3,4]. In the present patient, however, infliximab was neither effective nor safe, inducing an allergic reaction at re-infusion. Moreover, another drug, thalidomide, which is thought to act through the inhibition of TNF[5], had no effect on the disease. Thus, these data indicate that the use of other recently developed anti-TNF therapies, such as the humanized monoclonal antibody CDP-571[6] or the receptor antagonist etanercept[7], although most probably

Table 1 Outcomes of attempted treatments

Effective (partially)	*Ineffective*	*Serious adverse events*
Steroids	Methotrexate	Azathioprine
Interleukin-10	Infliximab	Infliximab
		Thalidomide

safer than infliximab, would be equally useless. Other biological agents that have been recently developed for the treatment of Crohn's or other disimmune diseases, such as IL-11 or GH, have been studied in single trials[8,9] and await confirmation of the results.

Immunosuppressive agents should also be taken into consideration. Cyclosporine A has a potentially rapid effect and may be used for long-term treatments. However, 3 large trials[10–12] using 5 mg kg^{-1} day^{-1} of oral cyclosporine failed to show significant therapeutic advantages over placebo. Tacrolimus showed positive results in several open studies[13,14] and the results of a randomized clinical trial are expected soon. A randomized trial has shown that mycophenolate mofetil has a similar therapeutic effect to that of azathioprine[15–17], with a slight advantage in patients with a high CDAI score at baseline.

'Older' therapeutic modalities, including enteral and parenteral nutrition and surgery, should also be considered. The use of nutritional therapy should be considered in this patient, also because of the probable malabsorption syndrome resulting from extensive involvement of the small bowel. As primary treatments, both parenteral and enteral nutrition have been proposed in Crohn's disease. The enteral route is preferred mainly on the basis of its superior safety profile. In the use of enteral diets, one should, however, bear in mind that enteral formulations are less effective than steroids, particularly on an intention-to-treat analyisis.

A surgical approach to the disease of this patient appears to be difficult, due to the diffuse inflammatory involvement of the small bowel, the previous surgical procedures and the high relapse rate observed in the history. Resection of the diseased bowel would certainly result in short bowel syndrome, leading to the need for life-long parenteral nutrition. An alternative surgical approach would be that of small bowel transplant, which would, however, be hampered by the high rate of rejection and the possibility of disease recurrence.[18]

CONCLUSIONS

In conclusion, a possible flow-chart for this case would include:

1. Diagnostic re-evaluation with particular reference to exclusion of gastrointestinal tuberculosis;
2. A course of traditional (or low-bioavailability) steroids to induce disease remission;
3. The use of mycophenolate mofetil as tentative maintenance treatment;
4. In case of failure of this approach, the use of continuous enteral or parenteral nutrition and, as a last opportunity, surgical resection could be performed followed by total parenteral nutrition.

References

1. Horvath KD, Whelan RL. Intestinal tuberculosis: return of an old disease. Am J Gastroenterol. 1998;93:692–6.
2. Papi C, Luchetti R, Gili L, Montanti S, Koch M, Capurso L. Budesonide in the treatment of Crohn's disease: a meta-analysis. Aliment Pharmacol Ther. 2000;14:1419–28.

3. Targan SR, Hanauer SB, van Deventer SJ *et al.* A short-term study of chimeric monoclonal antibody cA2 to tumor necrosis factor alpha for Crohn's disease. Crohn's Disease cA2 Study Group. N Engl J Med. 1997;337:1029–35.
4. Rutgeerts P, D'Haens G, Targan S *et al.* Efficacy and safety of retreatment with anti-tumor necrosis factor antibody (infliximab) to maintain remission in Crohn's disease. Gastroenterology. 1999;117:761–9.
5. McHugh SM, Rifkin IR, Deighton J *et al.* The immunosuppressive drug thalidomide induces T helper cell type 2 (Th2) and concomitantly inhibits Th1 cytokine production in mitogen- and antigen-stimulated human peripheral blood mononuclear cell cultures. Clin Exp Immunol. 1995;99:160–7.
6. Sandborn WJ, Feagan BG, Hanauer SB *et al.* CDP571 Crohn's Disease Study Group. An engineered human antibody to TNF (CDP571) for active Crohn's disease: a randomised double-blind placebo-controlled trial. Gastroenterology. 2001;120:1330–8.
7. Mikuls TR, Moreland LW. TNF blockade in the treatment of rheumatoid arthritis: infliximab versus etanercept. Exp Opin Pharmacother. 2001;2:75–84.
8. Sands BE, Bank S, Snisky CA *et al.* Preliminary evaluation of safety and activity of recombinant human interleukin 11 in patients with active Crohn's disease. Gastroenterology. 1999;117: 58–64.
9. Slonim AE, Bulone L, Damore MB, Goldberg T, Wingertzahn MA, McKinley MJ. A preliminary study of growth hormone therapy for Crohn's disease. N Engl J Med. 2000;342:1633–7.
10. Stange EF, Modigliani R, Peña AS *et al.* European trial of cyclosporine in chronic active Crohn's disease: a 12-month study. Gastroenterology. 1995;109:774–82.
11. Feagan BG, McDonald JWD, Rochon J *et al.* Low-dose cyclosporine for the treatment of Crohn's disease. N Engl J Med. 1994;330:1846–51.
12. Jewell DP, Lennard-Jones JE, the Cyclosporin Study Group of Great Britain and Ireland. Oral cyclosporin for chronic active Crohn's disease. A multicentre controlled trial. Eur J Gastroenterol Hepatol. 1994;6:499–505.
13. Ierardi E, Principi M, Francavilla R *et al.* Oral tacrolimus long-term therapy in patients with Crohn's disease and steroid resistance. Aliment Pharmacol Ther. 2001;15:371–7.
14. Sandborn WJ. Preliminary report on the use of oral tacrolimus (FK506) in the treatment of complicated proximal small bowel and fistulizing Crohn's disease. Am J Gastroenterol. 1997; 92:876–9.
15. Neurath MF, Wanitschke R, Peters M, Krummenauer F, Meyer zum Buschenfelde KH, Schlaak JF. Randomised trial of mycophenolate mofetil versus azathioprine for treatment of chronic active Crohn's disease. Gut. 1999;44:625–8.
16. Rampton DS, Neurath MF, Almer S, D'Haens G, Petritsch W, Stange EF. Mycophelonate mofetil in Crohn's disease. Lancet. 2000;356:163–4.
17. Miehsler W, Reinisch W, Moser G, Gangl A, Vogelsang H. Is mycophelonate mofetil an effective alternative in azathioprine-intolerant patients with chronic active Crohn's disease? Am J Gastroenterol. 2001;96:782–7.
18. Sustento-Reodica N, Ruiz P, Rogers A, Viciana AL, Conn HO, Tzakis AG. Recurrent Crohn's disease in transplanted bowel. Lancet. 1997;349:688–91.

25
Mechanisms of refractoriness in Crohn's disease

J. SCHÖLMERICH

INTRODUCTION

Although the overall prognosis of patients with inflammatory bowel disease has much improved in the second half of the last century, there are still patients who cannot be treated sufficiently with the drugs currently available. Although there are, rarely, patients in whom the disease is severe to such an extent that any treatment must fail, in most instances, a cause for refractoriness can be found and can be dealt with. Table 1 gives a list of possible causes of refractoriness which need to be considered when confronting a patient with treatment failure of any kind.

In this chapter, the possible different causes of refractoriness will be discussed using examples which can by no means be representative of the full array of studies available in IBD. Furthermore, this discussion will be focused on Crohn's disease, where the size of the problem seems to be much larger than in ulcerative colitis. In order to deal with refractoriness, we first have to define the size of this problem in Crohn's disease.

Table 1 Mechanisms of refractoriness in Crohn's disease

Wrong indication for treatment
Wrong symptom as target
Wrong patient/patient subgroup
Wrong drug
Wrong form of application
Wrong dose
Abnormal drug–receptor interaction
Wrong paradigm (concept)

SIZE OF THE PROBLEM

Patients with Crohn's disease are currently first treated using glucocorticosteroids either in a systemic or, more recently, in a topical way. A number of reviews have discussed this in more detail[1–3]. However, as is evident from a number of studies, the success rate of steroid treatment measured as long-lasting remission is less than 50%[4] (Figure 1) while 20% are primarily steroid resistant and another 36% become steroid dependent. These numbers are rather similar in different studies around the world; thus, for example, treatment with budesonide achieves between 50% and 70% remission[5–8] while treatment with systemic glucocorticosteroids in older trials achieved about 80% initial remission[9]. All these studies, however, indicate that long-term remission is in the range of that given in Figure 1, indicating that about 50% of patients with Crohn's disease cannot be treated sufficiently in the long term using glucocorticosteroids only. Furthermore, it needs to be mentioned that long-term steroid treatment is probably not a good choice in young patients due to side effects such as osteoporosis and others[10].

The size of the problem using other drugs is more difficult to define. Earlier studies have indicated that the potent immunosuppressant azathioprine or its metabolite 6-mercaptopurine achieve remission, even in patients not sufficiently responding to steroids, in about 66%[11]. However, more recent studies have shown that long-term effects of azathioprine in placebo-controlled trials are again in the range of less than 50%[12] (Table 2). Numbers for the alternative drug

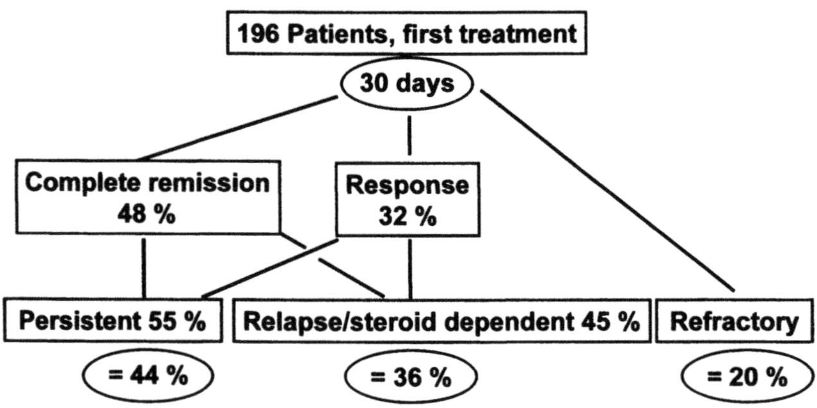

Figure 1 Steroid response rates in Crohn's disease[4]

Table 2 Azathioprine in active Crohn's disease – short- and long-term effects[12]

	Prednisolone (12 weeks, tapered)	
	+Placebo (n = 30)	*+AZA, 2.5 mg/kg (n = 33)*
Remission 12 weeks (%)	63	72
Remission 15 months (%)	7	42*

*Significant. From 12 weeks on only AZA!

Table 3 Infliximab for refractory CD[14]

	Placebo	*5 mg*	*10 mg*	*20 mg*	*All*
4 weeks					
Remission (%)	4	42	27	33	35
Response (%)*	17	81	50	64	66
12 weeks					
Response (%)	6	48	28	46	—
SE (%)	60 (4)	78 (4)	68 (7)	73 (7)	—

108 patients, >80% steroids, >30% AZA, CDAI ~300 (median).
*CDAI decrease of >70.

methotrexate are rather similar[13]. Finally, even the most recent drug innovation, i.e. infliximab used in patients refractory to steroids and in some cases to azathioprine, induces remission only in between 27% and 42% of patients and leads to a response in 50–81%[14] (Table 3). Thus, there is a considerable number of patients with Crohn's disease who seem to be resistant to our current treatment approaches when looking at controlled trials. This is, however, not in accordance with our daily experience. Most experts on IBD, even when working in tertiary referral centres, do not encounter so many patients who cannot be treated sufficiently when treatment is approached in an individualized way using all drugs available at appropriate doses or even in combination. This leads to the conclusion that probably results of clinical trials are not completely representative of daily practice or that there are causes of refractoriness which can be overcome using the conventional drugs and other means just by defining the cause and dealing with it.

POSSIBLE CAUSES OF REFRACTORINESS

Table 1 shows a number of possible causes which probably are not complete. The basic idea must certainly be that each patient needs individual treatment regardless of any claims of evidence-based medicine. This seems to be particularly true for patients with Crohn's disease where so many different expressions of the disease, variable symptoms and variable ways of dealing with symptoms exist.

Wrong indications

The first cause of refractoriness to be considered is the possibility that the indication for treatment is wrong, i.e. that the diagnosis is not correct. This is probably rare in patients with Crohn's disease; it seems to occur more often in patients with ulcerative colitis[15]. However, the lack of distinction between these two disorders may be the cause of frustrating treatment attempts when looking at the different immune reactions, and the transmural mucosal inflammatory involvement in Crohn's disease vs. ulcerative colitis. Even more important seems to be superinfection causing a flare which probably does not respond to steroids or any other anti-inflammatory treatment. It is not quite clear how many patients with a flare of Crohn's disease do indeed have an infectious cause of their complaints and maybe an infection as the starting event for a flare[16]. There are, however, several studies indicating that, for example, infections with *Giardia lamblia*[17] or many others can mimic Crohn's disease and can also mimic a flare of a pre-existent Crohn's disease which is well in remission[18]. Therefore, it is difficult to clarify how often a wrong indication is the cause of refractoriness in treatment of Crohn's disease but it may be more often than we all currently presume. In any case, the differentiation between Crohn's disease and ulcerative colitis is necessary since, for example, 5-aminosalicylic acid maintains remission in ulcerative colitis but does not do so in Crohn's disease[19].

Wrong symptoms

Patients with Crohn's disease, particularly when they have been operated or have extraintestinal symptoms or complications, may demonstrate a number of symptoms which are not due to activity of the disease and therefore cannot be treated successfully by conventional treatment. A recent study showed that prior intestinal resection or perianal disease actually led to a significantly higher frequency of steroid refractoriness[20]. While it is understandable that perianal disease with all its microbial and infectious complications may not be treated as well with steroids as just standard inflammation of the mucosa, the reason why prior resection was a cause of refractoriness remains somewhat obscure (Figure 2). However, analysis of the CDAI components in patients after resection revealed that the only factor different from patients without resection was the frequency of bowel movements. As a trend, the use of antidiarrhoeals was also increased in patients with prior resection (Figure 3). It therefore seems to be quite reasonable that surgery by itself caused the increased frequency of bowel movements, i.e. by the induction of chologenic diarrhoea which, by itself, is obviously not treatable with steroids but needs, in contrast, bile-acid-binding agents. Very similarly, patients with a short stricture leading to pain cannot be treated very successfully

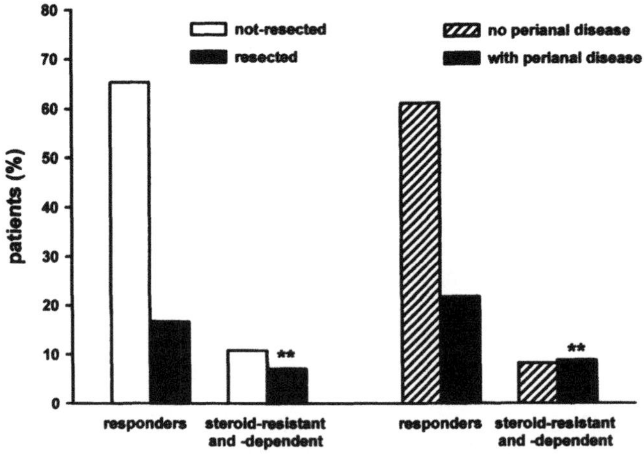

Figure 2 Factors determining steroid refractoriness in Crohn's disease

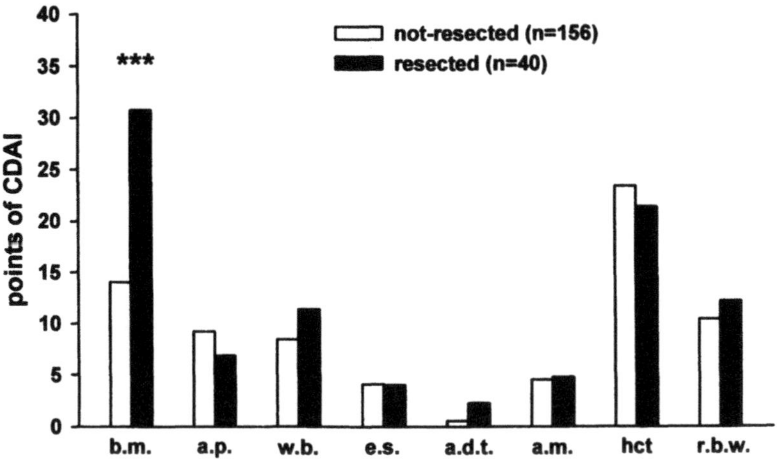

Figure 3 Influence of resection on CDAI components

b.m. – bowel movements; a.p. – abdominal pain; w.b. – well being; e.s. – extraintestinal symptoms; a.d.t. – antidiarrhoeals taken; a.m. – abdominal mass; hct – hematocrit; r.b.w. – relative body weight.

Table 4 Activity assessment in Crohn's disease – comparison of several parameters

CDAI		
– AI	$r = 0.505$	$p < 0.05$
– ESR	$r = 0.382$	N.S.
– CRP	$r = 0.060$	N.S.
AI		
– ESR	$r = 0.772$	$p < 0.01$
– CRP	$r = 0.391$	N.S.
ESR		
– CRP	$r = 0.608$	$p < 0.05$

CDAI – Crohn's disease activity index; AI – van Hees index; ESR – Erytrocyte sedimentation rate; CRP – C-reactive protein.

when this stricture is due to fibrosis and is just a scar due to prior inflammatory activity. These patients need to be treated with surgery or, for example, balloon dilatation[21]. The only problem is how to find out whether pain is really due to this type of stenosis. Probably, inflammation scintigraphy would be helpful for this purpose[22]. Finally a completely destroyed large bowel cannot be restored by any drug available and needs surgery as the only potential treatment. The fact that the activity of Crohn's disease, as measured by one activity index, does not correlate with activity measured by other activity indices, nor does it correlate with any parameter of inflammation, such as ESR or CRP (Table 4), further underlines that treatment of the symptoms is not by definition identical to treatment of inflammation. Thus, anti-inflammatory treatment with steroids or any other anti-inflammatory agent should only be used if there are clear signs of inflammation.

Table 5 Subtypes of Crohn's disease – effects of postoperative remission maintenance in 232 patients[24]

	Time to next operation (years)		
	Perforating	*Non-perforating*	*Perianal*
5-ASA/antibiotics	2.3 ± 2.2	12.9 ± 6.8	3.5 ± 3.3
Steroids/immunosuppressants	6.4 ± 7.5	3.8 ± 4.0	2.9 ± 1.7

Table 6 Response rates to infliximab – different TNF haplotypes[26]

Haplotype	*With haplotype % response (n)**	*Without haplotype % response (n)*
A	53 (19)	63 (40)
B	60 (15)	59 (44)
C	50 (12)	62 (47)
D	56 (9)	60 (50)
E	29 (7)	64 (52)

**n* = number of patients with or without haplotype. Greatest response with presence of s-ANCA; p-ANCA ⊕ and haplotype LTA Ncol TNFc-aa13L-aa26 associated with poor response.

Wrong patient/patient subgroup

Numerous studies in the last two decades have shown that Crohn's disease probably does not comprise a single disorder. It may be more like a syndrome and a number of different causes may result in inflammation in any part of the gut. Furthermore, it has been shown that location, behaviour and some other factors actually define the later course and therefore also the response to treatment in these subgroups[23]. A nice example is a study[24] which, although retrospective, showed that, for different behaviours of Crohn's disease, the response to postoperative relapse prevention was very different according to the type of drugs used. They showed that, while, in perforating disease, steroids and immunosuppressants were much better in prolonging the time to the second operation, the contrary was true for patients with non-perforating disease, where 5-aminosalicylic acid (5-ASA) and antibiotics were obviously superior to steroids and immunosuppressants (Table 5)[24].

It has to be assumed that the different phenotypes are related to different genotypes. Very few studies have thus far assessed the effect of genotyping on treatment response. One such study has shown that TNF-α gene polymorphism is associated with frequency of steroid dependency[25]. In a similar way, TNF haplotypes seem to have an influence on the response to infliximab (Table 6)[26].

Wrong drug

It is possible that the drug chosen to treat a patient is not appropriate. A good example is sulphasalazine for Crohn's disease. Since the active moiety of this drug is only released in the colon by cleaving of the azo-bond to sulphapyridine by bacterial enzymes in the colon, it is obvious that it cannot be very efficient in patients with small intestinal involvement. Furthermore, there have been data showing that the enzyme azoreductase which actually releases the active moiety is much less active in the faeces of patients with Crohn's disease as compared with healthy controls (Table 7)[27]. This may be explained by the fact that the bacterial flora in the gut of patients with Crohn's disease is different from that of healthy people, possibly due to different pH[28]. Recent studies showing that 5-ASA is indeed able to improve symptoms in patients with Crohn's disease indicate that prior failures of sulphasalazine might be indeed due to this fact (Table 8)[29].

Wrong form of application

Since many of the drugs used actually work in a topical way, i.e. from the lumen of the gut, it is obvious that the application form or galenic preparation plays a major role in efficacy and thereby refractoriness. For example, a patient with oral or oesophageal involvement probably could not be treated by a large- or small-bowel release preparation. Furthermore, the dose of a topical release formulation may be important in order to reveal a positive effect in a given location. This is clarified by the example of pH-dependent release budesonide which seems to be effective in colonic distal disease only if given at a higher dose. This is explained by the fact that it needs to reach that location without prior absorption (Table 9)[30]. This example also shows that different doses may be needed to treat patients with the same disease but varying activity.

Wrong dose of a given drug

This is very obvious when looking at the results of studies with 5-aminosalicylic acid. While earlier trials using this drug showed clear inefficacy when given at a

Table 7 Faecal azoreductase – release of 5-ASA from SASP in Crohn's disease?[27]

	Crohn's disease (n = 14)	*Control (n = 12)*
Azoreductase (mU/g) → Cause of reduced efficacy?	11.4 ± 7.9	51.1 ± 21.4

Table 8 Mesalamine (pH dependent) for mild-to-moderate active Crohn's disease[29]

12 weeks	*5-ASA*		*6-Methylprednisolone*
	4 g/d (tablets) (n=35)	*4 g/d (microgranular) (n=28)*	*40 mg (n = 31)*
Change in CDAI (median)	−113 (33–149)	−123 (77–155)	−154 (99–197)
Remission (%)	60	79	61
Withdrawal			
Failure (%)	31	9	13
AE (%)	0	4	16

CDAI, Crohn's disease activity index.

Table 9 Dose response for budesonide (pH dependent) in CD patients with different location and activity

6 weeks	*Remission (%) with*		
	6 mg	*9 mg*	*18 mg*
Initial CDAI			
<300 ($n = 79$)	47	71	64
≥300 ($n = 25$)	0	25	75*
Location			
Ileocolonic ($n = 57$)	30	60	59
Colonic distal ($n = 44$)	31	46	73*

*Significant.

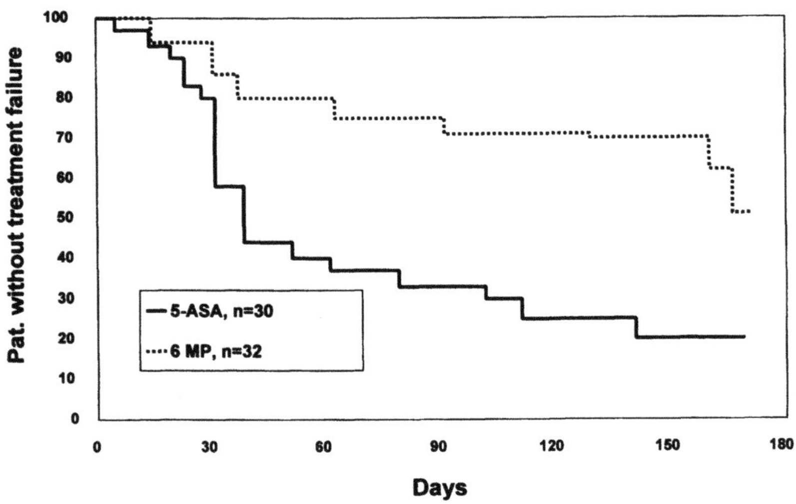

Figure 4 5-ASA, 2 g, vs. 6-methylprednisolone (MP) for active Crohn's disease

dose of 2 g/d which was recommended at that time (Figure 4)[31], later studies using higher doses revealed an efficacy somewhat comparable to that of 6-methylprednisolone (Figure 5)[32]. These data are in accordance with those found by others[33] and those mentioned before[29]. Recent studies, demonstrating that the mucosal concentrations of 5-ASA as well as its metabolite *N*-acetyl-5-aminosalicylic acid are identical after the application of 3 doses of 400 mg or 1 dose of 1200 mg per day[34] (Table 10), show that we still have much to learn about application modes in order to achieve the drug concentrations we want at a given place.

Another example of difficulties with dosing is a recent trial where 6-mercaptopurine was compared with 5-ASA for the prevention of postoperative relapse in Crohn's disease. While the results using a dose of 3 g/d 5-ASA

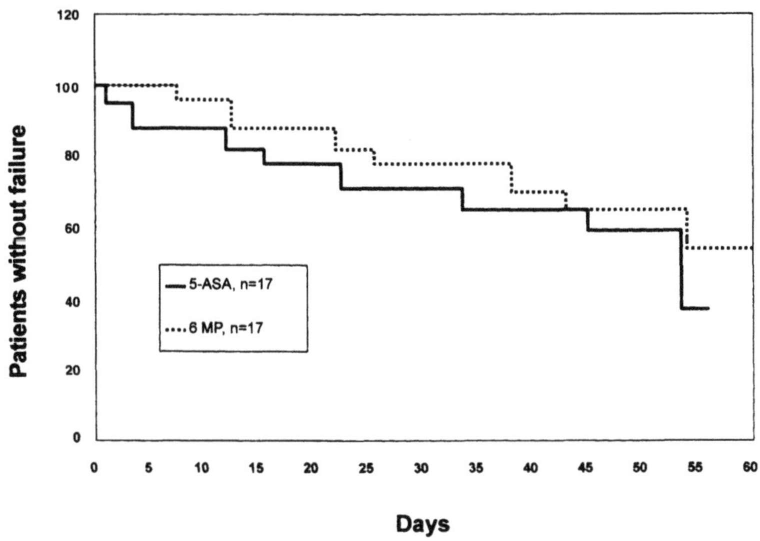

Figure 5 5-ASA, 4.5 g vs. 6-methylprednisolone (MP) for active Crohn's disease

Table 10 Divided doses of 5-ASA in IBD?[34]

	5-ASA/N-acetyl-5-ASA	
	3 × 400 mg	*1 × 1200 mg*
Faecal excretion (mg/24 h)	142/387	215/231
Mucosal concentration (ng/ml)	2.9/9.0	3.0/12.0

Serum AUC/peak and renal excretion not relevantly different!

Table 11 6-Mercaptopurine and Pentasa for prevention of postoperative relapse in CD[35]

24 months	*6-MP* *50 mg/d* ($n = 47$)	*Pentasa* *3 g/d* ($n = 44$)	*Placebo* ($n = 40$)
Clinical relapse (%)	53*	62	70
Endoscopic relapse (%)	83*	86*	98
Severe endoscopic relapse (%)	68**	80	90
Radiological relapse (%)	68*	82	85

*$p < 0.05$ vs. placebo. **$p < 0.05$ vs. placebo and Pentasa.

were in the range of those to be expected, as were those of placebo, the effect of 6-mercaptopurine given at 50 mg/d was somewhat disappointing, although better than those of the two other groups[35] (Table 11). That this may be a problem of the dose is demonstrated by a recent study where it was shown that the levels of

Table 12 Azathioprine metabolites and clinical effect in IBD[36]

	6-Thioguanine (nmol/L)	*6-TGN > 250 (n)*	*6-Methylmercaptopurine (nmol/L)*
Responders ($n = 10$)	305	8/10	1926
Non-responders ($n = 12$)	168	2/12	2075

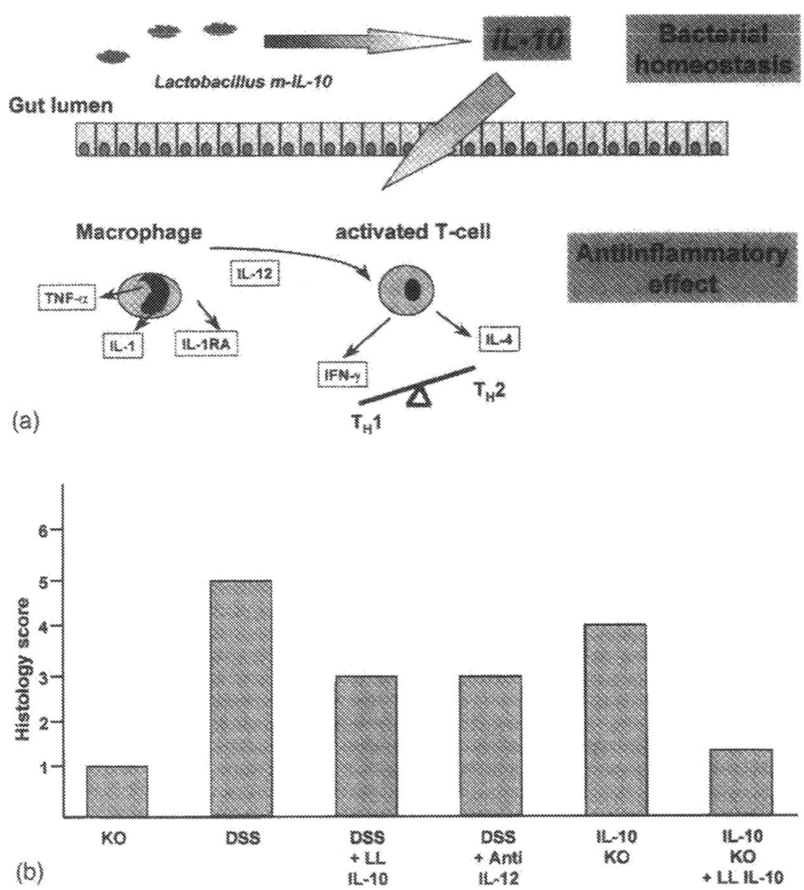

Figure 6 A combination of probiotics and immune modulation by IL-10 in experimental colitis (DSS and IL-10 knockout). (a) Model used. (b) Results in different forms of colitis

azathioprine metabolites to some extent correlate with the clinical effect in inflammatory bowel disease (Table 12)[36]. Thus, we may need to adjust doses more to specific patients and their specific problems and, furthermore, to the pharmacokinetics and -dynamics in a given patient.

Finally, this is exemplified by a very recent approach where lactobacilli producing interleukin-10 were used in an animal experiment with quite good success (Figure 6)[37]. In contrast to earlier studies with systemic application[38], this study demonstrates that the local dose may be much more important than we used to believe.

Abnormal interaction between the drug and its receptor

Several studies show that glucocorticocoid receptors are down-regulated in patients with chronic inflammatory disorders. This has been found regarding circulating blood cells in patients with collagen disorders regardless of their treatment status while, in patients with IBD, only those treated with steroids showed reduced receptors in circulating lymphocytes indicating that, in IBD, this is not a general problem. However, in the intestinal mucosa, glucocorticoid receptors were severely down-regulated compared with healthy controls, indicating that there may be an immanent problem which may cause refractoriness in some patients (Figure 7)[39]. We probably need more studies of all the drugs we use regarding this type of refractariety.

Wrong concept/wrong paradigm

Regarding the aetiology of IBD, there is a large number of proposals which range from abnormal barrier functions (mucins, permeability, epithelial integrity, motility, bacterial adhesion) via abnormal or lacking luminal components (bacteria, dietary factors, xenobiotics, bile acids) to an abnormal local immune

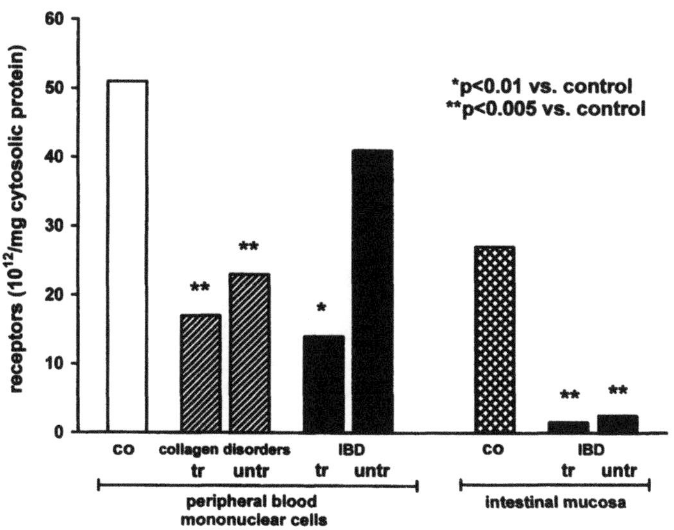

Figure 7 Glucocorticoid receptors in IBD and collagen disorders

tr – treated; untr – untreated; CO – healthy control; IBD – inflammatory bowel diseases.

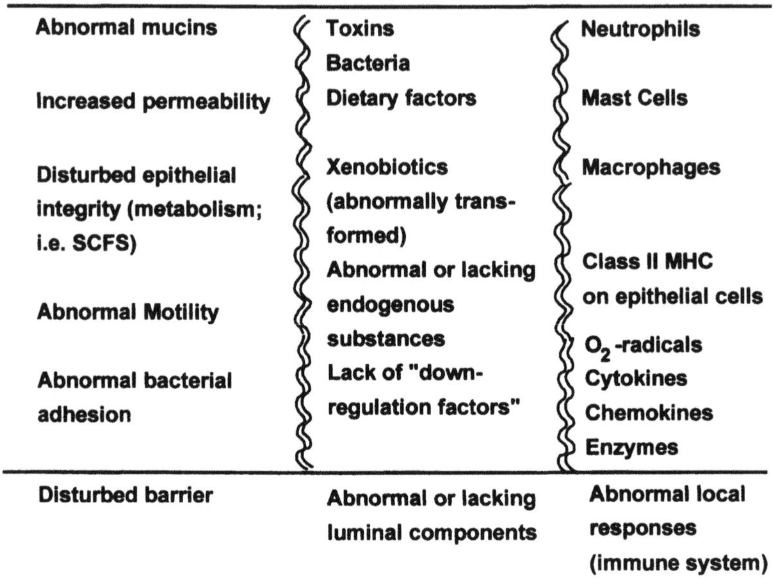

Figure 8 Aetiology of IBD – possibilities

response (Figure 8). All these disturbances lead to the pathophysiological changes generally recognized. These pathophysiological principles actually reflect general inflammatory pathways which are probably not specific for inflammatory bowel disease. All available treatments up to now have been shown to be pluripotent, i.e. acting on a vast number of mediators or cell types. All attempts to target single mediators have been futile as exemplified by the platelet activating factor antagonists or the leukotriene inhibitors[40,41]. Even infliximab may not work by inhibiting TNF but by driving TNF-expressing activated lymphocytes and monocytes into apoptosis[42]. The general paradigm of IBD as an inflammatory disorder has been questioned by a number of people[43] and most experts meanwhile agree that there is probably a variety of causes resulting in these chronic disorders. In particular, the fact that tolerance to resident intestinal flora is broken in IBD[44] (Table 13) leads to new approaches changing the luminal contents and in particular the gut flora[45]. Thus far, no specific bacteria have been found, in particular *Mycobacterium tuberculosis* and relatives have not been a successful proposal. This has been shown particularly by the lack of effect of long-term tuberculostatic treatment (Table 14)[46]. This is only one more example of a wrong paradigm which is the cause of the lack of efficacy for a given treatment.

CLINICAL CONSEQUENCES

As demonstrated with a number of clinical studies and clinical examples, there are many causes for refractariety towards currently available treatment in Crohn's

Table 13 Tolerance towards resident intestinal flora is broken in active IBD[44]

	BSA		*BSH*	
	Anaerobic	*Aerobic*	*Anaerobic*	*Aerobic*
Controls ($n = 9/6$)	751*	710	11756	12276
CD inactive ($n = 6/3$)	698	800	8719	12462
CD active ($n = 5/3$)	17533	13467	8109	8410

Tolerance can be restored (in mice) by IL-10 or anti-IL-12!
*Proliferation as ct/min.
BSA/H = bacterial sonicate autologous/heterologous.

Table 14 No effect of tuberculostatic therapy in active Crohn's disease[46]

2 Years	*Triple* (n=63)*	*Placebo (n=63)*
At least 12 months therapy (%)	76	77
Surgery (n)	15	14
Steroids necessary (%)	86	86

9 patients dropped out due to side effects (Verum), CDAI never different.
*Rifampicin, isoniazid, ethambutol.

disease. In many cases, there may be ways to deliver successful relief of the symptoms to many more patients if we learn to consider these different causes of refractoriness. In particular, the following should always be assured:

- The cause of symptoms, the patient type, and the indication for treatment should always be ascertained using appropriate methods.
- The drug used must be chosen according to the location of the disease and target the appropriate cells for drug action in a given patient.
- The form of application and the dose must be appropriate with respect to the location of the disease and available study results.
- There may be patients where the disease paradigm is not correct – pluripotent drugs may be superior while we do not understand disease paradigms.
- Changes in patients regarding their drug response over time need to be considered in most patients – this can be learned from other disciplines, i.e. rheumatology or even cardiology.

Fortunately, the survival of patients with IBD has improved much during the last century (Figure 9)[47]. However, the quality of life of those patients is still not satisfactory. This gives us reason to further improve current drug technologies and, in particular, to make sure that our approaches are appropriate for each individual patient.

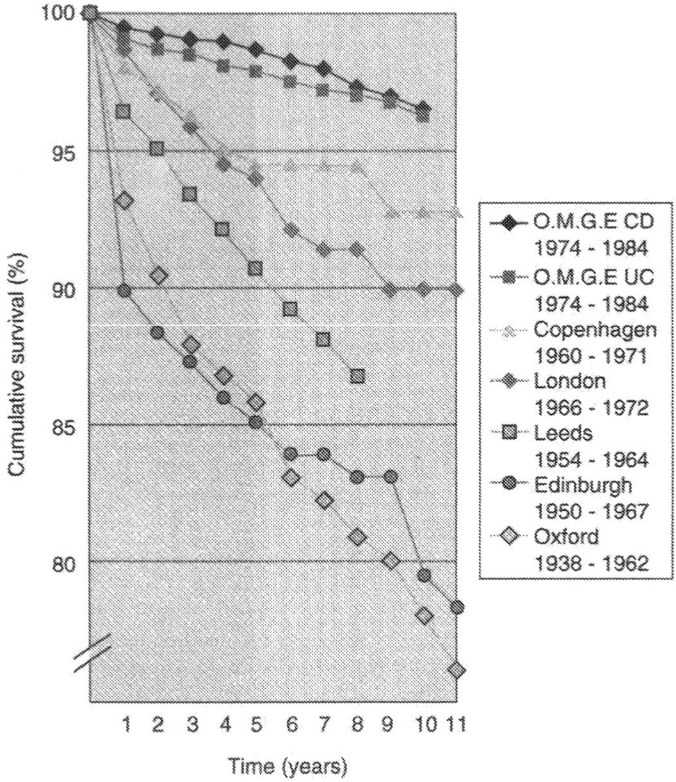

Figure 9 Ten-year survival in patients with IBD during the last century[47]

References

1. Schölmerich J, Andus T. Steroids in IBD: which steroids for what patient? In: Rachmilewitz D, editor, V International Symposium on Inflammatory Bowel Diseases. Dordrecht: Kluwer Academic Publishers, 1998:138–50.
2. Andus T, Targan SR. Corticosteroids. In: Targan S, Shanahan F, editors, Inflammatory Bowel Disease: From Bench to Bedside. Baltimore, MD: Williams & Wilkins, USA, 1993:487–502.
3. Gross V, Andus T, Caesar I, Schölmerich J. Steroids – new and old. In: Campieri M, Bianchi-Porro G, Fiocchi C, Schölmerich J, editors, Clinical Challenges in Inflammatory Bowel Diseases – Diagnosis, Prognosis and Treatment. Dordrecht: Kluwer Academic Publishers, 1998:127–40.
4. Munkholm P, Langholz E, Davidsen M, Binder V. Frequency of glucocorticoid resistance and dependency in Crohn's disease. Gut. 1994;35:360–2.
5. Bar-Meir S, Chowers Y, Lavy A *et al.* The Israeli Budesonide Study Group. Budesonide versus prednisone in the treatment of active Crohn's disease. Gastroenterology. 1998;115:835–40.
6. Rutgeerts P, Löfberg R, Malchow H *et al.* A comparison of budesonide with prednisolone for active Crohn's disease. N Engl J Med. 1994;331:842–5.
7. Gross V, Andus T, Caesar I *et al.* German/Austrian Budesonide Study Group. Oral pH-modified release budesonide versus 6-methylprednisolone in active Crohn's disease. Eur J Gastroenterol Hepatol. 1996;8:905–9.
8. Ostergaard-Thomsen O, Cortot A, Jewell D *et al.* International Budesonide–Mesalamine Study Group. A comparison of budesonide and mesalamine for active Crohn's disease. N Engl J Med. 1998;399:370–4.

9. Malchow H, Ewe K, Brandes JW *et al.* European Cooperative Crohn's Disease Study (ECCDS): results of drug treatment. Gastroenterology. 1984;86:249–66.
10. Bregenzer N, Erban P, Albrich H *et al.* Screening for osteoporosis in patients with inflammatory bowel disease by urinary *N*-telopeptides. Eur J Gastroenterol Hepatol, in press.
11. Present DH, Korelitz BI, Wisch N, Glass JL, Sachar DB, Pasternack BS. Treatment of Crohn's disease with 6-mercaptopurine. A long-term, randomized, double-blind study. N Engl J Med. 1980;302:981–7.
12. Candy S, Wright J, Gerber M, Adams G, Gerig M, Goodman R. A controlled double blind study of azathioprine in the management of Crohn's disease. Gut. 1995;37:674–8.
13. Feagan BG, Rochon J, Fedorak RN *et al.* The North American Crohn's Study Group Investigators. Methotrexate for the treatment of Crohn's disease. N Engl J Med. 1995;332: 292–7.
14. Targan SR, Hanauer SB, van Deventer SJ *et al.* Crohn's Disease cA2 Study Group. A short-term study of chimeric monoclonal antibody cA2 to tumor necrosis factor α for Crohn's disease. N Engl J Med. 1997;337:1029–35.
15. Robinson MG, Dorrough CA. Metamorphosis of mucosal ulcerative colitis to Crohn's disease with olsalazine and other 5-ASA analogs. Gastroenterology. 1988;94:A380 (abstract).
16. Tysk C, Järnerot G. Seasonal variation in exacerbations of ulcerative colitis. Scand J Gastroenterol. 1993;28:95.
17. Scheurlen C, Kruis W, Weinzierl M, Lamina J, Paumgartner G. Giardiasis in patients with Crohn's disease. Scand J Gastroenterol. 1988;23:833–9.
18. Sartor RB. Induction, perpetuation and exacerbation of inflammatory bowel diseases by viral and bacterial agents. In: Lembcke B, Kruis W, Sartor RB, editors, Systemic Manifestations of IBD: The Pending Challenge for Subtle Diagnosis and Treatment. Dodrecht: Kluwer Academic Publishers, 1988:289–99.
19. De Franchis R, Omodei P, Ranzi T *et al.* Controlled trial of oral 5-aminosalicylic acid for the prevention of early relapse in Crohn's disease. Aliment Pharmacol Ther. 1997;11:845–52.
20. Gelbmann CM. Prediction of treatment refractoriness in ulcerative colitis and Crohn's disease – do we have reliable markers? Inflamm Bowel Dis. 2000;6:123–31.
21. Couckuyt H, Gevers AM, Coremans G, Hiele M, Rutgeerts P. Efficacy and safety of hydrostatic balloon dilatation of ileocolonic Crohn's strictures: a prospective longterm analysis. Gut. 1995;36:577–80.
22. Schölmerich J, Schmidt E, Schümichen C, Billmann P, Schmidt H, Gerok W. Scintigraphic assessment of bowel involvement and disease activity in Crohn's disease using technetium-99m-HM-PAO as leukocyte label. Gastroenterology. 1988;95:1287–98.
23. Gasché C, Schölmerich J, Brynskow J *et al.* A simple classification of Crohn's disease: report of the Working Party for the World Congresses of Gastroenterology, Vienna 1998. Inflamm Bowel Dis. 2000;6:8–15.
24. Greenway SE, Buckmire MA, Rolandelli RH. Clinical subtypes of Crohn's disease according to surgical outcome. Gastroenterology. 1998;114:A1390 (abstract).
25. Louis E, Peeters M, Franchimon D *et al.* Tumour necrosis factor (TNF) gene polymorphism in Crohn's disease (CD): influence on diseases behaviour? Clin Exp Immunol. 2000;119:64–8.
26. Taylor KD, Plevy SE, Yang H *et al.* ANCA pattern and LTA haplotype relationship to clinical responses to anti-TNF antibody treatment in Crohn's disease. Gastroenterology. 2001;120: 1347–55.
27. Carrette O, Favier C, Mizon C *et al.* Bacterial enzymes used for colon-specific drug delivery are decreased in active Crohn's disease. Dig Dis Sci. 1995;40:2641–6.
28. Schölmerich J, Walz-Binninger U, Lock G. Patients with Crohn's disease have lower fecal pH and more often H_2 low excretors after oral lactulose. Submitted.
29. Prantera C, Cottone M, Pallone F *et al.* Mesalamine in the treatment of mild to moderate active Crohn's ileitis: results of a randomized, multicenter trial. Gastroenterology. 1999;116: 521–6.
30. Schölmerich J, Gross V, Andus T *et al.* The German/Austrian Budesonide Study Group. Dose finding study with oral pH-dependent release budesonide in patients with active Crohn's disease. Submitted.
31. Schölmerich J, Jenss H, Hartmann F, Döpfer H. The German 5-ASA Study Group. Oral 5-aminosalicylic acid versus methylprednisolone in active Crohn's disease. Can J Gastroenterol. 1990;4:446–51.

32. Gross V, Andus T, Fischbach W *et al.* German 5-ASA Study Group. Comparison between high dose 5-aminosalicylic acid and 6-methylprednisolone in active Crohn's ileocolitis. A multicenter randomized double-blind study. Z Gastroenterol. 1995;33:581–4.
33. Singleton JW, Hanauer S, Gitnick GL *et al.* Mesalamine capsules for the treatment of active Crohn's disease: results of a 16-week trial. Pentasa Crohn's Disease Study Group. Gastroenterology. 1993;104:1293–301.
34. Hussain FN, Ajjan RA, Kapur K, Moustafa M, Riley SA. Once versus divided daily dosing with delayed-release mesalazine: a study of tissue drug concentrations and standard pharmacokinetic parameters. Aliment Pharmacol Ther. 2001;15:53–62.
35. Korelitz B, Hanauer S, Rutgeerts P, Present D, Peppercorn M. Post-operative prophylaxis with 6-MP, 5-ASA or placebo in Crohn's disease: a 2 year multicenter trial. Gastroenterology. 1998;114:A1011 (abstract).
36. Cuffari C, Hunt S, Bayless TM. Enhanced bioavailability of azathioprine compared to 6-mercaptopurine therapy in inflammatory bowel disease: correlation with treatment efficacy. Aliment Pharmacol Ther. 2000;14:1009–14.
37. Steidler L, Hans W, Schotte L *et al.* Treatment of murine colitis by lactococcus lactis secreting interleukin-10. Science. 2000;289:1353–5.
38. Herfarth HH, Bocker U, Janardhanam R, Sartor RB. Subtherapeutic corticosteroids potentiate the ability of interleukin 10 to prevent chronic inflammation in rats. Gastroenterology. 1998;115:856–65.
39. Rogler G, Meinel A, Lingauer A *et al.* Glucocorticoid receptors are down-regulated in inflamed colonic mucosa but not in peripheral blood mononuclear cells from patients with inflammatory bowel disease. Eur J Clin Invest. 1999;29:330–6.
40. Malchow H, Ewe K, Goebell H, Wellmann W, Leimer HG, Kempe R. Failure of the specific PAF-antagonist apafant in the treatment of ulcerative colitis. Gastroenterology. 1994;106:A728 (abstract).
41. Hawkey C, Gassull M, Lauritsen K. Efficacy of zileuton, a 5-lipoxygenase inhibitor, in the maintenance of remission in patients with ulcerative colitis. Gastroenterology. 1994;96:A697 (abstract).
42. Wittig BM, Zeitz M. Zytokin- und Antizytokintherapien bei chronisch entzündlichen Darmerkrankungen. Dtsch Med Wsch. 2001;126:S52–8.
43. Crotty B. Ulcerative colitis and xenobiotic metabolism. Lancet. 1994;343:35–8.
44. Duchmann R, Neurath MF, Meyer zum Büschenfelde KH. Responses to self and non-self intestinal microflora in health and inflammatory bowel disease. Res Immunol. 1997;148:589–94.
45. Sartor RB, Rath HC, Sellon RK. Microbial factors in chronic intestinal inflammation. Curr Opin Gastroenterol. 1996;12:327–33.
46. Swift G, Srivastava ED, Stone R *et al.* Controlled trial of anti-tuberculous chemotherapy for two years in Crohn's disease. Gut. 1994;35:363–8.
47. Softley A, Clamp SE, Watkinson G, Bouchier IA, Myren J, de Combal FT. The natural history of inflammatory bowel disease: has there been a change in the last 20 years? Scand J Gastroenterol. Suppl. 1988;144:20–3.

26 The traditional immunosuppressors

E. F. STANGE

The traditional immunosuppressive agents in inflammatory bowel disease are azathioprine and 6-mercaptopurine. More recently, methotrexate, cyclosporin A, tacrolimus and mycophenolate have been introduced for steroid-dependent or refractory disease. The rationale for the use of these drugs lies in the multiple immunological abnormalities described in both types of disease. The role of these treatment alternatives will be reviewed in the present chapter.

AZATHIOPRINE AND 6-MERCAPTOPURINE

The precise mechanism of action of both azathioprine and 6-mercaptopurine remains enigmatic although some progress has been made in this regard. Azathioprine has been demonstrated to be converted to 6-mercaptopurine *in vivo*, suggesting that there is no difference in principle between the action of both these agents. 6-Mercaptopurine is subsequently metabolized to 6-thioguanine, the presumed active metabolite which becomes incorporated into developing strands of DNA. In lymphocytes, this substitution blocks critical gene activation of effector lymphocyte clones, not only inhibiting proliferation but also inducing lymphocyte apoptosis.

In Crohn's disease, eight reports on controlled trials of azathioprine or 6-mercaptopurine in active[1–8] and five in quiescent disease[1,4,7,9,10] have been fully published. An overview of these studies is given in the Cochrane Library. The two initial small trials[1,2] failed to show a significant benefit, probably due to insufficient statistical power (β-error) and the short treatment course. In the milestone study by Present *et al.*[5], 83 chronically ill patients were entered into a 2-year double-blind study comparing 6-mercaptopurine with placebo. Crossover data showed that improvement occurred in 26 of 39 courses of the drug (67%) as compared with 3 of 39 courses of placebo (8%, $p < 0.0001$). Non-crossover data also confirmed the superiority of 6-mercaptopurine. The drug was more effective in closing fistulae (31% vs. 6%) and in permitting discontinuation or reduction of steroid dosage (75% vs. 36%). It is important to note that the onset of response was often delayed, with 32% of the patients taking longer than 3 months to respond, and 19% taking longer than 4 months. The National Cooperative Crohn's Disease Study[4] gave a negative result but was biased against azathioprine for several reasons. Corticosteroids were withdrawn in a significant proportion of the patients immediately before the start of the trial so that many patients experienced an early relapse. Since azathioprine requires several months for its action, this design probably doomed the azathioprine arm of the trial. Thus, the treatment period of 4 months may simply have been too short and the data actually indicate an improved action after 7 weeks of treatment.

A more recent study examined whether azathioprine combined with standard prednisolone therapy improved the therapeutic outcome compared with monotherapy using prednisolone in active Crohn's disease[6]. At the end of the 4-month trial, 16 of 21 patients (76%) with combined therapy vs. 8 of 21 patients treated with corticosteroids alone (38%) were in remission ($p = 0.03$). The differences in activity indices became significant after 8 weeks. In addition, the average steroid dose was significantly lower in the combined treatment group. However, in the initial period of 3 months in the trial of Candy *et al.*, the difference between placebo and azathioprine was not significant[7], confirming the slow onset of its action. Thus, although a synergistic effect of azathioprine and corticosteroids is not yet proven, the combination of both agents during the initial phase of active disease is probably wise. A recent meta analysis of these trials by the Cochrane Collaboration[11,12] supports the significant advantage of azathioprine/6-mercaptopurine in active disease. It was also found that the response rate was dependent on treatment time and daily as well as cumulative dose. The interesting new approach to speed up the slow onset of action by use of high-dose intravenous therapy failed to prove superiority in a controlled trial[13]. Finally, the combined studies of the meta analysis[11,12] demonstrated a steroid-sparing effect both in active and quiescent disease with an odds ratio of 3.7 and 4.6, respectively. In addition, fistulae improved with azathioprine therapy with an odds ratio of 4.4.

The benefit of these immunosuppressive agents, which is now generally accepted, has to be weighed against eventual toxicity. In the large experience of Present *et al.*[14] in 396 patients treated with 6-mercaptopurine based on a mean period of follow-up of 5 years, toxicity included pancreatitis (3.3%), bone marrow depression (2%), allergic reactions (2%) and drug hepatitis (0.3%). All complications were reversible with no mortality. Infectious complications were seen in 7.4% of the patients in whom 1.8% were severe. Again, all infections were cured with no deaths. Of the cohort, 3.1% developed neoplasms but only one (0.3%), a diffuse histiocytic lymphoma of the brain, had a probable association with the drug. However, even when the lymphoma risk was considered in a decision analysis, azathioprine is of benefit with respect to survival.

It may be concluded that azathioprine and 6-mercaptopurine represent a reasonable and fairly safe medication in otherwise intractable chronic active inflammatory bowel disease, provided that surgery is not indicated. Most importantly, all patients have to be carefully monitored to detect potential side-effects early.

METHOTREXATE

Methotrexate, another cytotoxic immunosuppressant, is usually administered in refractory Crohn's disease as weekly intramuscular injections over a 12-week treatment period. Thereafter, the dosing may be switched to oral medication in tapered fashion if remission is achieved. The controlled trial of this drug in active Crohn's disease by Feagan *et al.* reported a therapeutic benefit of approximately 20%[15]. Prolonged administration of the drug in responders appears to maintain remission in some patients. The uncontrolled French study by Lémann *et al.*[16] confirmed an initial response to methotrexate but the relapse rate amounted to 60% after 10 months. Thus, methotrexate is a second-line drug for this indication, reserved for those not responding or intolerant to azathioprine/6-mercaptopurine.

CYCLOSPORINE A

Depite its revolutionary role in transplantation medicine and its well-known mechanism of action, cyclosporine A is of limited value in the field of inflammatory bowel diseases. This hydrophobic undecapeptide is obtained by extraction of the soil fungus *Tolypocladium infatum gams*. After entering the target cell, the drug binds to cyclophilin, inactivates calcineurin and prevents the nuclear factor of activated T cells (NFAT) induced transcription of messenger-RNA encoding for interleukin-2 and its receptor. In addition, cyclosporine interferes with B-cell activation indirectly by suppressing the formation of activating factors by helper T cells. These molecular mechanisms are responsible for the unique selectivity of cyclosporine which acts only on lymphocytes but not on granulocytes, monocytes or macrophages. Since the T cell is currently believed to play a pivotal role in the mucosal inflammatory process, the rationale for the use of the drug in these diseases is obvious.

The first fully reported controlled trial of cyclosporine A was that of Brynskov *et al.* in active chronic Crohn's disease[17]. Following a 3-month study period, 59% of cyclosporine-treated but only 32% of placebo patients had improved ($p = 0.032$). The effect became evident after 2 weeks. However, during the subsequent 3 months when the drug was gradually withdrawn, the proportion of patients with improvement dropped to 38% (29) and the benefit was essentially lost after 1 year (30). The study was criticized because response was measured by a grading score rather than the standard Crohn's disease activity index. Unfortunately, none of the subsequent three large controlled trials[18–20] confirmed these findings. Therefore, there is little long-term benefit of oral cyclosporine. It has been argued that this failure is due to the low dose used in the latter negative trials but that nephrotoxicity at higher doses appears to be prohibitive. Taken together, the data suggest that the use of cyclosporine should be a last resort and only in very severe disease, particularly in fistulating Crohn's disease, but even this has changed with the advent of infliximab.

It is possible that newer drug developments, like tacrolimus (FK 506), may further improve the therapeutic options. This drug is well absorbed, more potent than cyclosporine A and, at least in the transplant field, is associated with fewer infections. In our hands, using 1–2 weeks of iv therapy followed by a switch to the oral route, nine out of eleven patients responded[21]. It also seems possible to maintain remission during the oral phase in about half of the patients when azathioprine is coadministered. It should be emphasized that this represents only preliminary and uncontrolled experience and has to be confirmed by formal controlled trials. Most importantly, the caveat holds that the potential benefit of all immunosuppressive agents should be considered in the light of known and possibly unknown untoward effects of these aggressive and often long-term treatments.

NEW DEVELOPMENTS: MYCOPHENOLATE AND 6-THIOGUANINE

Mycophenolate-mofetil is an established drug in transplantation medicine but has also been tested in IBD patients. Unfortunately, the single controlled trial[22] in Crohn's disease was unblind and is therefore difficult to interpret. In this study, mycophenolate-mofetil proved to be at least equivalent to azathioprine with a more rapid action in cases with high inflammatory activity. We[23] and most other groups have had much less-promising experience with this immunosuppressant.

Finally, based on the traditional immunosuppressant, azathioprine, its major immunosuppressive metabolite, 6-thioguanine, has recently been introduced as a therapeutic agent in IBD. A small pilot study described a response or remission in 7 of 10 patients resistant to 6-mercaptopurine[24]. We have now used the drug in an ongoing open study in 30 Crohn's disease patients with good initial results. The 6-thioguanine levels in erythrocytes are at least 5-fold higher than during therapy with the parent immunosuppressants and the relevance of this finding with respect to short- or long-term toxicity is unclear. It has been suggested that the compound is better tolerated than its parent drugs, azathioprine or 6-mercaptopurine, and, hopefully, it acts more rapidly.

In conclusion, the field is moving but steroid-dependent and especially refractory Crohn's disease are still a major challenge. The major drawback of standard immunosuppressants like azathioprine and 6-mercaptopurine is their slow onset of action whereas that of infliximab is its poor potency in long-term maintenance, as evidenced by the ACCENT 1 trial. Thus, there is no perfect solution at hand and new ideas are welcome.

References

1. Willoughby JM, Beckett J, Kumar PJ *et al.* Controlled trial of azathioprine in Crohn's disease. Lancet. 1971;2:944–7.
2. Rhodes J, Bainton D, Beck P *et al.* Controlled trial of azathioprine in Crohn's disease. Lancet. 1971;2:1273–6.
3. Klein M, Binder HJ, Mitchell M *et al.* Treatment of Crohn's disease with azathioprine: a controlled evaluation. Gastroenterology. 1974;66:916–22.
4. Summers RW, Switz DM, Sessions-JT J *et al.* National Cooperative Crohn's Disease Study: results of drug treatment. Gastroenterology. 1979;77:847–69.
5. Present DH, Korelitz BI, Wisch N *et al.* Treatment of Crohn's disease with 6-mercaptopurine. A long-term, randomized, double-blind study. N Engl J Med. 1980;302:981–7.
6. Ewe K, Press AG, Singe CC *et al.* Azathioprine combined with prednisolone or monotherapy with prednisolone in active Crohn's disease. Gastroenterology. 1993;105:367–72.

7. Candy S, Wright J, Gerber M *et al.* A controlled double blind study of azathioprine in the management of Crohn's disease. Gut. 1995;37:674–8.
8. Oren R, Moshkowitz M, Odes S *et al.* Methotrexate in chronic active Crohn's disease: a double-blind, randomized, Israeli multicenter trial. Am J Gastroenterol. 1997;92:2203–9.
9. Rosenberg JL, Levin B, Wall AJ *et al.* A controlled trial of azathioprine in Crohn's disease. Am J Dig Dis. 1975;20:721–6.
10. O'Donoghue DP, Dawson AM, Powell TJ *et al.* Double-blind withdrawal trial of azathioprine as maintenance treatment for Crohn's disease. Lancet. 1978;2:955–7.
11. Sandborn WJ, Sutherland L, Pearson DC *et al.* Azathioprine or 6-mercaptopurine for inducing remission of Crohn's disease. The Cochrane Library. 2001;1:1–15.
12. Pearson DC, May GR, Fick GH *et al.* Azathioprine for maintaining remission of Crohn's disease. The Cochrane Library. 2001;1:1–10.
13. Sandborn WJ, Van OE, Zins BJ *et al.* An intravenous loading dose of azathioprine decreases the time to response in patients with Crohn's disease. Gastroenterology. 1995;109:1808–17.
14. Present DH, Meltzer SJ, Krumholz MP *et al.* 6-Mercaptopurine in the management of inflammatory bowel disease: short- and long-term toxicity. Ann Intern Med. 1989;111:641–9.
15. Feagan BG, Rochon J, Fedorak RN *et al.* Methotrexate for the treatment of Crohn's disease. The North American Crohn's Study Group Investigators. N Engl J Med. 1995;332:292–7.
16. Lémann M, Chamiot PC, Mesnard B *et al.* Methotrexate for the treatment of refractory Crohn's disease. Aliment Pharmacol Ther. 1996;10:309–14.
17. Brynskov J, Freund L, Rasmussen SN *et al.* A placebo-controlled, double-blind, randomized trial of cyclosporine therapy in active chronic Crohn's disease. N Engl J Med. 1989;321:845–50.
18. Feagan BG, McDonald JW, Rochon J *et al.* Low-dose cyclosporine for the treatment of Crohn's disease. The Canadian Crohn's Relapse Prevention Trial Investigators. N Engl J Med. 1994;330:1846–51.
19. Jewell DP, Lennard Jones JE and the Cyclosporine-Study Group of Great Britain and Ireland. Oral cyclosporin for chronic active Crohn's disease: a multicentre controlled trial. Eur J Gastroenterol Hepatol. 1994;6499–505.
20. Stange EF, Modigliani R, Pena AS *et al.* European trial of cyclosporine in chronic active Crohn's disease: a 12-month study. Gastroenterology. 1995;109:774–82.
21. Fellermann K, Ludwig D, Stahl M *et al.* Steroid-unresponsive acute attacks of inflammatory bowel disease: immunomodulation by tacrolimus (FK506). Am J Gastroenterol. 1998;93: 1860–6.
22. Neurath MF, Wanitschke R, Peters M *et al.* Randomised trial of mycophenolate mofetil versus azathioprine for treatment of chronic active Crohn's disease. Gut. 1999;44:625–8.
23. Fellermann K, Steffen M, Stein J *et al.* Mycophenolate-mofetil: lack of efficacy in chronic active inflammatory bowel disease. Aliment Pharmacol Ther. 2000;14:171–6.
24. Dubinsky M, Hassard PV, Seidman EG *et al.* An open-label pilot study using 6-thioguanine as a therapeutic agent in Crohn's disease patients resistant to mercaptopurine. Inflamm Bowel Dis. 2001;7:181–9.

27
Novel therapeutic options in Crohn's disease: targeting the MAP kinase pathways

B. VAN DEN BLINK, T. TEN HOVE, M. P. PEPPELENBOSCH and S. J. H. VAN DEVENTER

INTRODUCTION

Modern molecular biology has provided us with tools that rapidly enhance our insight into the pathogenesis of many inflammatory diseases, including Crohn's disease. In the past decade, the use of genetically modified mice in experimental models of colitis has shed light on the pivotal role of pro- and anti-inflammatory cytokines, such as TNF and IL-10 in this disease. Extending these data to the human situation has led to successful trials with e.g. anti-TNF. Apoptosis research has contributed to our knowledge of the determinants of deranged T-lymphocyte activation, as seen in Crohn's disease[1,2]. More recently, a gene for Crohn's disease was found encoding NOD-2, a protein involved in the recognition of microbes and signalling events leading to an immune response[3,4]. These and other lines of research are extending our grasp of the pathogenesis of Crohn's disease and may eventually lead to aetiology-based therapy.

Despite these exciting advances, current treatment modalities are still insufficient for many patients. Although remission induction can be achieved in many instances, using conventional (immunosuppressives) and new therapeutics (e.g. anti-TNF), medication side-effects and disease relapse remain unsurpassable problems.

In recent years, the focus of attention in Crohn's disease research has been shifting from known *inter*cellular mediators, such as TNF, IL-10, IFNγ, and IL-12, towards the *intra*cellular signals they invoke. Transduction of these signals, their regulation and their possible therapeutic value is thought to be of great interest. An important group of signal transduction proteins involved in regulating many inflammatory processes is the mitogen-activated protein kinase (MAPK) family. Recently, the first successful trial in Crohn's disease was reported using a new class of small molecules that inhibits the MAPK pathway[5].

In this chapter, we will describe the involvement of MAPK family members in processes governing Crohn's disease pathogenesis and discuss their possible therapeutic value.

THE MITOGEN-ACTIVATED PROTEIN KINASE PATHWAYS

MAPK family members can be found in all eukaryotic cells. They are evolutionarily well conserved and regulate a wide variety of cellular functions by mediating extracellular signals into intracellular responses. Their activity is controlled in a three-tiered cassette that consists of a MAPK, which is activated upon phosphorylation of both a threonine and tyrosine residue by a MAPK kinase (MKK). MKK is in turn activated by an upstream MKK kinase (MKKK). Once activated, MAPKs can phosphorylate and activate other kinases or transcription factors. Altered transcription factor activity in turn will lead to a different gene expression profile. On the other hand, MAPKs can also have an effect on translation by phosphorylation of factors involved in protein synthesis[6]. Three major MAPK pathways have been described: the p38 MAPK, p42/44 MAPK and c-Jun N-terminal kinase (JNK) pathways (Figure 1). Together with nuclear factor-κB (NFκB), these MAPKs largely control the cells' response to inflammation and stress.

p38 MAPKs are 38-kDa signal transduction proteins comprising four variants: p38α, β, γ and δ. p38 MAPK was first described as a protein that was activated in response to lipopolysaccharide (LPS)[7]. Independently, p38 MAPK was found to be the protein that was targeted by a novel class of medication, the cytokine-suppressive anti-inflammatory drugs[8]. Besides LPS, many other cellular stresses (e.g. UV, osmotic shock) and inflammatory stimuli (TNF, IL-1β, PMA) activate p38 MAPK, via upstream kinases MKK3/6, leading to phosphorylation of downstream transcription factors, e.g. ATF-2, and kinases such as MAPKAPK-2. Inhibition of p38 MAPK, for example with the commonly used SB203580,

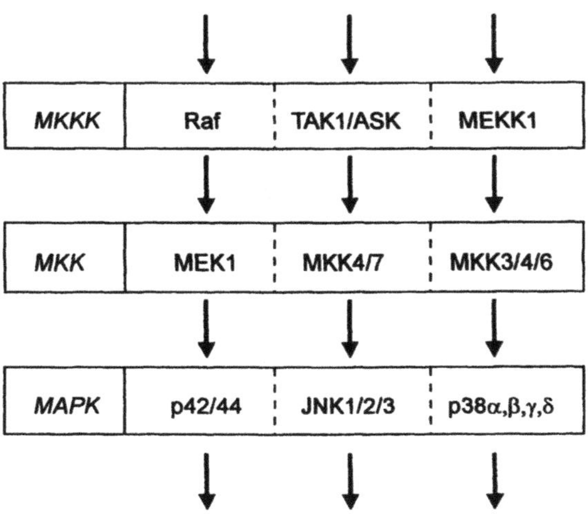

Figure 1 The three major MAPK pathways

reduces pro-inflammatory cytokine production in monocytes/macrophages, neutrophils and T lymphocytes. Furthermore, p38 MAPK is involved in various other inflammation-related events, such as neutrophil activation[9,10], apoptosis[11], and NO synthase induction[12]. Hence, p38 MAPK is thought to be a prime candidate for new anti-inflammatory/anticytokine therapies.

p42/44 MAPK consist of two isoforms, p44 MAPK (or extracellular regulated kinase (ERK)-1) and p42 MAPK (or ERK-2). These kinases are activated by mitogenic stimuli, such as growth factors (EGF, PDGF), phorbol esters and insulin. Typically, upon binding of the mitogen to its receptor, the signal is transduced into the cell via sequential activation of the small GTPase Ras, Raf, MEK1/2 (MAPK or ERK kinase, a MKK). Activated p42/44 MAPK in turn phosphorylates downstream transcription factors, such as Elk-1/Ets. Furthermore, p42/44 MAPK can also influence translation by directly phosphorylating p90RSK[13]. p42/44 MAPK is involved in normal cell growth, differentiation and survival. However, involvement of p42/44 MAPK was also observed in malignant disease, often accompanied by Ras mutations[14]. High levels of activated p42/44 MAPK have been found in acute myelogenous leukaemia cells and breast cancer cells, and therapeutic targeting of the p42/44 MAPK pathway in these conditions is being suggested[14,15]. Alongside the classic role of p42/44 MAPK in mitogen-induced growth and differentiation, p42/44 MAPK is also involved in inflammatory cytokine production. Active p42/44 was observed to be a prerequisite for T lymphocyte IL-10 production[16], and LPS induced TNF production in monocytes[17].

JNK consist of at least three isoforms (JNK1/2/3) that each have 2–4 different splice variants, resulting in 46-kDa and 54-kDa proteins[6]. Whereas JNK1 and 2 are ubiquitously expressed, JNK3 is mainly expressed in the brain. Like p38 MAPK, JNK is activated by cellular stress (UV, osmoshock, ionizing radiation) and inflammatory cytokines (TNF, IL-1) and together they have been dubbed the stress-activated protein kinases (SAPKs). Upon activation through upstream kinases MKK4/7[18], JNK controls, among others, AP-1 transcription activity through phosphorylation of c-Jun[19]. In contrast to p38 MAPK and p42/44 MAPK, specific JNK inhibitors are not readily available, and, so far, the role of JNK in inflammation remains enigmatic. However, targeted disruption of JNK1 and 2 in mice showed that they play an important role in T-cell growth and differentiation[20,21]. The role of JNK in T-cell proliferation and differentiation will be discussed more extensively further on.

TUMOUR NECROSIS FACTOR

Crohn's disease is characterized by chronic inflammation leading to destruction of normal tissue integrity. Tumour necrosis factor (TNF), a prototype pro-inflammatory cytokine, plays a central role in the initiation and amplification of the inflammatory reaction seen in Crohn's disease[22]. Altering the regulation of TNF production or its efficacy thus seems attractive in Crohn's disease. Indeed, monoclonal antibodies against TNF have proven effective in inducing both clinical remission and endoscopic healing[23,24]. Several MAPK members are involved in transcriptional and post-transcriptional regulation of TNF production in monocytes/macrophages and T lymphocytes. Lee *et al.* reported that

LPS-induced TNF production in monocytes could be blocked with a p38 MAPK inhibitor[8]. Inhibition of p42/44 MAPK also leads to decreased levels of TNF in monocytes[17]. In a T-cell line, TNF gene transcription was found to be dependent on all three MAPK pathways[25]. Similarly, full TNF gene induction relies on activation of all three major MAPK pathways in macrophages[26]. A co-operative effect of p38 MAPK and p42/44 MAPK was also found in TNF and IL-6 production in alveolar macrophages[27]. On the other hand, inhibition of p42/44 MAPK in primary murine peritoneal macrophages did not inhibit LPS-induced TNF production[28]. Furthermore, inhibition of p38 MAPK increased TNF production in primary murine peritoneal macrophages, suggesting that MAPK-regulated cytokine production is cell-type dependent[29]. *In vivo*, inhibition of p38 MAPK was found to inhibit endotoxic shock-induced TNF production and mortality in mice[30]. In a model for pulmonary inflammation, TNF accumulation appeared to be dependent on active p38 MAPK[31]. Mice deficient in MAPKAPK-2, a target downstream from p38 MAPK, are endotoxin tolerant, although this resistance seems to depend on reduced TNF translation rather than transcription[32]. Thus it seems that TNF release from monocytes/macrophages and T lymphocytes can be inhibited, at least in part, by inhibiting the p38 MAPK or p42/44 MAPK pathway.

INTERLEUKIN 12 AND 18

Poorly controlled activation of Th-1-biased CD4+ T lymphocytes is believed to be a major pathogenic mechanism in Crohn's disease. IL-12 and IL-18 play an important role in activating naive T cells and driving them into a Th-1 phenotype, leading to increased IFNγ and TNF release. Indeed, elevated levels of IL-12 and IL-18 (initially described as IFNγ-inducing factor) have been measured in intestinal lesions from patients with Crohn's disease[33,34], and stimulation of lamina propria cells with IL-18 and IL-12 resulted in an increased IFNγ production[35].

IL-12 was shown to induce MKK3/6 and p38 MAPK, but not JNK or p42/44 activation in T cells[36,37], suggesting involvement of the p38 MAPK pathway in IL-12 signalling. A well-known component of IL-12 signalling, signal transducer and activator of transcription (STAT)-4, can be phosphorylated on serine 721 by MKK6 and p38 MAPK, and this p38 MAPK pathway-dependent phosphorylation was shown to be necessary for STAT4-mediated IL-12 activity[37]. However, IL-12 can also induce effects such as IFNγ production in a STAT4-independent manner[38]. Zhang *et al.* described that IL-12-induced, STAT4-independent IFNγ production depends on functional p38 MAPK[36]. Finally, T cell stimulation through TLR4, which preferentially induces a Th-1 response, induces IL-12p70 in a p38 MAPK-dependent fashion[39]. These data are in line with *in-vivo* experiments. Mice with a targeted MKK3 disruption, resulting in diminished p38 MAPK activation, show defective IL-12 production in antigen-presenting cells (macrophages and dendritic cells), leading to decreased IFNγ production by naive T cells[40]. In a murine model of colitis (TNBS-induced colitis), inhibition of p38 MAPK with SB203580 significantly decreased the amount of IL-12p70 in colon homogenates, although no beneficial effect of p38 MAPK inhibition was observed, correlating with an increased TNF level[41]. Contrasting these data is a report describing p38 MAPK inhibition-induced augmentation of

IL-12 production by human monocytes/macrophages upon stimulation with LPS and IFNγ[42]. These data again suggest that p38 MAPK function in cytokine production is cell-type specific.

So far, little is known about IL-18 signal transduction in Th cells. Similar to IL-1, IL-18 utilizes an IL-1R-associated kinase (IRAK)-mediated pathway, and thus MAPK involvement is very conceivable. Indeed, IL-18 induces activation of p38 MAPK and JNK in a T cell line[43], and p42/44 MAPK in an NK cell line[44]. IL-18-induced NK cytolytic activity was shown to be dependent on p42/44 MAPK activation, and IL-18 induced IFNγ production could be inhibited with p38 and p42/44 MAPK inhibitors[44].

Th-1 DIFFERENTIATION AND INTERFERON γ PRODUCTION

IL-2 is an important factor in driving T-cell proliferation and activation. Signal transduction events in CD4+ T cells following exposure to IL-2 include p38 MAPK and JNK phosphorylation[45]. However, reports concerning the functional significance of p38 MAPK and JNK activity in IL-2 signalling are contradictory[45,46], and it is unclear whether MAPKs are critically involved in IL-2-induced T-cell proliferation. Whether IL-2 production in T cells is under the control of JNK is under debate[47]. JNK1- and JNK2-deficient T cells produce normal levels of IL-2[21,20]. In contrast, JNK1/2 and MKK4-deficient T cells were observed to produce reduced levels of IL-2 upon CD28 costimulation[48,49].

Differentiation of naive CD4+ T cells into Th-1 is regulated by JNK1/2. JNK1-deficient naive CD4+ T cells preferentially differentiate into Th-2 cells, and thus JNK1 seems to be a negative regulator of Th-2 differentiation[20]. T cells defective in JNK2 produced less IFN and differentiation into Th-1 was impaired, while differentiation into Th-2 was not[21]. For Th-2 differentiation and IL-4 production, p42/44 MAPK activation seems to be a prerequisite[50].

Th-1 differentiation is also under the control of p38 MAPK. Using a specific inhibitor of p38 MAPK and by generating transgenic mice that overexpress a dominant-negative p38 MAP kinase, Rincon *et al.* showed that inactivation of p38 MAPK led to reduced IFNγ production in Th-1 cells, but had no effect on IL-4 production in Th-2 cells[51]. In line with these results, Th-1 cells from transgenic mice overexpressing MKK6, leading to constitutively activated p38 MAPK, showed increased IFNγ production[51]. Furthermore, Zhang *et al.* observed that p38 MAPK, but not p42/44 MAP or JNK, is required for IL-12-induced IFNγ production in activated T cells and Th-1 cells[36]. Correlating with these studies, CD4+ T cells from MKK3-deficient mice exhibit impaired IFNγ production[40]. Recently, it was shown that TCR-dependent and -independent IFNγ production in Th-1 cells depend on p38 MAPK and JNK via GADD45, a protein involved in cell cycle and differentiation[52–54]. Thus, both p38 MAPK and JNK are critical determinants of Th-1 differentiation.

CONCLUDING REMARKS

Involvement of the MAPK family members in the pathogenesis of Crohn's disease seems very likely. Many known mediators and derailed immune functions that are critical in the pathogenesis in Crohn's disease are under the regulatory control of one or more MAPK pathways. Indeed, recently, activation of several MAPK members was reported in biopsies from inflamed mucosa from Crohn's disease patients[55]. Furthermore, a trial using a JNK/p38MAPK inhibitor (CNI-1493) showed significant clinical benefit and rapid endoscopic ulcer healing in patients with severe Crohn's disease (mean CDAI before treatment: 380; after treatment: 146.5), correlating with decreased JNK activation in intra-epithelial lymphocytes and lamina propria cells[5]. Furthermore, in a murine model of rheumatoid arthritis, a disease with many similarities with Crohn's disease, inhibition of JNK or p38MAPK was shown to be beneficial[30,56].

One must keep in mind that a great deal of our current knowledge concerning normal and stress-induced MAPK function comes from cell-based and murine models. This obviously limits extrapolation of these data to the human situation and calls for caution in the use of MAPK inhibitors in patients. Indeed, inhibition of p38 and 42/44 MAPK impairs normal bactericidal mechanisms in neutrophils[57,58], and, in a murine pneumonia model, inhibition of p38 MAPK decreased bacterial clearing[29].

Nevertheless, MAPK inhibition seems an attractive new avenue for treatment of Th-1-mediated inflammatory conditions such as Crohn's disease. Whether MAPK inhibition should be selective rather than general is a point for discussion. So far, MAPK inhibition-related side-effects (mainly hepatotoxicity) and adverse events are limited[5]. However, the ubiquitous presence of the MAPK pathways and their widespread involvement in a vast array of processes suggests that selective inhibition of isoforms of MAPK is preferable. On the other hand, in Crohn's disease, inhibition of both JNK1 and 2, preventing Th1 differentiation, and p38 MAPK(α), preventing pro-inflammatory cytokine production, seems attractive.

References

1. Bu P, Keshavarzian A, Stone DD *et al.* Apoptosis: one of the mechanisms that maintains unresponsiveness of the intestinal mucosal immune system. J Immunol. 2001;166:6399–403.
2. ten Hove T, van Montfrans C, Peppelenbosch MP, van Deventer SJH. Infliximab treatment induces apoptosis of lamina propria T lymphocytes in Crohn's disease. Gut. 2002;50:206–11.
3. Hugot JP, Chamaillard M, Zouali H *et al.* Association of NOD2 leucine-rich repeat variants with susceptibility to Crohn's disease. Nature. 2001;411:599–603.
4. Ogura Y, Bonen DK, Inohara N *et al.* A frameshift mutation in NOD2 associated with susceptibility to Crohn's disease. Nature. 2001;411:603–6.
5. Hommes D, van den Blink B, Plasse T *et al.* Inhibition of stress-activated MAP *kinases* induces clinical improvement in moderate to severe Crohn's disease. Gastroenterology. 2002;122:7–14.
6. Kyriakis JM, Avruch J. Mammalian mitogen-activated protein kinase signal transduction pathways activated by stress and inflammation. Physiol Rev. 2001;81:807–69.
7. Han J, Lee JD, Bibbs L, Ulevitch RJ. A MAP kinase targeted by endotoxin and hyperosmolarity in mammalian cells. Science. 1994;265:808–11.
8. Lee JC, Laydon JT, McDonnell PC *et al.* A protein kinase involved in the regulation of inflammatory cytokine biosynthesis. Nature. 1994;372:739–46.
9. Read MA, Whitley MZ, Gupta S *et al.* Tumor necrosis factor alpha-induced E-selection expression is activated by the nuclear factor-kappaB and c-JUN N-terminal kinase/p38 mitogen-activated protein kinase pathways. J Biol Chem. 1997;272:2753–61.
10. Nick JA, Avdi NJ, Young SK *et al.* Selective activation and functional significance of p38alpha mitogen-activated protein kinase in lipopolysaccharide-stimulated neutrophils. J Clin Invest. 1999;103:851–8.

11. Mackay K, Mochly-Rosen D. An inhibitor of p38 mitogen-activated protein kinase protects neonatal cardiac myocytes from ischemia. J Biol Chem. 1999;274:6272–9.
12. Chen CC, Wang JK. p38 but not p44/42 mitogen-activated protein kinase is required for nitric oxide synthase induction mediated by lipopolysaccharide in RAW 264.7 macrophages. Mol Pharmacol. 1999;55:481–8.
13. Sale EM, Atkinson PG, Sale GJ. Requirement of MAP kinase for differentiation of fibroblasts to adipocytes, for insulin activation of p90 S6 kinase and for insulin or serum stimulation of DNA synthesis. EMBO J. 1995;14:674–84.
14. Milella M, Kornblau SM, Estrov Z *et al.* Therapeutic targeting of the MEK/MAPK signal transduction module in acute myeloid leukemia. J Clin Invest. 2001;108:851–9.
15. Gee JM, Robertson JF, Ellis IO, Nicholson RI. Phosphorylation of ERK1/2 mitogen-activated protein kinase is associated with poor response to anti-hormonal therapy and decreased patient survival in clinical breast cancer. Int J Cancer. 2001;95:247–54.
16. Egerton M, Fitzpatrick DR, Kelso A. Activation of the extracellular signal-regulated kinase pathway is differentially required for TCR-stimulated production of six cytokines in primary T lymphocytes. Int Immunol. 1998;10:223–9.
17. van der Bruggen T, Nijenhuis S, van Raaij E, Verhoef J, van Asbeck BS. Lipopolysaccharide-induced tumor necrosis factor alpha production by human monocytes involves the raf-1/MEK1-MEK2/ERK1-ERK2 pathway. Infect Immun. 1999;67:3824–9.
18. Tournier C, Dong C, Turner TK, Jones SN, Flavell RA, Davis RJ. MKK7 is an essential component of the JNK signal transduction pathway activated by proinflammatory cytokines. Genes Dev. 2001;15:1419–26.
19. Davis RJ. Signal transduction by the JNK group of MAP kinases. Cell. 2000;103:239–52.
20. Dong C, Yang DD, Wysk M, Whitmarsh AJ, Davis RJ, Flavell RA. Defective T cell differentiation in the absence of Jnk1. Science. 1998;282:2092–5.
21. Yang DD, Conze D, Whitmarsh AJ *et al.* Differentiation of CD4+ T cells to Th1 cells requires MAP kinase JNK2. Immunity. 1998;9:575–85.
22. van Deventer SJ. Immunotherapy of Crohn's disease. Scand J Immunol. 2000;51:18–22.
23. Targan SR, Hanauer SB, van Deventer SJ *et al.* A short-term study of chimeric monoclonal antibody cA2 to tumor necrosis factor alpha for Crohn's disease. Crohn's Disease cA2 Study Group. N Engl J Med. 1997;337:1029–35.
24. Van Dullemen HM, van Deventer SJ, Hommes DW *et al.* Treatment of Crohn's disease with anti-tumor necrosis factor chimeric monoclonal antibody (cA2). Gastroenterology. 1995;109:129–35.
25. Hoffmeyer A, Grosse-Wilde A, Flory E *et al.* Different mitogen-activated protein kinase signaling pathways cooperate to regulate tumor necrosis factor alpha gene expression in T lymphocytes. J Biol Chem. 1999;274:4319–27.
26. Zhu W, Downey JS, Gu J, Di Padova F, Gram H, Han J. Regulation of TNF expression by multiple mitogen-activated protein kinase pathways. J Immunol. 2000;164:6349–58.
27. Carter AB, Monick MM, Hunninghake GW. Both Erk and p38 kinases are necessary for cytokine gene transcription. Am J Resp Cell Mol Biol. 1999;20:751–8.
28. Means TK, Pavlovich RP, Roca D, Vermeulen MW, Fenton MJ. Activation of TNF-alpha transcription utilizes distinct MAP kinase pathways in different macrophage populations. J Leuk Biol. 2000;67:885–93.
29. van den Blink B, Juffermans NP, ten Hove T *et al.* p38 mitogen-activated protein kinase inhibition increases cytokine release by macrophages in vitro and during infection in vivo. J Immunol. 2001;166:582–7.
30. Badger AM, Bradbeer JN, Votta B, Lee JC, Adams JL, Griswold DE. Pharmacological profile of SB 203580, a selective inhibitor of cytokine suppressive binding protein/p38 kinase, in animal models of arthritis, bone resorption, endotoxin shock and immune function. J Pharmacol Exp Ther. 1996;279:1453–61.
31. Nick JA, Young SK, Brown KK *et al.* Role of p38 mitogen-activated protein kinase in a murine model of pulmonary inflammation. J Immunol. 2000;164:2151–9.
32. Kotlyarov A, Neininger A, Schubert C *et al.* MAPKAP kinase 2 is essential for LPS-induced TNF-alpha biosynthesis. Nat Cell Biol. 1999;1:94–7.
33. Parronchi P, Romagnani P, Annunziato F *et al.* Type 1 T-helper cell predominance and interleukin-12 expression in the gut of patients with Crohn's disease. Am J Pathol. 1997;150:823–32.
34. Pizarro TT, Michie MH, Bentz M *et al.* IL-18, a novel immunoregulatory cytokine, is up-regulated in Crohn's disease: expression and localization in intestinal mucosal cells. J Immunol. 1999;162:6829–35.

35. Siegmund B, Fantuzzi G, Rieder F *et al.* Neutralization of interleukin-18 reduces severity in murine colitis and intestinal IFN-gamma and TNF-alpha production. Am J Physiol Regul Integr Comp Physiol. 2001;281:R1264–73.
36. Zhang S, Kaplan MH. The p38 mitogen-activated protein kinase is required for IL-12-induced IFN-gamma expression. J Immunol. 2000;165:1374–80.
37. Visconti R, Gadina M, Chiariello M *et al.* Importance of the MKK6/p38 pathway for interleukin-12-induced STAT4 serine phosphorylation and transcriptional activity. Blood. 2000;96: 1844–52.
38. Verhagen CE, de Boer T, Smits HH *et al.* Residual type 1 immunity in patients genetically deficient for interleukin 12 receptor beta1 (IL-12Rbeta1): evidence for an IL-12Rbeta1-independent pathway of IL-12 responsiveness in human T cells. J Exp Med. 2000;192:517–28.
39. Re F, Strominger JL. Toll-like receptor 2 (TLR2) and TLR4 differentially activate human dendritic cells. J Biol Chem. 2001;26:26.
40. Lu HT, Yang DD, Wysk M *et al.* Defective IL-12 production in mitogen-activated protein (MAP) kinase kinase 3 (Mkk3)-deficient mice. EMBO J. 1999;18:1845–57.
41. ten Hove T, van den Blink B, Pronk I, Drillenburg P, Peppelenbosch MP, van Deventer SJ. Inhibition of p38 MAPK with SB 203580 in experimental colitis. Gut. 2001; (in press).
42. Marriott JB, Clarke IA, Dalgleish AG. Inhibition of p38 MAP kinase during cellular activation results in IFN-gamma-dependent augmentation of IL-12 production by human monocytes/ macrophages. Clin Exp Immunol. 2001;125:64–70.
43. Thomassen E, Bird TA, Renshaw BR, Kennedy MK, Sims JE. Binding of interleukin-18 to the interleukin-1 receptor homologous receptor IL-1Rrp1 leads to activation of signaling pathways similar to those used by interleukin-1. J Interferon Cytokine Res. 1998;18:1077–88.
44. Kalina U, Kauschat D, Koyama N *et al.* IL-18 activates STAT3 in the natural killer cell line 92, augments cytotoxic activity, and mediates IFN-gamma production by the stress kinase p38 and by the extracellular regulated kinases p44erk-1 and p42erk-21. J Immunol. 2000;165:1307–13.
45. Crawley JB, Rawlinson L, Lali FV, Page TH, Saklatvala J, Foxwell BM. T cell proliferation in response to interleukins 2 and 7 requires p38MAP kinase activation. J Biol Chem. 1997;272:15023–7.
46. Hunt AE, Lali FV, Lord JD *et al.* Role of interleukin (IL)-2 receptor beta-chain subdomains and Shc in p38 mitogen-activated protein (MAP) kinase and p54 MAP kinase (stress-activated protein kinase/c-Jun N-terminal kinase) activation. IL-2-driven proliferation is independent of p38 and p54 MAP kinase activation. J Biol Chem. 1999;274:7591–7.
47. Rincon M. MAP-kinase signaling pathways in T cells. Curr Opin Immunol. 2001;13:339–45.
48. Nishina H, Bachmann M, Oliveira-dos-Santos AJ *et al.* Impaired CD28-mediated interleukin 2 production and proliferation in stress kinase SAPK/ERK1 kinase (SEK1)/mitogen-activated protein kinase kinase 4 (MKK4)-deficient T lymphocytes. J Exp Med. 1997;186:941–53.
49. Sabapathy K, Kallunki T, David JP, Graef I, Karin M, Wagner EF. c-Jun NH2-terminal kinase (JNK)1 and JNK2 have similar and stage-dependent roles in regulating T cell apoptosis and proliferation. J Exp Med. 2001;193:317–28.
50. Yamashita M, Kimura M, Kubo M *et al.* T cell antigen receptor-mediated activation of the Ras/mitogen-activated protein kinase pathway controls interleukin 4 receptor function and type-2 helper T cell differentiation. Proc Natl Acad Sci USA. 1999;96:1024–9.
51. Rincon M, Enslen H, Raingeaud J *et al.* Interferon-gamma expression by Th1 effector T cells mediated by the p38 MAP kinase signaling pathway. EMBO J. 1998;17:2817–29.
52. Lu B, Yu H, Chow C *et al.* GADD45gamma mediates the activation of the p38 and JNK MAP kinase pathways and cytokine production in effector TH1 cells. Immunity. 2001;14:583–90.
53. Yang J, Zhu H, Murphy TL, Ouyang W, Murphy KM. IL-18-stimulated GADD45 beta required in cytokine-induced, but not TCR-induced, IFN-gamma production. Nat Immunol. 2001;2:157–64.
54. Nakanishi K. Innate and acquired activation pathways in T cells. Nat Immunol. 2001;2:140–2.
55. Waetzig GH, Seegert D, Nikolaus S *et al.* Differential activity and expression of mitogen-activated protein kinases in inflammatory bowel disease. Proc Dig Dis Week. 2001:Abstract 2657.
56. Han Z, Boyle DL, Aupperle KR, Bennett B, Manning AM, Firestein GS. Jun N-terminal kinase in rheumatoid arthritis. J Pharmacol Exp Ther. 1999;291:124–30.
57. Zu YL, Qi J, Gilchrist A *et al.* p38 mitogen-activated protein kinase activation is required for human neutrophil function triggered by TNF-alpha or FMLP stimulation. J Immunol. 1998;160:1982–9.
58. Downey GP, Butler JR, Tapper H *et al.* Importance of MEK in neutrophil microbicidal responsiveness. J Immunol. 1998;160:434–43.

28
Refractory Crohn's disease – when is the time for surgery?

R. S. McLEOD and E. D. KENNEDY

Crohn's disease is a chronic inflammatory disease which may involve any part of the gastrointestinal tract. It tends to manifest in young adults and is characterized by periods of activity followed by periods of inactivity. Although most patients' life spans are not shortened by the disease, their health-related quality of life may be severely impaired during flareups. While recent advances in elucidating the pathogenesis of Crohn's disease are exciting, as yet, the aetiology of Crohn's disease is unknown and, therefore, there is no cure for the disease. The disease is chronic in nature and treatment is palliative. Thus, the goal of therapy should be to minimize both the frequency and severity of flareups in order to minimize the impact of the disease on patients' wellbeing and maximize quality of life. To do so, various treatment modalities including medication, nutrition and surgery are used to treat the disease when it is active and to maintain remission of the disease. Despite the introduction of new classes of drugs, approximately 80% of patients with Crohn's disease will ultimately require surgery at some point in their disease[1]. Thus, surgical therapy should be considered another treatment option and not be considered a last resort when all other forms of treatment have failed.

Although surgery should be part of the treatment considerations of clinicians treating patients with the disease, it is often difficult to know when to continue with medical therapy and when to opt for surgery. Surgery is usually very successful in alleviating complications and improving quality of life. However, because Crohn's disease is a panintestinal disease, there is the potential for progression of the disease, the need for further resections and the possibility of complications related to short bowel syndrome following surgery. Thus, a conservative approach to surgery is warranted. On the other hand, it must also be recognized that most medical therapies also are associated with side-effects and long-term, sometimes irreversible, toxicity. Also, patients' quality of life may be severely impaired by continuous disease activity.

Sandborn *et al.* have defined refractory Crohn's disease as a score of 150–450 on the Crohn's Disease Activity Index despite treatment with prednisone at a dose of 20 mg/day or more for at least 4 weeks[2]. Modigliani has defined chronic active Crohn's disease as: a form of Crohn's disease giving rise to virtually permanent symptoms; or acute outbreaks which occur close together (2–3 times per year) in spite of maintenance treatment with salicylates; or steroid-dependent Crohn's disease either requiring continuous steroid therapy for over 6 months, in excess of 10 mg/day of prednisone, or relapsing after at least two successive attempts at withdrawal of steroids[3]. Munkholm *et al.* have reported that 35% of patients with Crohn's disease will become steroid dependent after a course of steroids[4]. Despite this, as an indication for surgery it is relatively uncommon. Farmer and colleagues from the Cleveland Clinic reported on the indications for surgery in 500 patients[5]. The indications varied depending on the site of disease. However, failure of medical management was the indication for surgery in only 7–9% of patients with predominantly small bowel or ileocolic disease, respectively, whereas it was the indication for surgery in 26% of patients with colonic disease. More often, in patients with small bowel or ileocolonic disease, the indication was obstruction (35–55% of patients) or fistulizing disease (32–47%). It is likely that this discrepancy is due to the fact that, while these complications were the primary reason for surgery, many patients probably had some associated disease activity and, although not stated, were also steroid dependent.

In deciding on whether patients should have surgery rather than continue with other forms of medical therapy, it is prudent to consider such issues as the morbidity, quality of life, long-term outcome and cost of surgery. These will be reviewed in the following section.

OUTCOME FOLLOWING SURGERY

Morbidity of surgery

Various surgical procedures may be performed in Crohn's disease because of the variable manifestations and sites of the gastrointestinal tract affected by the disease. A full discussion of the various operations is beyond the scope of this chapter. However, resection is the preferred option in most situations whether there is small or large bowel involvement. Generally, all of the grossly involved disease is removed and primary anastomosis performed. Although a large proportion of patients will require surgery for Crohn's disease, only a small proportion (those with rectal or perianal involvement) will require a permanent ileostomy. In emergent situations, or where the patient's nutritional status is impaired, a temporary ileostomy may be necessary.

Strictureplasty is used in select patients who have had multiple previous resections or have multiple skip lesions. Bypass procedures (the so-called Eisenhower procedure) were popular in the 1960s but they are rarely performed now because of the high rate of recrudescence of the disease in the short term and the increased risk of small bowel cancer in the long term. At present, the only indication for a bypass procedure would be a gastrojejunostomy for duodenal Crohn's disease.

Surgery today is very safe in patients with Crohn's disease. The operative mortality is extremely low in patients having surgery for Crohn's disease with many large series not reporting any deaths. However, to achieve optimal results, the gastrointestinal tract should be fully evaluated, the patient's medical status should be optimized and other measures, such as correction of fluid and electrolyte abnormalities, administration of antibiotic and thromboembolic prophylaxis, should be taken. Percutaneous drainage of intra-abdominal abscesses is an important component of the preoperative management of Crohn's disease patients. Doing so may avoid a multiple staged operation and a temporary stoma.

One of the most significant changes in the surgical approach to Crohn's disease has been the introduction of laparoscopic techniques[6]. Crohn's disease is an ideal indication for the laparoscopic approach since it is a benign disease and the concerns related to cancer recurrence do not apply. In addition, an improved cosmetic result is an important consideration in this often young patient population. There tends to be less pain and higher patient satisfaction with laparoscopic procedures. On the other hand, the patient may have multiple adhesions from previous operations, or a large inflammatory mass, abscess or fistula or obstructed bowel which may preclude a laparoscopic approach. The other issues related to a laparoscopic approach are that it may be more difficult to assess the extent of the disease, particularly small bowel skip lesions, and that operative time tends to be longer. However, these issues are of less concern now as more surgeons attain greater experience generally with laparoscopic techniques. On the other hand, there is no consistent evidence that hospital stays are shortened significantly or that return to work occurs earlier following laparoscopy.

As laparoscopic techniques have become more widely adopted, the indications have widened. It is well accepted that the laparoscopic approach for performing defunctioning stomas offers real advantages over an open approach. It can be performed easily with the stoma being brought out through one of the port sites. Also, terminal ileal and right colon resections, segmental resections of the small and large bowel, proctectomy, reconstruction of the gastrointestinal tract following a Hartmann procedure and even total proctocolectomy are being performed.

Most proponents advocate performing laparoscopic assisted resections so the bowel is exteriorized through a small incision at one of the port sites, and the mesentery, which is often thickened, is divided extracorporeally. However, with the introduction of the ligature, intracorporeal division of the vessels is possible. Also, fistulizing disease is no longer a contraindication for the laparoscopic approach and several reports have documented successful completion of such resections laparoscopically in up to 80% of patients[7,8].

The early experience suggests that laparoscopic resections are safe although patient selection is important. Milsom and colleagues performed a randomized controlled trial of 60 patients randomized to either open or laparoscopic ileocolic resection[9]. The operative time in the laparoscopic group was significantly longer. Although the overall complication rate was lower in the laparoscopic group, there was no significant difference in the rate of major complications, with one observed in each group. There were no significant differences in the analgesia requirements or return of bowel function although time to discharge was earlier in the laparoscopic group.

Aleali and Milsom summarized the world literature on laparoscopic resections for Crohn's disease[10]. Data came from retrospective case series. In total, there were 578 resections of which 376 were ileocolic resections. The conversion rate ranged from 0% to 33%. Overall, the complication rate varied from 0% to 18% and, where series compared the results with historical controls, there was no significant differences. The mean operative times ranged from 105 to 200 min for ileocolic resections and the average hospital stay ranged from 4.2 to 7 days.

Thus, surgery is an attractive option for patients with limited Crohn's disease. It can be performed safely and, with the introduction of laparoscopy, patient acceptance is extremely high.

Quality of life following surgery

Several series have measured outcome in patients preoperatively and postoperative using validated instruments following surgery. All have consistently reported significantly improved outcome postoperatively compared with the preoperative status.

Thirlby and colleagues studied 63 patients who had surgery for inflammatory bowel disease[11]. Of these, 36 had Crohn's disease and all had intractable disease as the indication for surgery. Outcome was measured preoperatively and at 3 months postoperatively using the Medical Outcomes Health Status Questionnaire (SF-36). In this cohort, health-related quality of life (HRQL) was low preoperatively with scores in all 8 scales below the general population whereas scores were significantly improved postoperatively and equal to the general population in most scales.

Yazdanpanah and colleagues examined HRQL in 26 patients who had an elective ileocolonic resection for Crohn's disease[12]. They used a questionnaire comprised of the SF-36 to which was added the Rating Form of Inflammatory Bowel Disease Patients' Concerns (RFIPC), a sleep module and 3 questions of pertinence to the French population. This was administered immediately preoperatively and 3 months postoperatively. Again these investigators found that HRQL was significantly better postoperatively although patients' concerns about having an ostomy bag, surgery, energy level, uncertainty of the disease and pain or suffering were unchanged.

Tillinger and colleagues studied 16 patients preoperatively, and at 3, 6 and 24 months postoperatively using the time trade-off technique and direct questioning of objectives (DQO) to ascertain utilities for their HRQL as well as administering the Crohn's Disease Activity Index (CDAI), RFIPC, and Beck Depression Index[13]. Again, using these instruments, there was significant improvement in all patients at 3 and 6 months preoperatively. However, at 24 months, 4 patients had developed recurrent disease and their scores were similar to those obtained preoperatively whereas the other 12 patients continued to have significantly improved scores.

Casellas and colleagues performed a cross-sectional study which included four cohorts of individuals: 29 patients in remission following surgical resection; 48 patients with a medically induced remission; 42 patients with clinically active disease; and a control group of 63 healthy individuals[14]. HRQL was measured using the Inflammatory Bowel Disease Questionnaire (IBDQ), the Psychological General Well Being Index (PGWBI) and the EuroQol. Patients with active Crohn's disease had significantly poorer scores on the IBDQ, PGWBI and EuroQol. Both cohorts of patients with inactive disease (whether it was surgically or medically induced) had better scores on the three instruments than those with active disease and there was no significant difference between the two cohorts.

Thus, these studies indicate that quality of life is consistently improved following surgery for Crohn's disease. However, quality of life appears to correlate with disease activity. Thus, patients appear to have equally good HRQL whether they are in remission due to surgery or to medical treatment. Furthermore, patients who have had a surgical resection continue to have excellent HRQL until the disease recurs when their quality of life again deteriorates.

Long-term outcome following surgery

While surgery is often successful in treating the complications of the disease and improving patients' quality of life initially, it is important to consider the long-term outcome in these patients since it is a chronic disease. The major consideration in this regard is disease recurrence. The reported recurrence rates are quite variable depending on the criteria used to define recurrence. Although endoscopic recurrence rates varying from 29% to 93% at 1 year have been reported, the reported clinical or symptomatic recurrence rates, which are probably most relevant, range from 6% to 16% per year[15–18]. At 5 years, the recurrence rate approaches 50% and thereafter plateaus. Thus, while approximately 50% of patients will have a recurrence at 5 years, one can also state that a similar proportion will be free of disease and, as discussed previously, will enjoy an excellent quality of life.

Recurrence rates vary with the site of disease so that patients with mainly colonic disease have a lower risk of recurrence[19]. Those who have had previous resections appear to have a higher risk of recurrence. There is some evidence that the risk of recurrence may vary with the pattern of disease. However, it is controversial whether the course of the disease follows a predictable pattern[20]. There is less evidence that the age of onset and duration of disease affect the risk of recurrence. On the other hand, smoking, especially in women, increases the risk of recurrence[21].

One of the concerns with advising surgery in patients with Crohn's disease is that the disease may recur, further resections may be required and the patient may be left with a short gut, requiring permanent total parenteral nutrition. However, despite the propensity to recur and the need for further operations, the risk of short gut syndrome is extremely rare in patients with Crohn's disease. Thus, generally, it should not be a consideration in deciding on whether a patient should have surgery with the exception of those occasional patients with extensive disease or multiple skip lesions.

Cost of surgery

Several studies have addressed the long-term health care costs of patients with Crohn's disease. Silverstein and colleagues from the Mayo Clinic used data from a cohort of 174 patients in Olmsted County in Minnesota who were followed for a median duration of 10 years[22]. These data were then used to model the lifetime costs of care for a representative patient. The projected median total cost of care was $39,906 US and the mean cost of care was $125,404. Of this, $17,526 or 44% of the median costs were incurred by surgical therapy. However, although the costs of surgery accounted for a large part of the total costs, in fact, surgery also was the most effective treatment with 40% of the cohort being in the postsurgical remission state over the subsequent 20 years and, in this state, being well and not taking medication. This analysis was performed using data up to December 1993 and thus did not include the costs of treatment with infliximab and other new therapies. Thus, surgery might now be an even more cost-effective alternative.

SURGERY VERSUS CONTINUED MEDICAL THERAPY IN PATIENTS WITH REFRACTORY CROHN'S DISEASE

Although there is a range of new medications, including infliximab, for use in the steroid-dependent patient, most commonly, the decision in patients deemed to have refractory disease is whether to institute immunosuppressive therapy, usually azathioprine or 6-mercaptopurine, or recommend surgery. Decision analysis is useful in situations which involve complex decision making because this method explicitly models tradeoffs between the risks and benefits of each treatment option taking into consideration all clinically important variables and patient preferences for them. Decision analysis can also be helpful in determining which variables are most important in treatment decisions and therefore may assist in clinical decision making. Our group performed a decision analysis to determine whether initial azathioprine treatment or initial ileocolic resection without a trial of azathioprine is the preferred treatment option in steroid-dependent short-segment terminal ileal Crohn's disease[23].

We based the model on a hypothetical 30-year-old patient with a short segment of terminal ileal Crohn's disease with a 5-year history of disease. He had an acute flareup 6 months ago and, since then, has had one unsuccessful attempt at tapering prednisone. The patient, therefore, has been taking prednisone 10 mg/day to control his symptoms for the past 3 months. The question is whether the patient should be advised to have an ileocolic resection or be placed on azathioprine therapy and, if that fails, have an ileocolic resection.

A Markov model was performed with the time horizon set at 36 months. Those in the azathioprine cohort receive azathioprine, 2 mg/kg/day. If a side-effect develops, the patient is treated with methotrexate. If the patient responds to azathioprine, then he remains on azathioprine until he relapses at which time he is treated with high-dose prednisone. If the patient responds, he again receives azathioprine. If there is only a partial or no response to prednisone, or if a second relapse on azathioprine occurs, patients are started on methotrexate plus high-dose prednisone. Patients remain in this state unless there is no initial response to methotrexate, until a major side-effect from methotrexate develops or a relapse occurs on methotrexate. If any of these events occurs, then patients enter the surgery state and subsequently follow the same path as patients initially in the surgery cohort.

All patients in the surgery cohort initially undergo ileocolic resection. Patients who die postoperatively enter the postop death state. Those who survive are placed on 5-ASA maintenance therapy and continue in the well postop state until they develop a recurrence. Patients who develop a recurrence are treated with high-dose prednisone. Those who respond to prednisone continue in the well postrecurrence state and are treated again with prednisone if a flareup occurs subsequently. Those who do not respond are treated with methotrexate.

Patients in the methotrexate state continue to cycle in this state unless there is no initial response to methotrexate or a major side-effect or relapse occurs while on methotrexate. If so, then they have another surgical resection. Probabilities and utilities for each state were derived from the literature and by consulting with experts.

Based on this model, the expected value for quality-adjusted life months (QALMs) is 30.56 months for azathioprine and 29.96 for ilocolic resection over the 36-month time frame. Thus, azathioprine offers a 0.60 QALM relative to ileocolic resection. This is equivalent to 18 quality-adjusted life days. It was not considered significant.

Various sensitivity analyses were performed, adjusting the variables through the plausible ranges. The model was sensitive to relatively small changes in only two variables: the utility for being symptom free on azathioprine and the utility for being symptom free postoperatively. In the base case, the utility for being symptom free on azathioprine was 0.86 and similarly the utility when the patient was symptom free postoperatively was set at 0.86. Changes of 0.02 in either of these variables changed the model so that initial ileocolic resection would be the preferred strategy. Interestingly, the model was not sensitive to the risk of postoperative recurrence. However, the model was probably affected indirectly by this variable as the utility of the patient postoperatively would vary depending on the disease status.

Thus, this model confirms that early surgery compared with initial azathioprine therapy followed by ileocolic resection result in fairly equal outcomes. Either option appears to be an acceptable alternative. However, quality of life after surgery and while taking azathioprine are key to which treatment strategy is preferred. Thus, clinicians must base the decision of which treatment alternative to recommend based on their best prediction of how the patient may respond to the two treatment alternatives. Unfortunately, predicting response to therapy and which patient is likely to develop an early postoperative recurrence may be difficult. A second key consideration in making decisions should be the patients' preferences. It is likely that the patient himself will have a preference for one or the other treatment alternatives.

WHO SHOULD HAVE SURGERY?

Failure of medical management or refractory Crohn's disease is an uncommon indication for surgery. Thus, before labelling patients with disease refractory to medical therapy, it is important to exclude obstructive symptoms due to fibrostenotic disease, or ongoing septic symptoms in patients with fistulizing disease. For patients in whom steroid therapy has failed, surgery is an excellent alternative especially for those patients with limited disease who have not had previous resections. Surgery can be performed safely, has a high patient acceptance and most patients have an excellent quality of life. However, the beneficial effects of surgery may be negated if there is recurrence of disease and symptoms. Thus, those patients at high risk of recurrence, who have long segments of disease or have had multiple previous operations are probably better treated with medical therapy, such as immunosuppressive agents or possibly the newer biological agents, before being referred for surgery.

References

1. Binder V, Both H, Hansen PK, Hendriksen C, Kreiner S, Torp-Pedersen K. Incidence and prevalence of ulcerative colitis and Crohn's disease in the county of Copenhagen 1962 to 1978. Gastroenterology. 1982;83:563–8.
2. Sandborn WJ, Tremaine WJ, Wolf DC *et al.* for the North American Azathioprine Study Group. Lack of effect of intravenous administration on time to respond to azathioprine for steroid-treated Crohn's disease. Gastroenterology. 1999;117:527–35.
3. Modigliani R. Chronic active Crohn's disease: an update on prevention and treatment. Res Clin Forums. 1998;20;171–7.
4. Munkholm P, Langholz E, Davidsen M, Binder V. Frequency of glucocorticoid resistance and dependency in Crohn's disease. Gut. 1994;35:360–2.
5. Farmer RG, Hawk WA, Turnbull RB. Indications for surgery in Crohn's disease. Analysis of 500 cases. Gastroenterology. 1976;71:245–50.
6. Aleali M, Milsom JW. Laparoscopic surgery in Crohn's disease. Surg Clin N Am. 2001;81: 217–30.
7. Wu JS, Birnbaum EH, Kodner IJ, Fry RD, Read TE, Fleshman JW. Laparoscopic-assisted ileocolic resections in patients with Crohn's disease: Are abscesses, phlegmons, or recurrent disease contraindications? Surgery. 1997;122:682–9.
8. Poulin EC, Schlachta CM, Mamazza J, Seshadri PA. Should enteric fistulas from Crohn's disease or diverticulitis be treated laparoscopically or by open surgery? Dis Colon Rectum. 2000;43:621–7.
9. Milsom JW, Hammerhefer KA, Bohm B *et al.* Prospective randomized trial comparing laparoscopic to conventional surgery in refractive ileocolic Crohn's disease. Dis Colon Rectum. (in press).
10. Aleali M, Milsom JW. Laparoscopic surgery in Crohn's disease. Surg Clin North Am. 2001;81:217–230.
11. Thirlby RC, Land JC, Fenster LF, Lonborg R. Effect of surgery on health-related quality of life in patients with inflammatory bowel disease; a prospective study. Arch Surg. 1998;133:826–32.
12. Yazdanpanah Y, Klein O, Gambiez L *et al.* Impact of surgery on quality of life in Crohn's disease. Am J Gastroenterol. 1997;92:1897–1900.
13. Tillinger W, Mittermaier C, Lochs H, Moser G. Health-related quality of life in patients with Crohn's disease. Dig Dis Sci. 1999;44:932–8.
14. Casellas F, Lopez-Vivancos J, Badia X, Vilaseca J, Malagelada JR. Impact of surgery for Crohn's disease on health-related quality of life. Am J Gastroenterol. 2000;95:177–82.
15. McLeod RS, Wolff BG, Steinhart AH *et al.* Prophylactic mesalamine treatment decreases post-operative recurrence of Crohn's disease. Gastroenterology. 1995;109:404–13.
16. Rutgeerts P, Geboes K, Vantrappen G, Kerremans R, Coenegrachts JL, Coremans G. Natural history of recurrent Crohn's disease at the ileocolonic anastomosis after curative surgery. Gut. 1984;25:665–72.
17. Olaison G, Smedh K, Sjodahl R. Natural course of Crohn's disease after ileocolic resection: endoscopically visualized ileal ulcers preceding symptoms. Gut. 119;33:331–5.
18. McLeod RS. Resection margins and recurrent Crohn's disease. Hepatogastroenterology. 1990; 37:63–5.
19. Williams JG, Wong WD, Rothenberger DA, Goldberg SM. Recurrence of Crohn's disease after resection. Br J Surg. 1991;78:10–19.
20. Steinhart AH, Girgrah N, McLeod RS. Reliability of a Crohn's disease clinical classification scheme based on disease behavior. Inflamm Bowel Dis. 1998;4:228–234.
21. Sutherland LR, Ramcharan S, Bryant H, Fick G. Effect of cigarette smoking on recurrence of Crohn's disease. Gastroenterology. 1990;98:1123–1128.
22. Silverstein MD, Loftus EV, Sandborn WJ *et al.* Clinical course and costs of care for Crohn's disease: Markov model analysis of a population-based cohort. Gastroenterology. 1999;117: 49–57.
23. Kennedy ED, Urbach DR, Krahn MD, Steinhart AH, Cohen Z, McLeod RS. Azathioprine or ileocolic resection for steroid dependent terminal ileal Crohn's disease? Decision Anal. (in press).

Section VI
Fistulizing CD

29
Fistulizing CD: a case report

G. RIEGLER, F. SELVAGGI, A. GIULIANI and L. CASERTA

In December 1990, we observed a fifteen-year-old female who had been suffering from diarrhoea and anal incontinence for six months. The history of her disease had begun one year before with diarrhoea, four or five bowel movements per day without blood or mucus from the anus. Abdominal examination was normal; fissure, skin tags and multiple perianal and anovaginal fistulas were present on examination of the anal canal with a fungal infection too (see Figure 1).

The presence of diarrhoea for twelve months associated with perianal lesions led to the diagnosis of Crohn's disease (CD). In the clinical course of CD, perianal lesions are present in 75% of patients with colonic disease and in about 25% of those with small bowel involvement (furthermore, 5% of patients with anorectal CD have no other localization in the proximal bowel)[1,2]. The most frequent perianal lesions are fissures, abscesses, fistulas, stenosis and the presence of skin tags[3].

The presence of perianal fistulas can be the first manifestation of CD in 10% of the patients[2].

Twenty-three per cent of females with anorectal CD suffer from a rectovaginal fistula[4,5]. Patients often complain of the passage of flatus, stools or pus from the vagina; however, 20% of patients have no symptoms and they suffer only due to the presence of rectal CD and not the presence of a rectovaginal fistula[4,5].

In this case report, the patient had chronic diarrhoea without serious abdominal involvement. The perianal localization of the disease, on the contrary, was particularly aggressive. The clinical examination of the patient led to a diagnosis of CD with a primary recto-anal localization and with subsequent perianal involvement. Furthermore, the patient had no fever, mucus or blood leakage from the anus but she suffered from flatus and faecal incontinence.

The presence of rectovaginal or extrarectal fistulous tracts that reach the perineum can determine some interruptions in the anal sphincter with consequent anal incontinence.

The presence of multiple fistulas, skin tags and fissures led to a need to make a differential diagnosis with other perianal diseases, such as perianal tuberculosis and hidradenitis suppurative (see Table 1). However, scarification of the lesions with a culture showed the presence of an infection from *Candida* spp.

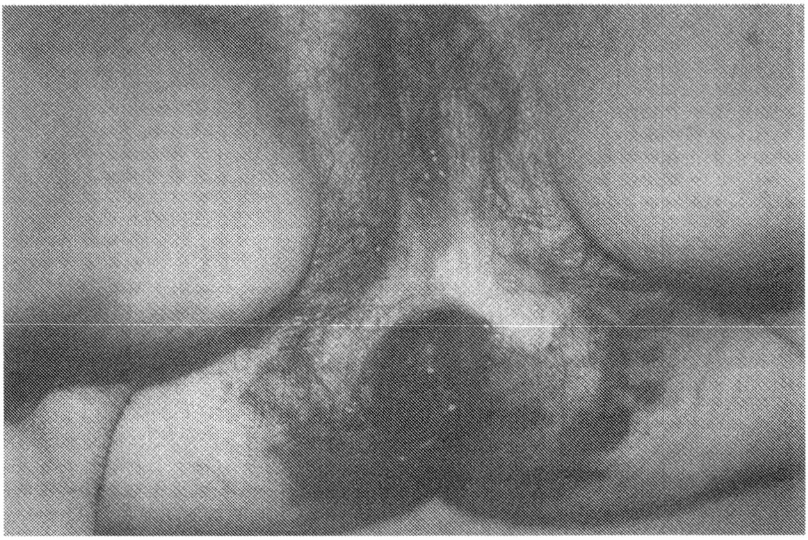

Figure 1 Fissure, skin tags and multiple perianal and anovaginal fistulas

Table 1 Differential diagnosis

	Yes	*No*
Anal Crohn's disease	Type of lesions, chronic diarrhoea	No abdominal symptoms
Hidradenitis suppurative	Presence of complex fistulas	Age, absence of leakage
Perianal tuberculosis	Type of lesions, chronic diarrhoea	No abdominal symptoms
Perianal candidiasis	Type of lesions	Absence of exudate

In particular, the most difficult differential diagnosis was between CD and intestinal tuberculosis in which the clinical presentation and the aspect of the perianal lesions can be similar[6,7]. Then, we decided to proceed in the diagnosis of the case.

Anal resting pressure on digital examination was absent. A pancolonoscopy showed contact bleeding, granulosity and cavity ulceration in the rectum while the remaining colon was disease free. Rectal and skin tags biopsy showed granulomata and a pathological pattern, suggesting the diagnosis of Crohn's disease. Tine-test and cultural examination of perianal debris were negative for the presence of Kock bacillus. A small bowel enema was negative.

The absence of the resting anal pressure and voluntary contraction associated with the presence of complex fistulous tracts led to faecal incontinence, probably due to a double mechanism; there was a neuropathic and a myopathic aetiology, probably related to a primary sphincter lesion of fibrous nature[3]. Furthermore, the presence of about five bowel movements per day determines the clinic pattern of faecal incontinence. We did not perform a bimanual rectovaginal exploration to evaluate the rectovaginal fistulous tract; its presence was shown by the leakage of faeces from the vagina. We did not perform a manometric evaluation of the anal continence because the patient refused any invasive or manual manoeuvre on the anus.

We performed a pancolonoscopy under narcosis. There was massive rectal involvement while the remaining tract of the colon appeared to be spared from the disease.

Less than 50% of patients with CD localized in the colon are spared rectal disease[2]. Rectal involvement is present in about 5–10% of patients with CD. In CD, the inflammation of the rectal disease is not related to the activity of other tracts of the colon; for this reason, a pancolonoscopy is mandatory to evaluate the activity of the disease[1,2].

At the examination, we found many cavitary ulcers and granulosity that bled when touched with the instrument.

Histological examination of rectal and perianal skin tag specimens showed the presence of granulomas.

Several studies have reported the presence of granulomas in over than two thirds of anatomic specimens from CD patients who underwent surgery[8]. Microscopic examination of intestinal mucosal specimens from CD patients showed the presence of granulomas in about 28% and 14% of biopsies in patients with and without evidence of endoscopic mucosal involvement, respectively[9,10]. Granulomas are more frequently seen in colorectal CD than in the small bowel; furthermore, evidence of granulomas decreases over the years with a reduction of about 10% three years after the CD diagnosis[11,12].

Seventeen per cent of the patients with ulcerative colitis showed the presence of granulomas on histological examination[13]. However, non-caseous granulomas can be observed in patients with CD and tuberculosis[7]. For these reasons it is impossible to make a diagnosis of CD from histological evidence of granulomas alone.

Moreover, the rectal and perianal skin tags biopsies showed a characteristic CD aspect with transmural inflammation, submucosal oedema, deeply penetrating ulcers and preservation of goblet cell population.

Cutaneous tests for *Mycobacterium tuberculosis* and the culture of perianal debris for Kock bacillus were negative. The isolation of *Mycobacterium tuberculosis* in faecal culture is very difficult while the demonstration of Kock bacillus in biopsies or perianal debris is specific for the diagnosis of tuberculosis[14].

After the diagnosis of anorectal CD, we performed a small bowel enema to evaluate the presence of small bowel involvement.

Small bowel enema in patients with CD shows oedematous plication, superficial and deep ulcers, fistulas, stenosis, etc. However, the endoscopic examination of small bowel rarely demonstrates a lesion without evidence at small bowel enema, but a biopsy of lesions, seen at radiological study, rarely demonstrates the presence of CD[15]. Furthermore, small bowel enema failed to evaluate the gravity of stenosis instead of endoscopic examination[15].

In this case, the absence of clear small bowel involvement with a normal abdominal examination led us to start with drug therapy for the anorectal localization of CD.

The patient was treated with metronidazole 20 mg/kg iv for ten days and afterwards with metronidazole 250 mg *per os* three times daily for three months. She then took prednisolone 50 mg *per os* once daily and sulphasalazine 4.5 g daily.

Metronidazole is an antibiotic with a strong activity for some protozoa and many anaerobic bacteria[16].

A co-operative Swedish study compared the efficacy of metronidazole with that of sulphasalazine in patients with active CD. The activity index was reduced by both the drugs. Furthermore, metronidazole induced a reduction of the activity index in those patients in whom sulphasalazine failed but there was no evidence of the opposite. Patients with colorectal CD showed a more clear improvement in comparison with those with small bowel involvement[17,18].

Metronidazole induced an improvement in perianal CD in more than 80% of patients with a relapse of the disease when the administration of the drug is stopped[19]. Probably, the effect of metronidazole is due to an antibacterial and immunomodulating activity that leads to an improvement of anorectal disease. However, there are some adverse affects in long-term therapy, such as peripheral neuropathy with paraesthesia, and a mutagenic effect has been shown in experimental animals[19,20].

After an initial treatment with metronidazole 20 mg/kg i.v for ten days, an oral dose of 250 mg three times daily for three months was administrated without a clear improvement of perianal lesions; for this reason we introduced prednisolone and sulphasalazine to the therapy. Sulphasalazine shows efficacy in the superficial localization of CD limited to the bowel lumen but its efficacy decreases with transmural disease with fistulas and abscesses. Furthermore, sulphasalazine is more efficient in the colon because of better release at this site[21].

Although clinical evidence in the literature shows no clear advantage from an association of steroids with sulphasalazine[22–24], we introduced steroid therapy because of a decrease in the clinical status of the patient with an increase in ESV (110 mm/h), anaemia (Hb: 9.4 g/dl) and low serum albumin.

There was no clinical improvement, so azathioprine (1.5 mg kg^{-1} day^{-1}) was introduced with a gradual reduction in steroid dosage. Six months later, perianal disease had not improved so proctectomy and left colostomy was performed in February 1992.

We administered prednisolone and sulphasalazine for 30 days; after this period, we did not observe any improvement in general condition or perianal disease.

Many studies have shown an efficacy of azathioprine to heal CD fistulas in one third of patients after 90 days of therapy with 67% of rectovaginal and 50% of perianal fistulas closing[25,26]. A long-term study showed an efficacy of azathioprine to induce an interruption in steroid administration in about 66% of the patients, with 86.7% and 67.7% closure of recto-vaginal and perianal fistulas, respectively[27].

Thus, we introduced azathioprine with a 1.5 mg $kg^{-1}$$day^{-1}$ schedule followed by a gradual reduction in steroidal dosage.

The patient did not improve after treatment for six months although a small improvement in her health status with a decrease in the activity index was observed. Thus, we decided to start with surgical therapy. The decision about the most useful technique to use was very difficult; her age and the rarity of a rectal localization without evidence of more proximal involvement led us to use a less aggressive approach.

We decided to perform a proctectomy with a left colostomy. The presence of a rectal localization with more proximal colon involvement means that proctectomy alone should be avoided[28].

In this case, we performed an intra-operative colonoscopy with histological examination without finding evidence of any other localization of CD. Thus, we performed the proctectomy and the left colostomy.

Ritchie, in 24 patients with a rectal localization of CD, observed a relapse of the disease in 11% of patients after 10 years[29] while Stern *et al.* in a 5-year study of 7 patients with a similar localization, found no recurrence of the CD[30].

The perineal incision is open in about one third of patients 3 months after surgery with a 10% overall rate of developing a persistent perineal sinus[31,32].

We performed a wound closure with a suture of the pelvic floor muscles and with the apposition of drainage. The wound was closed about 2 months after the operation.

The patient was in good health until October 1995 when she developed complex peristomal fistulas. Endoscopy showed an involvement of the colon from the left tract to the hepatic flexure. A total colectomy with Brooke ileostomy was performed.

Her health condition improved after surgery; however, the patient developed complex peristomal fistulas on the site of the colostomy about 3 years after the operation. An endoscopic examination showed involvement of the remaining colon. Williams and Hughes reported 25% peristomal complications in patients with anorectal CD operated on with proctectomy and left colostomy[33].

After the colonoscopy, we decided to perform a total colectomy with a Brooke ileostomy. The patient was in a good health for about 5 years after this operation without any medical treatment.

In January 2001 the patient showed a recurrence of the disease with evidence of peristomal fistulas (see Figure 2). Because she refused surgical treatment, an anti-TNF-α protocol (infliximab) was started. A clear improvement of the local

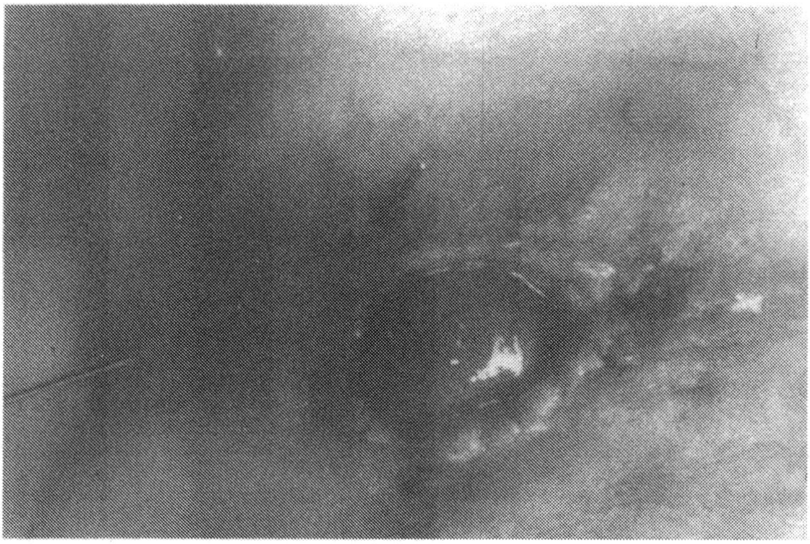

Figure 2 Fistulas peri-Brooke ileostomy

disease was observed soon after the first injection but no decrease in the number of open draining fistulas was achieved at the end of treatment.

After a proctocolectomy with Brooke ileostomy for CD, the rate of recurrence with the need for re-operation is 19% and 24%, respectively, 5 and 10 years after surgery, with a rate of recurrence at the site of the ileostomy of about 10–20%[34]. In 89% of patients the disease recurred within the first 25 cm of the ileostomy[34–36].

The optimal treatment of peristomal fistulas is surgery although many authors have tried a conservative approach[22]. Last *et al.* treated 17 patients with local drainage and curettage with a high percentage of local control after 3 months; results of long-term follow-up are unavailable[37].

However, our patient refused further surgical treatment so we decided to introduce medical treatment with infliximab although there were no clinical reports about this kind of treatment for peristomal fistulas in CD.

Infliximab was administered at a dosage of 5 mg/kg at weeks 0, 2 and 6. In a controlled study with infliximab vs. placebo, 94 patients with enterocutaneous and perianal fistulas were randomized into three groups. Thirty-one patients were treated with infliximab 5 mg/kg, 32 patients received 10 mg/kg and 31 received placebo. Sixty-eight per cent of the first group and 56% of the second group showed a clinical response to the treatment compared with 26% in the placebo group who reached a closure of 50% of fistulas observed before the treatment[38].

A clear improvement in both general health and local disease was observed soon after the first injection, but no decrease in the number of open draining fistulas was achieved at the end of treatment. The patient is now in discreet clinical conditions but her peristomal fistulas are still draining so a further surgical option has been suggested.

In this case report, a very aggressive anorectal Crohn's disease determined a very long clinical history with many medical and surgical approaches.

We started with a conventional therapy for perianal Crohn's disease, general therapy with sulphasalazine and prednisolone, and a more-aggressive approach with azathioprine. Then, we decided to operate on the patient with a proctectomy and a left colostomy.

A recurrence at the site of the colostomy led us to perform a total colectomy with Brooke ileostomy. Furthermore, there was another recurrence at the site of the ileostomy but the patient refused surgery so we tried a new approach for peristomal fistulas in CD with infliximab. When complex perianal fistulas are present, avoidance of surgery may be appropriate. Thus, in the presence of peristomal fistulas, probably a surgical approach is mandatory. New drugs, such as infliximab, tacrolimus and CDP 571, seem to achieve good results in our early experience but controlled trials, especially for patients with peristomal fistulas, are needed.

References

1. Lockhart-Mummery HE. Crohn's disease (regional enteritis) of the large intestine and its distinction from ulcerative colitis. Gut. 1960;1:87.
2. Wolff BG, Culp CE, Beart RW Jr *et al.* Anorectal Crohn's disease: anal lesions. Dis Colon Rectum. 1975;18:2000.
3. Nicholls RJ, Glass R. Inflammatory Bowel Diseases in Coloproctology: Diagnosis and Outpatient Management. Berlin: Springer-Verlag, 1985.

4. Radcliff AG, Ritchie JK, Hawley PR *et al.* Ano-vaginal and recto-vaginal fistulas in Crohn's diseases. Dis Colon Rectum. 1988;31:94–99.
5. Heyen F, Winslet MC, Andrews H *et al.* Vaginal fistulas in Crohn's disease. Dis Colon Rectum. 1989;32:379–383.
6. Morson BC, Dawson IMP, Day DW *et al.* Crohn's disease. In: Morson, Dawson, editors, Gastrointestinal Pathology, 3rd edn. London, Oxford: Blackwell Scientific, 1990.
7. Tandon HD, Prakash A. Pathology of intestinal tuberculosis and its distinction from Crohn's disease. Gut. 1972;13:260–269.
8. Chambers TJ, Morson BC. The histopathological evolution of Crohn's disease. In Pena AS, Weterman IT, Booth CC, Strober W, editors, Recent Advances in Crohn's Disease. The Hague: Martinus Nijhoff, 1981.
9. Surawicz CM, Meisel JL, Yivisaker T *et al.* Rectal biopsy in the diagnosis of Crohn's disease: value of multiple biopsies and serial sectioning. Gastroenterology. 1981;80:66–71.
10. Rotterdam H, Korelitz BL, Sommers SC. Microgranulomas in grossly normal rectal mucosal in Crohn's disease. Am J Clin Pathol. 1977;67:550–554.
11. Chambers TJ, Morson BC. Role of the granuloma in recurrent Crohn's disease. Gut. 1979;20:269–274.
12. Kelly JK, Sautherland KR. The chronological sequence in the pathology of Crohn's disease. J Clin Gastroenterol. 1988;10:28–33.
13. Glotzer DJ, Gardner RC, Goldman J *et al.* Comparative features and course of ulcerative colitis and granulomatous colitis. N Engl J Med. 1970;282:582–587.
14. Palmer KR, Patil DH, Basran GS *et al.* Abdominal tuberculosis in urban Britain – a common disease. Gut. 1985;26:1296–1305.
15. Zwas ER, Bonheim NA, Berken CA *et al.* Ileoscopy as an important tool for the diagnosis of Crohn's disease; a report of seven cases. Gastrointest Endosc. 1994;40:89–91.
16. Linn FV, Peppercorn MA. Drug therapy for inflammatory bowel disease: Part I. Am J Surg. 1992;164:178–185.
17. Rosen A, Ursing B, Alm T *et al.* A comparative study of metronidazole and sulfasalazine for active Crohn's disease: the Cooperative Crohn's Disease Study in Sweden. Part I. Design and methodologic considerations. Gastroenterology. 1982;8:541–549.
18. Ursing B, Alm T, Barany F *et al.* A comparative study of metronidazole and sulfasalazine for active Crohn's disease: the Cooperative Crohn's Disease Study in Sweden. Part II. Results. Gastroenterology. 1982;83:550–562.
19. Brandt LJ, Bernstein LH, Boley SS *et al.* Metronidazole therapy for perianal Crohn's disease: a follow-up study. Gastroenterology. 1982;8:383–387.
20. Stahlberg D, Barany F, Einarson K *et al.* Neurophysiologic studies of patients with Crohn's disease on long term treatment with metronidazole. Scand J Gastroenterol. 1991;26:219–224.
21. Dew MJ, Ebden O, Kidwai NS *et al.* Comparison of the absorption and metabolism of sulphasalazine and acrylic-coated 5-aminosalicylic acid in normal subjects and in patients with colitis. Br J Clin Pharmacol. 1984;17:474–476.
22. Lichtenstein GR. Treatment of fistulizing Crohn's disease. Gastroenterology. 2000;119:1132–1147.
23. Sparberg M, Kirsner JB. Long-term corticosteroid therapy for regional enteritis: an analysis of 58 courses in 54 patients. Am J Dig Dis. 1966;11:865–880.
24. Malchow H, Ewe EK, Brandes JW *et al.* European cooperative Crohn's disease study (ECCDS): results of drug treatment. Gastroenterology. 1984;86:249–266.
25. Korelitz BI, Present DH. Shortcomings of the National Cooperative Crohn's Disease Study: in the exclusion of azathioprine without adequate trial. Gastroenterology. 1981;80:193–196.
26. Korelitz BI, Present DH. Favorable effect of 6-mercaptopurine in fistulas of Crohn's disease. Dig Dis Sci. 1985;30:58–64.
27. Korelitz BI, Adler DJ, Mendelsohn RA. Long-term experience with 6-mercaptopurine in the treatment of Crohn's disease. Am J Gastroenterol. 1993;88:1198–1205.
28. Lockhart-Mummery HE, Ritchie JK. Surgical treatment: large intestine. In: Allan RN, Keighley MRB, Alexander-Williams J, Hawkins C, editors, Inflammatory Bowel Diseases. 1st edn. Edinburgh: Churchill-Livingstone, 1983.
29. Ritchie JK. The results of surgery for large bowel Crohn's disease. Ann R Coll Surg Engl. 1990;72:155–157.
30. Stern HS, Goldberg SM, Rothenberger DA *et al.* Segmental versus total colectomy for large bowel Crohn's disease. World J Surg. 1984;8:118–122.

31. Ritchie JK, Lockhart-Mummery HE. Non-restorative surgery in the treatment of Crohn's disease of the large bowel. Gut. 1973;14:263–269.
32. Goligher JC. Surgical treatment of Crohn's disease affecting mainly or entirely the large bowel. World J Surg. 1988;12:186–190.
33. Williams JG, Hughes LE. Abdomino-perineal resection for severe perianal Crohn's disease. Dis Colon Rectum. 1990;33:402–407.
34. Scammel BE, Andrews H, Allan RN *et al.* Results of proctocolectomy in Crohn's disease. Br J Surg. 1987;74:671–674.
35. Goligher JC. The long term results of excisional surgery for primary and recurrent Crohn's disease of the large bowel. Dis Colon Rectum. 1985;28:51–55.
36. Greenstein AJ, Dicker A, Mayers S *et al.* Peri-ileostomy fistulae in Crohn's disease. Ann Surg. 1983;197:179–182.
37. Last M, Fazio VV, Lavery I *et al.* Conservative management of para-ileostomy ulcers in patients with Crohn's disease. Dis Colon Rectum. 1984;27:779–786.
38. Present DH, Rutgeerts P, Targan S *et al.* Infliximab for the treatment of fistulas in patients with Crohn's disease. N Engl J Med. 1999;340:1398–1405.

30
Fistulizing Crohn's disease – discussion of the case

H. HERFARTH

INTRODUCTION

The lifetime risk of fistulizing Crohn's disease (CD) is reported to be 20–40%. Fistulizing disease can be categorized according to the location, number and complexity of tracts, concomitant complications, such as abscesses or obstructions, and the severity of clinical symptoms.

The presented case highlights the complicated disease course of a perianal fistulizing disease, which can be divided into three different stages of complications and medical or surgical treatments. First, the presentation of a complex perianal and anovaginal fistulizing disease, which was refractory to a whole variety of medical measures. Second the surgical approach, which ultimately resulted in a complete resection of the entire colon and rectum and creation of a Brook ileostomy. Finally the postoperative recurrence of CD with peristomal fistulas, which were treated with monoclonal antibodies against TNF (infliximab).

Each of the stages in this case will be briefly reviewed and discussed.

DISCUSSION OF THE MEDICAL APPROACH BEFORE SURGICAL INTERVENTION – ANTIBIOTICS AND IMMUNOSUPPRESSION IN FISTULIZING CD

The decision when and how to treat fistulas in CD depends on the location of the disease, the number and complexity of the tracts, the presence of complications, such as abscesses or bowel obstructions, and the severity of clinical symptoms. The described patient presented with a complex perianal fistulizing disease and was initially treated with metronidazole. Because of the clinical activity of the disease, systemic steroids were also given. After 9 months, immunosuppressive therapy was initiated due to the refractory course of the fistulizing disease.

Metronidazole is a widely accepted drug for the treatment of fistulas in CD. However, the experience with this drug is based on retrospective analyses of small numbers of patients treated with this drug; no prospective placebo-controlled trial has been performed. Bernstein *et al.*[1] and Brandt *et al.*[2] were the first to report the efficacy of metronidazole in a cohort of patients treated with a dose of 20 mg kg^{-1} day^{-1}. In 10 of 18 patients, a complete closure of the fistulas occurred (56%). Similar results were reported by Jakobovits *et al.*[3] and Schneider *et al.*[4] with 8 and 18 patients (50% and 40%, respectively). Improvement in fistula drainage and healing can be expected approximately 10 weeks after the initiation of therapy but can take up to 6 months[3]. It is important to note that the drug can only be successfully discontinued in a minority of patients (28%) and, in the majority, fistulizing CD is exacerbated again 3–4 months after discontinuation[2]. Due to the long-term treatment and the high doses (15–20 mg kg^{-1} day^{-1}), peripheral sensory neuropathy develops in up to 50% of patients, and is not always reversible[2,3,5].

Because of the antimicrobial activity of metronidazole against anaerobic bacteria and of ciprofloxacin against Gram-negative organisms, combination therapy with ciprofloxacin and metronidazole could further improve the healing of fistulas. However, only one retrospective study on 14 patients has been published so far, reporting an improvement in 9 patients and a complete healing in 3 patients[6].

6-Mercaptopurine (6-MP) and azathioprine, which is non-enzymatically converted to 6-MP, are widely accepted immunosuppressive agents for the treatment of fistulas. The effect of 6-MP (1.5 mg kg^{-1} day^{-1}) on fistulas was studied in a subgroup of patients with fistulizing CD ($n = 36$) in a placebo-controlled trial comparing the effectiveness of 6-MP vs. placebo in the treatment of CD[7]. Thirty-one per cent (9/29) of all fistulas closed in the 6-MP-treated group compared with 1/17 (6%) in the placebo group. Furthermore, a decrease of the symptoms (clinical response) was observed in 7/29 (24%) patients with 6-MP compared with 3/17 (18%) in the placebo group. Korelitz and Present published, in 1985, a follow-up study including 27 patients of the above-described trial and 7 additional patients[8]. All fistulas closed in 13 of the 34 patients (39%) and a clinical response was observed in 26% of the patients. The median time to response was 3.1 months. However, 5 of 7 patients who were taken off 6-MP, relapsed, indicating the need for continuous therapy.

A recently published retrospective analysis including 20 paediatric patients with fistulizing CD (mean age at start of treatment 13.9 years; mean age at CD onset 10.2 years) probably better reflects the presented case[9]. After 6 months of treatment, the fistulas resolved in only 7% of the cases, a decrease in size was observed in 33%, and 60% of all fistulas remained clinically unaltered. These results may indicate a more aggressive and therapeutically resistant course of fistulizing CD in paediatric patients.

THE SURGICAL APPROACH – RISK FACTORS FOR PERMANENT ILEOSTOMY

In this patient, due to resistant fistulizing perianal disease, a colostomy and proctectomy was performed in February 1992.

The factors influencing the healing of perianal fistulas were analysed prospectively in 90 patients by Makowiec *et al.* In 42/90 patients (47%), the fistulas

Table 1 Risk factors for requiring a permanent stoma in CD. The data represent a single-centre experience[12]

	n (Total = 746)	*RR for stoma (CI)*
Site of disease		
Small intestine	581	0.2 (0.1–0.3); $p < 0.001$
Colon	423	1.0 (0.6–1.6)
Rectum	130	4.6 (2.9–7.3); $p < 0.001$
Abscess		
Abdominal	100	0.1 (0.0–0.7); $p < 0.05$
Perianal	94	2.9 (1.7–5.0); $p < 0.05$
Fistulas		
Intra-abdominal	309	0.7 (0.4–1.2)
Genital	53	1.5 (0.7–3.3)
Perianal	185	3.8 (2.3–6.0); $p < 0.01$

CI, confidence interval.

closed after a median time of 11.4 months[10]. Multiple regression analysis revealed that the presence of a stoma and the absence of rectal disease enhanced the healing process ($p < 0.005$ and $p < 0.017$, respectively), whereas immunosuppression had no influence on the healing rate.

Due to severe peristomal fistulizing disease, 3 years after the first operation, a colectomy and Brooks ileostomy was performed. The cumulative risk for a permanent ileostomy in patients with colorectal CD increases over time and is 16%, 25% and 38% 5, 10 and 25 years, respectively, after diagnosis[11]. Fistulas present an additional risk factor (relative risk 2.1). The individual risk factors requiring a permanent stoma were analysed in large cohort of 746 CD patients (Table 1)[12]. Whereas sex, age of onset, duration of disease and the time of the first operation had no influence, rectal disease or perianal fistulas increased the risk significantly.

POSTOPERATIVE RECURRENCE OF DISEASE – BLOCKING TNF IN FISTULIZING DISEASE

Due to severe peristomal fistulization, the patient was treated with anti-TNF (infliximab).

Anti-TNF therapy is probably the best evaluated therapy in fistulizing CD. In a placebo-controlled trial, 94 patients (90% perianal fistulas, 10% abdominal fistulas) were included and treated subsequently with three infusions of infliximab (5 or 10 mg/kg on weeks 0, 2 and 6) or placebo[13]. A complete closure of all fistulas was achieved in 55% of the patients in the 5 mg/kg group and in 38% of the patients in the 10 mg/kg group compared with 13% in the placebo arm ($p < 0.001$). The best effects were observed in patients with perianal disease. However, the fistulas stayed closed for a median of 3 months only, indicating the need for repeated administrations of infliximab. Furthermore, more abscesses were observed in the infliximab-treated patients (11% vs. 3% in the placebo group).

Table 2 Effect of infliximab in patients with fistulizing disease according to the location of fistulas[14]

	n	*Complete healing n (%)*	*Partial healing n (%)*	*Non-response n (%)*
Total patients	39	18 (46.2)	9 (23.1)	12 (30.7)
Total fistulas	74	36 (48.6)	9 (12.2)	29 (39.2)
Type of fistula				
Perianal	50	28 (56.0)	6 (12.0)	16 (32.0)
Rectovaginal	15	5 (33.4)	1 (6.6)	9 (60.0)
Enterocutaneous	6	2 (33.0)	—	4 (67.0)
Peristomal	3	1 (33.5)	2 (66.5)	—

Ricart *et al.* analysed the effects of infliximab on the different types of fistulas[14]. Again, better effects of infliximab were found in patients with perianal fistulas than in patients with enterocutaneous or rectovaginal fistulas (Table 2). In this study, only 2/39 (5%) patients developed abscesses (compared with 11% in the study of Present *et al.*[13]). However, of the 39 patients, 3 had abscess incision and drainage before the start of infliximab and 6 had placements of setons. Eight of these 9 patients were additionally treated with metronidazole and/or ciprofloxacin. The authors of this study suggested that, by combining perianal surgery, antibiotics and immune modifiers with infliximab, a reduction in abscess formation may be achieved. However, infliximab should only be used in fistulizing CD if all other conservative medical (antibiotics, immunosuppression) as well as surgical approaches (e.g. seton placement) have been exhausted[15,16].

THERAPEUTIC PERSPECTIVE – MONITORING IMMUNOSUPPRESSIVE THERAPY

Despite successful therapy with infliximab, there is still a high probability of recurrence of peristomal fistulas in this patient[13,17]. Therefore, the patient should be placed on additional immunosuppressive therapy for maintenance of the remission. Currently, an interesting new concept of individually adapting azathioprine therapy by monitoring of 6-thioguanine nucleotides (6-TGN) in patients with CD is evolving[18]. The metabolism of azathioprine and 6-MP comprises several steps (Figure 1). Azathioprine is a prodrug and is non-enzymatically converted to 6-MP. 6-MP is metabolized by several enzymes. The enzymes, xanthine oxidase and thiopurine methyltransferase, break 6-MP down into inactive metabolites. The enzyme hypoxanthine phosphoribosyl transferase, followed by several other enzymatic processes, converts 6-MP into the active metabolite 6-TGN. Two studies so far have reported higher median 6-TGN concentrations in patients responding to therapy of azathioprine or 6-MP than in patients failing to respond[19,20]. In a recently published study including 63 patients with CD, significantly more clinical remissions were observed in patients with 6-TGN levels higher than 250 pmol/8×10^8 red blood cells (RBC) than in patients with levels below this value[21]. Six patients with fistulizing CD were also included in

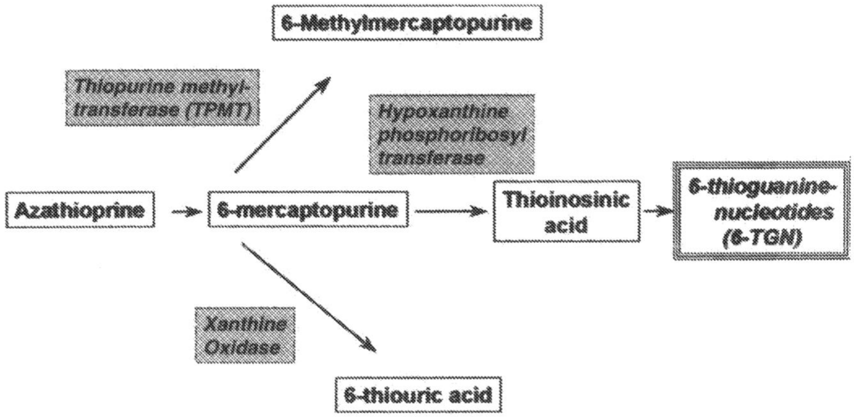

Figure 1 Metabolism of azathioprine and 6-mercaptopurine (6-MP)

Table 3 Association of 6-TGN levels and clinical efficacy in patients with CD[21]

	6-TGN > 250 pmol/ 8 × 10⁸ RBC	*6-TGN <250 pmol/ 8 × 10⁸RBC*	*p-value*
Behaviour	Remission	Non-remission	
n	33	30	
Fistulizing	2/2	0/6	<0.01
Colonic	12/15	1/11	<0.01
Ileocolonic	6/16	2/13	NS

this study. The fistulas closed in only 2 patients. Both patients had 6-TGN levels above 250 pmol/8×10^8 (Table 3). Of 22 patients who did not respond to the initial treatment, 18 went into remission after the dose of azathioprine or 6-MP was increased. In 12 of these 18 patients the 6-TGN levels were, at this point, above 250 pmol/8×10^8. These results seem to indicate the novel possibility of an individually adapted immunosuppressive therapy in CD. Further trials are currently underway.

References

1. Bernstein LH, Frank MS, Brandt LJ, Boley SJ. Healing of perineal Crohn's disease with metronidazole. Gastroenterology. 1980;79:357–65.
2. Brandt LJ, Bernstein LH, Boley SJ, Frank MS. Metronidazole therapy for perineal Crohn's disease: a follow-up study. Gastroenterology. 1982;83:383–7.
3. Jakobovits J, Schuster MM. Metronidazole therapy for Crohn's disease and associated fistulae. Am J Gastroenterol. 1984;79:533–40.
4. Schneider MU, Laudage G, Guggenmoos-Holzmann I, Riemann JF. Metronidazole in the treatment of Crohn disease. Results of a controlled randomized prospective study. Dtsch Med Wochenschr. 1985;110:1724–30.
5. Duffy LF, Daum F, Fisher SE *et al.* Peripheral neuropathy in Crohn's disease patients treated with metronidazole. Gastroenterology. 1985;88:681–4.

6. Solomon M, McLeod R, O'Connor B, Steinhart A, Greenberg GR, Cohen Z. Combination ciprofloxacin and metronidazole in severe perianal Crohn's disease. Can J Gastroenterol. 1993;7:571–3.
7. Present DH, Lorelitz N, Wisch N, Glass JL, Sachar DB, Pasternack B. Treatment of Crohn's disease with 6-mercaptopurine. A long term randomized, double blind study. N Engl J Med. 1980;302:981–7.
8. Korelitz BI, Present DH. Favorable effect of 6-mercaptopurine on fistulae of Crohn's disease. Dig Dis Sci. 1985;30:58–64.
9. Jeshion WC, Larsen KL, Jawad AF *et al.* Azathioprine and 6-mercaptopurine for the treatment of perianal Crohn's disease in children. J Clin Gastroenterol. 2000;30:294–8.
10. Makowiec F, Jehle EC, Starlinger M. Clinical course of perianal fistulas in Crohn's disease. Gut. 1995;37:696–701.
11. Lapidus A, Bernell O, Hellers G, Lofberg R. Clinical course of colorectal Crohn's disease: a 35-year follow-up study of 507 patients. Gastroenterology. 1998;114:1151–60.
12. Post S, Herfarth C, Schumacher H, Golling M, Schurmann G, Timmermanns G. Experience with ileostomy and colostomy in Crohn's disease. Br J Surg. 1995;82:1629–33.
13. Present DH, Rutgeerts P, Targan S *et al.* Infliximab for the treatment of fistulas in patients with Crohn's disease. N Engl J Med. 1999;340:1398–405.
14. Ricart E, Panaccione R, Loftus EV, Tremaine WJ, Sandborn WJ. Infliximab for Crohn's disease in clinical practice at the Mayo Clinic: the first 100 patients. Am J Gastroenterol. 2001;96:722–9.
15. Schreiber S, Campieri M, Colombel JF *et al.* Use of anti-tumour necrosis factor agents in inflammatory bowel disease. European guidelines for 2001–2003. Int J Colorectal Dis. 2001;16:1–11.
16. Lochs H, Adler G, Beglinger C *et al.* Anti-TNF antibody in Crohn's disease – status of information, comments and recommendations of an international working group. Z Gastroenterol. 1999;37:509–12.
17. Present DH. Review article: the efficacy of infliximab in Crohn's disease – healing of fistulae. Aliment Pharmacol Ther. 1999;13:23–8.
18. Sandborn WJ. Rational dosing of azathioprine and 6-mercaptopurine. Gut. 2001;48:591–2.
19. Dubinsky MC, Lamothe S, Yang HY *et al.* Pharmacogenomics and metabolite measurement for 6-mercaptopurine therapy in inflammatory bowel disease. Gastroenterology. 2000;118:705–13.
20. Cuffari C, Theoret Y, Latour S, Seidman G. 6-Mercaptopurine metabolism in Crohn's disease: correlation with efficacy and toxicity. Gut. 1996;39:401–6.
21. Cuffari C, Hunt S, Bayless T. Utilisation of erythrocyte 6-thioguanine metabolite levels to optimise azathioprine therapy in patients with inflammatory bowel disease. Gut. 2001;48:642–6.

31 Fistulizing Crohn's disease – medical treatment

D. H. PRESENT

Unlike ulcerative colitis, which primarily affects the mucosa, in Crohn's disease there is transmural inflammation. As a result, fissuring may occur in which the inflammatory process penetrates into adjacent organs or most commonly around the perianal area. Review of the literature suggests that fistulization can range from as low as 17% to as high as 85% of Crohn's patients. Fistulization in the perianal area may be represented by a mild single fistula or multiple sites of penetration of the skin requiring a proctectomy in about 10% of cases. In a large series in which fistulas were observed in one third of patients, half proved to be enteroenteric.

Therefore, transmural inflammation produces fissuring and fistulization through the bowel wall and causes internal fistula, such as ileoileal, ileocolic, ileovesical and gastrocolic. External fistulization can occur in the perianal area or through the abdominal wall, the latter occurring most often after a prior surgical resection.

Most recently in the era of colonoscopy, fistulization may be missed since radiographic evaluation provides the best opportunity to determine internal fistulization. CT scanning may be suggestive but, in my experience, barium small bowel series and/or barium enema, are still the procedures of choice in determining fistulization.

A common presentation with perianal fistula is development of an abscess which is then drained surgically or spontaneously leading to a resulting fistula. Internal fistulas often present as severe abdominal pain, chills and fever. This requires a CT scan which may detect the abscess that will subsequently lead to fistulization.

The purpose of this presentation is to review the medical management of Crohn's fistula. We will review 5-aminosalicylates, steroids, antibiotics and immunomodulatory drugs.

5-AMINOSALICYLATES

Sulphasalazine has been available for over seventy years and there have been multiple mesalamine derivatives. These agents have shown efficacy in induction and maintenance of remission in both ulcerative colitis and Crohn's disease. However, thus far, there have been no control trials looking at the efficacy of aminosalicylates in the treatment of either internal or external fistula.

STEROIDS

Throughout the majority of the world, steroids are considered to be first-line therapy for moderate to severe Crohn's disease. However, there has never been a controlled trial to look at the efficacy of steroids in the treatment of Crohn's fistula. In uncontrolled series there has been a suggestion that steroids may increase the need for surgery although this may have been because steroids were used in the more severe cases. On the other hand, in the controlled trials looking at steroid efficacy, the only deaths that occurred were in those patients who had an abdominal mass secondary to internal fistulization and subsequently developed an abscess, became septic and died[1,2]. Of great interest is that the newest available steroid is budesonide which has first-pass metabolism through the liver. Studies have shown efficacy almost equal to that of prednisolone with less toxicity. However, all patients with fistula were excluded from these control trials and we do not have data on whether or not to use this agent in patients with internal and/or external fistula.

I personally have had the experience of patients who, never having been on steroids, are subsequently exposed to these agents and who rapidly go on to develop a fistula, abscess and require surgery. I believe that these are probably genetically predisposed Crohn's patients and, unfortunately, I cannot determine in advance in which patients steroids may trigger a fistula and an abscess. I therefore avoid steroids whenever possible.

ANTIBIOTICS

Ciprofloxacin, which has a broad spectrum of bacterial coverage, has been used extensively in the treatment of Crohn's disease. However, there are few clinical reports and the studies were quite small, encompassing eight and five patients, respectively. A positive response was observed but larger control trials are required.

Metronidazole has been evaluated in controlled trials and has been shown to be clinically more effective than sulphasalazine in one study[3] whereas, in another study, both low and high doses appeared to be clinically somewhat more effective than placebo, especially in colonic disease, but, once again, no mention is made of fistulization.

In 1980, Bernstein reported clinical response in 20 of 21 patients with fistula treated with 20 mg/kg daily of metronidazole[4]. Complete healing was observed in 10 of the 18 patients (56%) if metronidazole was continued. The same centre reported a follow-up in 1982 on 26 patients who had more than three months of therapy[5]. Lowering the dose or stopping the metronidazole resulted in 6 out of 6 patients relapsing, and, with long-term observation, only 5 of 18 patients could successfully discontinue metronidazole without experiencing opening of the fistula.

A high percentage of patients (about 50%) experienced significant toxicity, especially peripheral neuropathy. Patients may clinically have no neuropathy but, when tested with nerve conduction studies, about 85% will have some abnormal finding. Gastrointestinal upset with a metallic taste in the mouth often results in patients discontinuing the medication despite clinical response.

In practice, ciprofloxacin and metronidazole are often used together and, in a 14-patient retrospective study. Improvement was noted in nine and healing in three patients when 1–1.5 g Cipro daily was added to 500–1500 mg metronidazole daily. In my personal experience, I have had some success maintaining patients on low-dose metronidazole (500–750 mg daily) once fistula have closed.

6-MERCAPTOPURINE AND AZATHIOPRINE (6 MP/AZA)

The first agent to demonstrate prolonged efficacy in the closure of fistula has been 6 MP/AZA. In our two-year multi-centre double-blind crossover study, we demonstrated efficacy in clinical response, as well as steroid sparing in about 70% of patients. In those patients who had been randomized for fistula, we saw closure in 9 of 29 (31%) compared with 1 of 17 (6%) with placebo[6]. Response of fistula with improvement occurred in 24% of 6 MP patients and 18% of placebo patients. Overall response seen with 6 MP was 55% compared to 24% with placebo. Unfortunately, the studies were not large enough to demonstrate statistical efficacy. A follow-up study was reported in 34 patients in whom closure was seen in 39% and improvement in another 26%[7]. A dose of 1.5 mg/kg was used with a mean time to respond of 3.1 months, although some patients took as long as eight months to close their fistula. Response was maintained if the patient remained on 6 MP; however, relapse occurred if the drug was discontinued. Several other centres have reported similar results. It is our practice to treat patients with 6 MP long-term and to use a concordant aminosalicylate, especially sulphasalazine, which tends to block TPMT and therefore provide more active drug (6TG). We have also had good response in closing enterovesical fistulas, with a response rate of approximately 58%, and long term almost 40% maintained their response. Once again, there are no control trials on the closure of internal fistula, such as gastrocolic and enterovesical.

METHOTREXATE

Recently, there have been control trial reports looking at methotrexate, in terms of both inducing and maintaining remission[8,9]. Treatment consisted of intramuscular methotrexate at a dose of 25 mg weekly with 39% induction of remission compared with 19% for placebo. A subsequent study used 15 mg weekly for maintenance and approximately two thirds of patients stayed well. In neither of these control trials, as well as several other smaller control trials, was there any mention of closure of fistula. We have presented data in abstract form in 33 patients who were treated in a similar manner with intramuscular methotrexate (25 mg daily)[10]. Clinical remission was observed in 62% of patients and 4 of 16 fistulas (25%) closed with this regimen. In another 5 of the 16 patients (31%), there was clinical response with an overall response rate of 56%. We observed frequent relapse when the dose was lowered or when patients were switched to oral methotrexate.

CYCLOSPORINE

Cyclosporine was initially shown to be effective in a controlled trial in active disease using a dose of 7.5 mg/kg per day. Three subsequent studies using lower doses of 5 mg/kg per day showed no benefit in treating active disease or maintaining remission. Fistulas were not specifically studied. We have had significant experience administering intravenous cyclosporine at a dose of 4 mg/kg daily. This is comparable to doses of 8–10 mg/kg given orally. A small series of five patients showed rapid response when treated with a 4 mg/kg intravenous dose[11]. A larger series of 16 patients showed 88% response in the acute phase[12]. When combining these two studies, 24 of 28 patients (86%) showed response with closure in 17 of the 28 (61%). The mean time to respond was four to seven days; however, relapse occurred in 10 of 24 (42%) patients when switched to oral cyclosporine.

Because of the high relapse rate, we treat all of our patients with 6 MP/azathioprine to try to obtain maintenance. We continue the cyclosporine for three to nine months before stopping it, to allow the 6 MP/AZA to be effective.

INFLIXIMAB

The largest placebo-controlled trial looking at fistulas in Crohn's disease has been carried out using infliximab[13]. This mouse–human antibody which binds to TNF-α was studied in 94 patients who had single or multiple draining enterocutaneous fistulas. All other medications were allowed but maintained at stable doses. This included aminosalicylates, steroids, 6 MP/AZA and antibiotics. Three infusions were given at weeks 0, 2 and 6, and the primary endpoint was response which was defined as a decrease of 50% or more from baseline in the number of open draining fistulas. This improvement had to be observed over at least two visits (one month). Doses of 5 mg/kg and 10 mg/kg were used and compared with placebo. Sixty-eight per cent of patients responded to 5 mg/kg and 56% responded to 10 mg/kg compared with 26% in the placebo group. Complete closure was observed in 55% of patients receiving 5 mg/kg and 38% of patients receiving 10 mg/kg; placebo response was observed in approximately 13% of patients, and this was statistically significant. A review of the odds ratio showed no differentiating factor predicting response looking at prior surgery, site of disease, medical treatment or the number of fistulas. There was a strong trend towards maintenance of response in the patients who were receiving concomitant 6 MP/azathioprine[14]. Subsequent follow-up open-label studies have shown similar response, and, in my personal experience, in another 38 patients there was closure in 39% and partial closure in another 39%. In three large series, each with over 100 patients, overall fistula response was observed in 58–78% and closure in 24–64%.

Many questions remain unanswered as regards Crohn's fistula patients and treatment with infliximab. How many infusions are required to close the fistula and how frequently should maintenance infusions be given? Can steroids prevent healing and are antibiotics required to prevent an abscess secondary to premature closure of a fistula? Should all patients receive 6 MP/azathioprine to prevent relapse? At this point we are not sure whether infliximab is truly a first-line therapy and we cannot predict who will respond. However, a large study is currently being conducted (ACCENT II) in order to try to answer these questions.

OTHER AGENTS

A recent placebo-control trial has been completed using CDP-571, which is a more humanized monoclonal antibody against TNF-α[15]. This agent has approximately 5% mouse tissue compared with 25% of infliximab. CDP-571 showed efficacy in both clinical response and steroid sparing and 45% of fistulas closed compared with 12% in placebo patients ($p = 0.026$).

In a recent uncontrolled study using thalidomide to treat Crohn's disease, response of fistula was observed in 9 of 13 (69%) patients. Closure of fistula was observed in 5 of 13 (38%) patients[16]. However, toxicity, including lethargy and peripheral neuropathy, has proven excessive and limits the use of this agent for this complication.

Tacrolimus, a fungus-derived macrolide which has shown a similar therapeutic profile to cyclosporine, has been shown in uncontrolled studies to be effective in the treatment of fistula[17]. A double blind placebo-control trial has recently been completed using this agent. However, the data are currently unavailable for review.

In summary, immunological agents appear to be most effective in the management of Crohn's fistula[18]. At the present time, we are still not certain which are the agents of first choice and which combinations may be required in the future to close fistula and maintain the response.

References

1. Summers RW, Switz DM, Sessions JT *et al.* National Cooperative Crohn's Disease Study: Results of drug treatment. Gastroenterology. 1979;77:847–69.
2. Malcow H, Ewe K, Brandes JW *et al.* European Cooperative Crohn's Disease Study: Results of drug treatment. Gastroenterology. 1984;86:249–66.
3. Ursing BO, Alm T, Barant F. A comparative study of metronidazole and sulfasalazine for active Crohn's disease: The Cooperative Crohn's Disease Study in Sweden. Gastroenterology. 1982;83:550–62.
4. Bernstein LH, Frank MS, Boley SJ *et al.* Healing of perineal Crohn's disease with metronidazole Gastroenterology. 1980;79:357–65.
5. Brandt LJ, Bernstein LH, Boley SJ *et al.* Metronidazole therapy for perineal Crohn's disease: A follow-up study. Gastroenterology. 1982;83:383–7.
6. Present DH, Korelitz BI, Wisch BI *et al.* Treatment of Crohn's disease with 6 mercaptopurine: A long term randomized, double-blind study. N Engl J Med. 1980;302:981–7.
7. Korelitz BI, Present DH. Favorable effect of 6-mercaptopurine on fistula of Crohn's disease. Dig Dis Sci. 1985;1:58–64.
8. Feagan BG, Rochon J, Fedorak RN *et al.* Methotrexate for the treatment of Crohn's disease. N Engl J Med. 1995;332:292–7.
9. Feagan BG, Fedorak RN, Irvine ES *et al.* A comparison of methotrexate with placebo for the maintenance of remission in Crohn's disease. N Engl J Med. 2000;342:1627–32.

10. Mahadevan U, Marion J, Present DH *et al.* The place for methotrexate in the treatment of refractory Crohn's disease. Gastroenterology. 1997;112A:1031.
11. Hanauer, SB, Smith MB. Rapid closure of Crohn's disease fistulas with continuous intravenous cyclosporine. Am J Gastroenterol. 1993;88:646–9.
12. Present DH, Lichtiger S. Efficacy of cyclosporine in treatment of fistula of Crohn's disease. Dig Dis Sci. 1994;39:374–80.
13. Present DH, Rutgeerts P, Targan S *et al.* Infliximab treatment of fistulas in patients with Crohn's disease. N Engl J Med. 1999;340:1398–405.
14. Rutgeerts P, D'Haens GR, Targan S. Efficacy and safety of retreatment with anti-tumor necrosis factor antibody to maintain remission in Crohn's disease. Gastroenterology. 1999;117:761–9.
15. Feagan BG, Sandborn WJ *et al.* A randomized, double-blind placebo controlled multicenter trial of the engineered human antibody to TNF (CDP 571) for steroid sparing and maintenance of remission in patients with Crohn's disease. Gastroenterology. 2000;118:A655.
16. Ehrenpreis ED, Kane SV, Cohen LB, Cohen RD, Hanauer SB. Thalidomide therapy for patients with refractory Crohn's disease: An open-label trial. Gastroenterology. 1999;117:1271–7.
17. Lowry PW, Weaver AL, Tremaine WJ, Sandborn WJ. Combination therapy with oral tacrolimus (FK506) and azathioprine or 6 mercaptopurine for treatment refractory Crohn's disease perianal fistula. Inflamm Bowel Dis. 1999;5:239–45.
18. Lichtenstein GR. Treatment of fistulizing Crohn's disease. Gastroenterology. 2000:119:1132–47.

32
Fistulizing Crohn's disease

V. W. FAZIO

INTRODUCTION

Most patients with Crohn's disease will require surgical treatment for their illness within 10 years of diagnosis. The most common anatomic clinical pattern that leads to a need for surgery is the ileocolitis patient. Not coincidentally, it is with this pattern that most perforated or septic complications arise. Frequently, there is an associated obstructive element to the clinical presentation.

PATHOGENESIS

The most accepted mechanism for septic/fistula complications from small and large intestinal sources is that the mucosal/submucosal ulceration progresses in a transmural fashion through the entire bowel wall, with penetration of the serosal cover of the intestinal segment. As sepsis progresses, there is a containment mechanism which walls off colon, covers or seals the impending or real perforation with adjacent omentum, colon, small bowel loops, other intestinal or internal viscera or parietes. The 'walling off' structure is usually an organ in the immediate proximity and this structure is usually *not* involved in the primary disease. Thus a 'source-target' phenomenon occurs, this concept being the basis for almost all modern surgical treatment. Thus the source resected, e.g. terminal ileal Crohn's disease, and the target, e.g. adjacent normal valve, sigmoid colon or urinary bladder, are treated by 'simple' repair, i.e. closure of the defect.

FISTULA CLASSIFICATION

For the purposes of discussion, fistulas in Crohn's disease are subclassified as *internal*, meaning the source of origin occurs in the abdomen (above the peritoneal reflection of the rectum) and external–perianal. This is somewhat artificial in that other internal fistulas may occur, e.g. oesophagopleural–tracheal. External fistulas also include parastomal, enterocutaneous and enteroperineal types. These three latter examples are discussed with internal fistulas since the basic management strategies are similar, namely resection of the source. Some authorities use 'enterocutaneous' as a third subclassification of fistulas.

There are many varieties of internal fistulas. On the *source* side of the ledger, Crohn's disease may arise from ileum, colon, jejunum and, rarely, duodenum or stomach. On the *target* side, in decreasing order of frequency, are the ileum, sigmoid colon, ascending colon, transverse colon, jejunum, urinary bladder and vagina. Rarely seen targets may include fallopian tubes, common bile duct, ureter, seminal vesicles, and gallbladder. In any series, complex fistulas with multiple targets (skin, sigmoid colon, bladder and small bowel) may be seen but they usually have just a single source, namely the bowel segment affected by Crohn's disease.

Another variety of internal fistula may be seen in which the source organ is *not* affected by Crohn's disease. This is seen in the early postoperative period when a bowel defect arises, e.g. overlooked enterotomy, inadvertent (by cautery, abdominal suture closure) injury, or anastomotic suture line breakdown occurs with extravasation of bowel contents through the point of least resistance. This is usually the abdominal wound or drain site, although the vagina or urinary bladder can be affected. Rarely, after an ileocaecal resection for Crohn's disease with associated psoas abscess, a patient may present many months later with an exacerbation of occult sepsis. This is secondary to an anastomotic defect that was contained in the early postoperative period.

INTERNAL FISTULAS

Investigation

The principles of work up for a patient with fistulas are similar to those generally applied to Crohn's disease. The anatomic distribution of the Crohn's disease is assessed by contrast radiography of the small and large bowel. This will often localize the fistula site. However, some fistulas remain occult and are only discovered at operation. *Colonoscopy* is sometimes useful in showing an ileosigmoid or ileoascending colon fistula. A characteristic patch of 'diseased' bowel is about 1–3 cm in circular distribution, reflecting granulation tissue along the fistulous tract that protrudes into the lumen. Biopsies are usually done.

There is often some incompletely drained septic focus associated with fistulas. It is suspected because of a general systemic inflammatory response, e.g. fever, chills, tachycardia and leukocytosis. These patients may benefit from *computerized tomographic scanning* to document the septic focus and to provide a means of needle aspiration or drainage, which will allow for specific antibiotic prescription based on culture and sensitivities.

Fistulography is used for enterocutaneous fistulas, e.g. abdominal wound, peristomal or via the perineum in the case of suspected ileoperineal fistula. The latter is often overlooked, with the patient being managed for many months as having an unhealed perineal wound – something which affects 10–30% of patients with Crohn's disease who undergo proctectomy. Although diagnosis by fistulography is key, and the patient's symptoms are improved by consequent resection of small bowel, the now long-established tract to the perineum will often be problematic with residual pain and sinus drainage. Frequently, a further procedure (gracilis or rectus abdominus flap) is required or this may be done synchronously with abdominal perineal wound incision with or without an omental pedicle graft.

Other investigations that are done relate to general assessment of the patient for possible surgery: blood count and chemistries, nutritional assessment, chest X-ray and coagulation profile.

INDICATIONS FOR SURGERY FOR INTERNAL FISTULAS

The general guideline applied to management of Crohn's disease is that surgery is an alternative when the patient and/or the surgeon perceives that the situation has reached a critical level of disability or is likely to do so in the near future, when the patient has already been treated with optimal therapy and when the advantages of surgery outweigh the disadvantages. This optimal therapy includes the appropriate choice and dosing schedules of medical treatment as well as ensuring patient compliance in taking the medication.

There is evidence that certain internal fistulas may have few, if any, symptoms and that there is zero disability. Enteroenteric, and ileosigmoid fistulas are but two of these. Broe and colleagues[1] reported on 64 patients with Crohn's disease enteroenteric fistulas. Of 24 patients managed without surgery, 10 required operation within one year and the remaining 14 went for three years without surgery. There was no added morbidity or mortality due to delaying such surgery.

The indications for surgery include:

1. Associated obstruction;
2. Symptoms refractory to medical treatment;
3. Malnutrition;
4. Significant side-effects of medication/dependency on steroids;
5. Abdominal or associated urinary infection;
6. Related morbidity, e.g. anaemia.

The contraindications to surgery include:

1. Low level of disease–fistula activity;
2. Fistula-induced bypass with relief of the patient's symptoms;
3. Crohn's disease is easily controlled;
4. Poor operative risk.

Thus patients with minimal symptoms of rectovaginal fistula are best observed as the surgical treatment, i.e. advancement flap, may not only fail, but may make the defect even larger and, therefore, more symptomatic than before. Likewise, caution or conservative management is appropriate for the multi-operated patient who now has a postoperative enterocutaneous fistula that can be managed by simple dressings.

Goals of surgery for Crohn's disease fistulas

Abdominal

- Resect fistula-bearing segment;
- Drain infection;

- Minimize risk of recurrence of fistulas;
  —Quarantine/drain sepsis;
  —Quarantine anastomosis;
  —Consider temporary diversion;
  —Chemoprophylaxis.

Perineal

- Drain sepsis;
- Minimize recurrence;
- Preserve anorectal function;
- Consider adjuvant medical therapy especially if reconstructive surgery has been used.

Principles of surgery

These are goal directed:

- Pre-operative stoma site marking;
- Drainage of sepsis;
- Resection of fistula origin;
- Assessment of secondary opening for:
  (a) Presence of Crohn's disease;
  (b) Associated phlegmon of target organ;
  (c) Decision to repair vs. resection and anastomosis of target intestine.
- Faecal diversion
  (a) If there is a high risk of leakage, e.g. adjacent abscess wall;
  (b) If an anastomotic leak will produce a significant mortality risk;
  (c) Location proximal to anastomosis;
- Quarantine the anastomotic site.

SPECIFIC INTERNAL FISTULAS

Ileosigmoid fistula

This is perhaps the most common important internal fistula. These include: ileo-ileal fistulas, ileo-transverse/ascending colon fistulas, and ileorectal fistulas, an uncommon variant. The principles of management for this lesion are similar for all enteroenteric fistulas.

Patient symptoms relate to the activity of Crohn's disease of the ileum with elements of obstruction, due to associated ileal narrowing and sepsis. In some series, as much as 25% of patients have an associated abscess, frequently on the right leaf of the mesorectum. In some cases, symptoms are absent as the fistula has acted as an 'auto bypass' of the obstructing ileal disease. Others will have profound diarrhoea secondary to bypass of a large amount of colon.

Diagnosis may be made on Gastrografin enema per rectum or by sigmoidoscopy. In the Cleveland Clinic series, contrast X-rays were valuable in making the diagnosis in only 20% of cases. Most fistulas were first diagnosed at operation. The importance of pre-operative diagnosis rests with pre-operative positioning of the patient in stirrups so that a sigmoid resection and transanal stapled colorectal anastomosis can be done easily.

The technical management of the fistula is open to some debate with those favouring simple closure (predicated on the absence of intrinsic sigmoid colon disease) and those favouring a short segmental resection and end-to-end anastomosis. The 'simple' closure is favoured if the fistula is easily identified, affecting the anti-mesenteric aspect of the colon and is not associated with phlegmonous inflammation or septic changes. This might lead to less long-term suture security. A biological analogue is the perforated peptic ulcer where suture closure may be very tenuous and omental patch-grafting is used.

On the other hand, in the presence of adverse indicators, e.g. a multiplicity of associated fistulas, a phlegmonous rind of inflammation affecting the colon, or particularly an *anti-mesenteric* location of the colon defect (the most common site in my own personal experience), segmental resection and anastomosis is done. This is facilitated by circular stapling techniques. A temporary stoma may be added depending on the merits of the case.

An unusual but important variant of this type of fistula is ileorectal fistula. A track may be identified passing from distal terminal ileum to right mesorectum, dissecting down to the presacral space with or without a secondary abscess. From here, perforation of the 'mesenteric' (posterior) aspect of the mid- to low-rectum may occur. This entity requires extensive presacral mobilization of the rectum down to the levators with resection of almost all of the rectum and a colo–low rectal or colo–anal anastomosis. The presacral space is drained and a temporary stoma is placed above the ileo-ascending colon anastomosis after resection of the source problem.

Another technical dilemma faced by the surgeon is when an ileosigmoid fistula is suspected but not found. The terminal ileum has to be sharply or bluntly dissected off the sigmoid colon where attachment of varying degrees is found. There is no defect found on the sigmoid and even after inspection, probing or even air or Betadine insufflation of the rectum, no leak is observed. Yet the surgeon is concerned because of residual induration over the right side of the sigmoid, often at the rectosigmoid junction. In this case, it is tempting to let things go. However, late development of sigmoid–cutaneous fistula is a common result. The message is, if you have any concerns, *resect the segment*, even if an overt fistula cannot be demonstrated.

Ileocoloduodenal fistula

This usually occurs after recurrence at ileotransverse colon anastomosis. The pancreas and second part of the duodenum may be involved in the phlegmon. Resection of the primary source is done, the duodenal defect is examined and the indurated area is trimmed. Options for closure include simple transverse closure of the duodenum, duodenojejunostomy, or onlay patch of vascularized free jejunal segment. After the repair, omentum is interopposed between the duodenum and the ileoneo–colic anastomosis. Prevention of the problem is possible by avoiding formal right colectomy and anastomosis to treat ileocaecal Crohn's disease. An omental wrap of the ileocolic anastomosis also helps prevent the problem.

Gastroduodenal fistulas

These may occur as for the above entity but also in combination with gastric fistulas. Also, ileogastric or colicgastric fistulas occur. In the series of Greenstein *et al.* of 1480 Crohn's disease patients, identified between 1960 and 1983, six gastric fistulas were identified. Five of the six had a colonic source; wedge resection of the stomach and colectomy were the preferred treatments of choice[2].

Enterovesical fistulas

The patient usually presents with both intestinal and urinary symptoms. In the Cleveland Clinic series[3] thirty-nine of the 63 patients were men. The patterns of disease were as follows: ileal 35%; colonic 8%; ileocolic 57%. Dysuria was present in 94% and pneumaturia in 80%. Half of the patients ($n = 43$) had other internal fistulas, most commonly ileosigmoid. Twenty-one patients had an associated intra-abdominal abscess. Treatment is usually surgical with medical management reserved for early postoperative occurrences of the fistula and serious comorbidity or high surgical risk. There has been increasing interest in definitive management with medical therapy involving antibiotic treatment and intermittent use of regularly scheduled infliximab and long-term immunosuppression. For surgeons, the observation that continued urosepsis may pose a threat to the upper urinary tracts and that medical treatment rarely cures the situation, especially when the drugs are withdrawn, has led to the view that resection of the fistula source and oversew-repair of the bladder defect is the treatment of choice.

Pelvic pouch fistulas

Fistulas arising from an ileopelvic pouch, affected by Crohn's disease, are more recent problems for clinicians to deal with. They may arise from the ileo pouch–anal anastomosis itself, from the midpouch at a staple line, or from the tip of the J-pouch. Also, cryptoglandular sepsis may be the source of a perianal, gluteal or even vaginal fistula. These occur distal to a stapled anastomosis of the pouch to the top of the anal columns. Since 'source resection' is a major and perhaps Draconian alternative – albeit, often needed – the focus of management is identification of Crohn's disease, mapping the rest of the intestine for other sites affected by Crohn's disease, identification of the fistula source (exactly) and then treatment.

Sepsis is controlled by antibiotics initially and fistula drainage by seton or mushroom catheter. In some patients, long-term setons for trans-sphincteric or suprasphincteric fistula is the preferred management. This is because the goals of therapy, mainly relief of pain, preservation of anal–rectal function and prevention of recurrent sepsis, are met. For others where the pouch looks to be unaffected or only mildly affected by Crohn's disease, the histology of resected colon, for example, is positive for Crohn's disease. Transanal ileo or pouch flaps and even repeat ileopouch–anal anastomosis with disconnection may be successful in 2/3 of cases[4]. Patients are generally managed with long-term immunosuppression.

ENTEROCUTANEOUS FISTULAS

These are discussed under the headings:

- Abdominal wall fistulas (wound, drain site);
- Peristomal;
- Enteroperineal;
- Extrasphincteric fistulas.

Abdominal wall

Principles of management are as for general management of any fistula, i.e. make the patient optimally fit for surgery, identify the fistula source and exclude distal bowel obstruction. One should wait a minimum of 4–6 months from the last laparotomy before reoperation is done.

The preferred management is resection of the affected bowel segment with anastomosis, debridement–excision of the septic component of the fistula tracts, and, in very high-risk cases, adding a temporary diverting stoma.

Peristomal fistulas

These may arise remotely from, or soon after, ileostomy construction. Remotely occurring fistulas are almost always associated with recurrent Crohn's disease at the stoma site and adjacent interabdominal recurrence of Crohn's disease. There is often extensive sepsis locally, but the patient rarely exhibits features of systemic sepsis.

In the early ostomy period, resection is indicated with or without relocation depending on how salvageable the local stoma is.

Fistulas arising in the peristomal region soon after ileostomy construction are usually associated *with* a technical mishap, i.e. injury to the ileal wall within the abdominal wall aperture. Avoidance of suturing ileum to the fascia is recommended. Usually, revision of the ileostomy with laparotomy is required, which can be a very difficult operation at this particular time so soon after major surgery.

Ileoperineal fistula

Similar principles apply as for abdominal fistula. Also, see earlier comments about persistent perineal sinus.

Extrasphincteric fistula

These may arise from ileum, sigmoid or rectum (rare). Treatment is source excision with bowel anastomosis and drainage of the tract.

PERIANAL, RECTAL AND PERIRECTAL FISTULAS

These are discussed under:

- Rectovaginal;
- Rectourethral;
- Anoperineal types.

Rectovaginal fistula

'She came for relief, not because of pain, but because she was ashamed of herself and ashamed for her husband. She was prepared to do away with herself if no relief could be given to her; she became very melancholy and felt that life meant nothing to her if she had to go on with this condition.' These words are attributed to J. F. Saphir, who discussed this type of fistula at the American Proctology Society Meeting, May 13, 1929 in Detroit, Michigan. Few descriptions can match the emotive and visual images conjured up in this quotation – which captures the essence of how devastating this complication can be. Traditional management has been a type of ileostomy construction usually with proctectomy or proctocolectomy. However, with selective reconstructive surgery, repair may be achieved in selected cases with or without adjuvant use of immunosuppressants.

Clinical presentation and assessment

The term rectovaginal covers both fistulas arising from the rectum (rare) and those arising from the anal canal (common). There are often associations with rectal involvement of Crohn's disease and with perianal fistulas – but not always! Patients may be asymptomatic apart from the occasional passage of vaginal gas or they may have overt passage of stool per vagina. The patient is assessed by studying the small and large bowel with colonoscopy and biopsy of the colon and rectum. Assessment is made regarding:

- Rectal involvement with active, quiescent or no disease;
- Sphincter status;
- Other fistulas, strictures or perianal tags;
- Degree of disability;
- Associated perineal sepsis;
- Distensibility of rectum.

Examination under anaesthesia is often required.

Treatment

Medical management. Medical management has included 5 aminosalicylic acid, imuran, cyclosporin A, antibiotics and infliximab.

Surgical management. The goals of treatment are discussed with the patient. For those with extensive rectal disease, there may be few alternatives to an immediate ileostomy with or without resection. In brief, the goals are to maintain normal function wherever possible and to render the patient able to cope with the results of treatment. In many cases, this is well achieved with fistula healing. In others, patients may live with degrees of disability but this disability is preferable, in their minds, to having an ileostomy.

Sepsis drainage by seton is occasionally valuable when septal thickening and discharge is apparent. Setons help to demarcate the defect, allowing for a well-planned flap. As a rule, long-term seton use is to be avoided as the 'wearing down effect' tends to enlarge the defect making the fistula more symptomatic.

A variety of repairs has been advocated. Transanal is the preferred approach although the trans-sphincteric approach is valuable for the patient affected by associated sphincter injury or cloaca. In that case, simultaneous repair of the sphincter muscles is carried out.

Transanal sleeve repair is appropriate for failed flaps and for patients with anal canal ulceration. Rarely, rectal resection and coloanal pull-through procedures are used. This may be done when the proximal colon is free of overt disease[5].

Of 40 patients with rectovaginal fistulas, 9 of 13 patients with severe rectal disease had a proctocolectomy. Four others had seton drainage. Thirty patients with mild rectal disease underwent flap advancement. Twenty had healing of rectal–vaginal fistula (four following repeat flap). Four failures were treated by TPC and ileostomy. Seven were living with their fistulas after failed repair. Five patients with anal ulceration and stricture underwent sleeve repair with success in four.

Thus, 68% of patients undergoing repair of rectovaginal fistula ultimately had successful healing. Therefore, in selected cases, these repairs are valuable.

Recto-urethral Fistulas

These are rare. Frequently, these require permanent ileostomy. Some reports exist on limited numbers of patients where advancement rectal flap operations have been successful.

Anoperineal fistulas

These occur in 10–80% of patients with Crohn's disease and are most common in those with Crohn's colitis.

Associated features

These include hypertrophic skin tags, anal ulceration, stricture and abscesses. Usually, there is proximal bowel disease which may or may not precede the development of anal fistula. Rarely is perianal disease the sole manifestation of Crohn's disease. The findings on examination may be similar to those of non-Crohn's-related fistulas. The internal os may be *above* the dentate line, but usually is not. Goodsall's rule is usually applicable although Crohn's disease is a recognized entity where departure from this rule may occur. There are often complex problems with multiple openings, perianal skin changes, or extension into the scrotum, inguinal regions or vulva.

Investigation

Apart from with simple, relatively asymptomatic fistulas, examination under anaesthesia and rectal assessment is required. This is complemented by a work-up of the intestine with small bowel series and colonoscopy with biopsy with particular focus on the rectum.

Sinography is usually reserved for fistulas that are recurrent or resistant to what would be considered adequate medical or surgical treatment. CT or MRI, likewise, is used in this situation. Endoluminal ultrasound is often used during examination under anaesthesia if branching tracks or cavities are suspected. Hydrogen peroxide will enhance the diagnostic accuracy.

Functional studies are important in that even low fistulas often treated by simple fistulotomy may be best treated by a conservative approach, for, if the resting sphincter pressures are low, fistulotomy may lead to incontinence.

Treatment

This is symptom-directed. The goals of treatment are explained to the patient. Abscesses are drained, conservatively, close to the anal verge. Mushroom catheters are left in place for 3 weeks and then removed. Up to 50% of abscesses resolve without resulting fistulas.

In most cases, setons are used if a fistula is deemed high or problematic, i.e. likely to produce incontinence if fistulotomy is performed. The fistula type is assessed, and then an assessment of the patient's tolerance of long-term setons is made. The seton is usually removed after 1–2 years and the patient observed for the possibility of recurrence.

Medical treatment is beyond the scope of this particular document but, in patients with rectal Crohn's disease, immunotherapy is commonly used where curative treatment is otherwise impossible. Similarly, previous results with anti-TNF-α medication have shown some utility although withdrawal of the drug seems to be associated with recurrence[6].

With respect to surgical treatment, apart from the use of setons, definitive treatment has included rectal advancement flap procedures, simple fistulotomy for low-lying fistulas, advanced rectal sleeve operations and staged fistulotomies. For those patients with normal-appearing rectum, simple fistulotomies are used for low-lying fistulas, i.e. intersphincteric or low trans-sphincteric fistulas. For those fistulas that are higher and associated with a risk of incontinence, it is questionable whether fistulotomy should be done. In this case, an advancement rectal flap operation is favoured. For patients who are treatment failures, a repeat flap operation can often be performed with a measure of success. However, this is recognized as being associated with ultimate treatment failure in a number of patients who subsequently require ileostomy as a final treatment option.

With respect to carcinoma and fistula, this complication is something that has to be considered, especially in patients who have had long-standing, relatively asymptomatic perianal fistulas. Often, there is induration out of proportion to the fistula appearance. In addition, glary, mucoid discharge is very suspicious for an underlying mucinous carcinoma. Superficial biopsies are usually negative and often require a high index of suspicion by the clinician to make the diagnosis based on true-cut needle biopsies. Such patients are usually treated by preoperative chemo–radiation, followed by radical Miles' resection after work-up for metastases.

References

1. Broe PJ, Bayless TM, Cameron JL. Crohn's disease. Are enteroenteral fistulas an indication for surgery? Surgery. 1982;91:249.
2. Greenstein A, Present DH, Sachar D *et al.* Gastric fistulas in Crohn's. Dis Colon Rectum. 1989;32:888–92.

3. MacNamara MJ, Fazio VW, Lavery IC, Weakley FL, Farmer RG. Surgical treatment of enterovesical fistulas in Crohn's disease. Dis Colon Rectum. 1990;33:271–6.
4. Fazio VW, Wu JS, Lavery IC. Repeat ileal-pouch anal anastomosis to salvage septic complications of pelvic pouches: Clinical outcome and quality of life assessment. Ann Surg. 1998; 228:588–97.
5. Hull TL, Fazio V. Surgical approaches to low anovaginal fistula in Crohn's disease. Am J Surg. 1997;173:95–8.
6. Present DH, Rutgeerts P, Targan S *et al.* Infliximab for the treatment of fistulas in patients with Crohn's disease. N Engl J Med. 1999;340:1398–405.

33 Alternative therapies in inflammatory bowel disease

D. RACHMILEWITZ

INTRODUCTION

The aetiology of ulcerative colitis and Crohn's disease in not yet known and this is why the available therapeutic modalities are far from being satisfactory. The current modalities include anti-inflammatory agents in which 5-aminosalycilic acid is the active agent, steroids and immunosuppressive drugs. Even the exciting new development of biologics, such as anti-TNF antibodies for the treatment of Crohn's disease, is far from being satisfactory, not to mention that a similar comparable biologic modality does not even exist for the treatment of ulcerative colitis.

However, in the last two decades, our understanding of the pathogenesis of IBD has significantly increased. The roles of the various cytokines, inflammatory mediators and free radicals in the propagation of the inflammatory cascade, even though its trigger is unknown, are now well recognized. Moreover, it was clearly established that the therapeutic modalities used at present are all directed to decrease the generation of the pro-inflammatory cytokines and mediators, and to block their receptors or to scavenge free radicals if their generation was not successfully decreased or totally prevented.

The better understanding of the pathogenesis of IBD stimulated and provoked several novel therapeutic approaches. These novel approaches take into consideration epidemiological observations, are directed against inflammatory mediators and free radicals or aim to change the intestinal flora. All the new innovative modalities have been evaluated in experimental models of colitis and several have also been evaluated in human IBD.

In this chapter the unconventional modalities are reviewed. Several can be regarded as complementary to the conventional therapeutic regimes already and others definitely deserve evaluation in clinical IBD.

MODALITIES AIMED TO AFFECT INFLAMMATORY MEDIATORS

These modalities take into consideration the established role of inflammatory mediators and especially eicosanoids in the pathogenesis of IBD. These novel approaches include specific inhibition of COX-2, the isoenzyme responsible for the stimulated generation of prostanoids in IBD, diversion of leukotriene generation towards LTB_5 instead of LTB_4 and prevention of the release of mediators from inflammatory cells, as well as non-specific anti-inflammatory effects of low-molecular-weight heparin.

Inhibition of COX-2 activity

More than 20 years ago, prostanoids were shown to be involved in the pathogenesis of IBD as well as in experimental colitis. Both in IBD and in experimental colitis, mucosal generation of prostanoids is increased. Moreover, inhibition of prostanoid generation by the 5-ASA compounds and steroids is considered as one of the mechanisms responsible for their therapeutic effects in IBD.

Nimesulide is an example of an inhibitor of COX activity with selectivity of COX-2 over COX-1. Inhibition of COX-2 is associated with anti-inflammatory activity and reduced incidence of adverse events in the upper gastrointestinal tract. The effect of nimesulide on the extent and severity of colonic inflammation was recently assessed in two models of experimental colitis[1].

Colitis was induced in rats either by injection of 2 ml 5% acetic acid into the lumen of the colon or by intracolonic administration of 0.1 ml 3% iodoacetamide in 1% methylcellulose. The acetic acid model represents superficial damage resembling the type of damage present in UC, whereas iodoacetamide, a sulphydryl blocker, induces chronic inflammation with large amounts of granuloma more similar to the damage observed in Crohn's disease. Rats were treated intragastrically with nimesulide (10 mg/kg) twice daily after induction of colitis and sacrificed 24 h after acetic acid or 3 days after iodoacetamide. The colon was isolated and weighed, mucosal lesions measured and mucosal scrapings were processed for determination of myeloperoxidase (MPO) and nitric oxide synthase (NOS) activities, as well as eicosanoid generation.

Nimesulide was found to reduce the lesion area induced by acetic acid and iodoacetamide by 61% and 78%, respectively. In nimesulide-treated rats, PGE_2 generation and MPO and NOS activities were significantly decreased. The amelioration of both types of experimental colitis, therefore, suggests that COX-2 inhibitors may be used for the treatment of IBD.

Modulation of the arachidonic acid cascade

The generation of arachidonic acid metabolites is enhanced in experimental colitis and in IBD. Prostanoids and leukotrienes, being pro-inflammatory agents, may therefore amplify tissue injury in IBD and attempts to interfere with their generation were therefore advocated. Moreover, the anti-inflammatory effect of steroids and 5-ASA compounds are ascribed, at least in part, to their inhibition of eicosanoid generation.

Whereas the results of clinical trials, several uncontrolled, with non-selective inhibition of COX, 5-lipoxygenase and thromboxane synthase activities were not encouraging, the results of the trial conducted with fish oil were different. The most convincing trial was conducted for a period of 1 year in patients with Crohn's disease in remission[2]. Patients received either 2.7 g of N-3 fatty acids or placebo daily. The relapse rate in the N-3 fatty acids treatment group was 28% as opposed to a 69% relapse rate in the control group. In ulcerative colitis patients the results were less impressive. In a large study conducted by Stenson *et al.*[3], 4 months treatment with a fish oil preparation induced significant improvement in the histological score and reduced LTB_4 generation but, apparently, the clinical response was less obvious. Diversion of arachidonic acid metabolism toward the less pro-inflammatory leukotriene, LTB_5, is the hypothesized mechanism responsible for the beneficial effects of fish oil. An additional mechanism is a reduction in the level of TXB_2. Enriching the diets of IBD patients with fish oil preparations is definitely another possible supplement to the conventional drug treatment available for IBD treatment.

Preventing the release of mediators from inflammatory cells

Increased numbers of activated mast cells and eosinophils are present at the active site of the gut involved in IBD and experimental colitis. Upon activation, mast cells generate and release mediators, among them eicosanoids and free radicals. Ketotifen is an anti-asthmatic drug that inhibits mediator release, especially from mast cells and eosinophils. Ketotifen was therefore given intragastrically (100 μg/100 g body weight) twice daily 48 h prior to intracolonic administration of 5% acetic acid.

Ketotifen was found to significantly decrease the extent of the damage by 68%. The effect of ketotifen was accompanied by a significant decrease in LTB_4 generation and NOS activity[4]. The effective modulation of experimental colitis by ketotifen, which is used in several parts of the world as an anti-asthmatic drug, justifies conducting a clinical trial to maintain remission in IBD patients. Unfortunately, drug companies are not interested in ketotifen, which is no longer under patent, and therefore, so far, it has been impossible to get sponsorship for such a trial.

Heparin as an anti-inflammatory drug

Heparin has recently been proposed as a new modality for the treatment of ulcerative colitis. In addition to its anticoagulant properties, clexane, low-molecular weight heparin, was reported to decrease inflammation in experimental hepatitis and in rheumatoid arthritis.

Recently, the effect of clexane on modulation of TNB colitis was assessed in rats[5]. Following induction of colitis, treated rats received clexane 80 μg/kg sc once. In clexane-treated rats, 3 and 7 days after induction of colitis, the lesion area was significantly reduced. The reduction in the lesion area is accompanied by significant decreases in PGE_2 generation, and MPO and NOS activities.

These observations, together with the results of the preliminary trials conducted in UC patients, suggest that low-molecular-weight heparin may also be regarded as an anti-inflammatory modality. This may be useful, especially in patients with refractory disease not responding to the conventional therapeutic approaches.

MODALITIES AIMED TO DECREASE THE EFFECTS OF FREE RADICALS

Free radicals, oxygen-derived active species and NO, are the agents that, in inflammatory settings irrespective of their trigger, as well as in IBD, induce tissue damage.

Decreasing the generation of free radicals, or their sequestration, provides protection and amelioration of the inflammatory response. This approach has encouraged the evaluation of several modalities.

Sequestration of oxygen-derived free radicals by nitroxides

Nitroxides are stable non-toxic radicals which block biological damage by breaking chain reactions through selective termination reactions with deleterious free radicals. Intragastric administration of the nitroxide Tempol immediately after induction of colitis by intracolonic injection of acetic acid provided impressive protection. This protection was reflected by decrease in the lesion area which was accompanied by decreased levels of inflammatory mediators. Tempol provided less remarkable protection of TNB-induced colitis[6].

The mechanism which underlies the protection provided by Tempol entails interception of paramagnetic species. Tempol reacts with O_2^--yielding O_2 and H_2O_2 and its advantage over superoxide dismutase is its penetration into cells, thus protecting also against the deleterious effect of intracellular O_2^-. Nitroxides also compete with H_2O_2 for oxidation-reduction active transition metal ions, to maintain iron and copper as Fe(III) and Cu(II) and pre-empt the injurious Fenton reaction. The protection provided by Tempol provides a novel approach to the possible treatment or prevention of inflammatory bowel disease, or both.

Antioxidant activity of allicin

Allicin is the main biologically active component of garlic clove extract and its biological effects have been attributed to its antioxidant activity.

The possible amelioration of experimental colitis by allicin has been evaluated[7]. Intragastric administration of a single dose of allicin (11.6 mg/kg) immediately after induction of colitis by intracolonic instillation of DNB decreased the lesion area by 93%. It is of interest that, in allicin-treated rats, colonic NOS activity was 50% of its activity in rats treated with DNB only. These observations suggest that decrease in NO generation may be among the mechanisms responsible for the anti-inflammatory effect of allicin and that allicin may be regarded as a possible supplement for the treatment of IBD.

Inhibition of NO generation

NO has been implicated in diverse biological functions and, when actively produced in large amounts, being a free radical, may induce tissue injury also due to its combination with superoxide-yielding peroxynitrite. In patients with active IBD, colonic NO generation and NOS activity are stimulated. Stimulation of colonic NOS activity was also reported in models of experimental colitis. Inhibition of NOS activity may therefore ameliorate the extent of tissue inflammation and may be used as a novel modality in IBD patients.

There are several compounds that inhibit NOS activity. L-NAME is an analogue of L-arginine, the substance from which NO is generated, and is a potent inhibitor of NOS activity. L-NAME (0.1 mg/ml) was added to the drinking water at the time of colitis induction either by intrarectal administration of TNB or, 7 days prior to colitis induction, by acetic acid in capsaicin-pretreated rats[8]. L-NAME was found to significantly decrease the lesion area by 55% in TNB-treated rats when sacrificed one week after colitis induction. The lesion area in acetic acid-treated rats was also significantly decreased by 61% when L-NAME was added to the drinking water. The administration of L-NAME induced a significant decrease in colonic NOS activity in both models. The amelioration of colitis by L-NAME was also demonstrated in iodoacetamide-induced colitis in rats and also in models in other species. Modulation of NO generation is definitely a possible important modality to treat IBD. It is, however, of great interest to use specific inhibitors of i-NOS, the isoenzyme responsible for the stimulated NOS activity in inflammation and to preserve the activity of c-NOS, the isoenzyme responsible for the generation of NO which is essential in the maintenance of tissue integrity.

Modulation of experimental colitis by iron chelation

Iron has a role in the generation of oxygen free radicals due to its participation in the Fenton reaction: $Fe^{2+} + H_2O_2 \rightarrow Fe^{3+} + OH^- + OH^*$ Substances that chelate iron may disrupt the inflammatory cascade, hence ameliorating the extent of mucosal damage in experimental colitis. Deferiprone (L_1) is an oral iron chelator used for the treatment of iron overload situations. Deferiprone possesses many advantages by virtue of its oral route of administration and its low price relative to that of the classical iron chelator, desferrioxamine. Recently, deferiprone was found to be effective in the modulation of iodoacetamide- and acetic acid-induced colitis[9]. In both models, deferiprone was given intragastrically in four separate doses to a total of 16.5 mg/100 g immediately after and at 2-h intervals after the induction of colonic inflammation with iodoacetamide or acetic acid. Twenty-four hours after induction of colitis in deferiprone-treated rats, the lesion area was decreased by 67% and 69%, respectively. The protective effect of deferiprone was accompanied by a significant decrease in colonic MPO and NOS activities and in colonic PGE_2 generation. Decreasing the generation of iron-dependent oxygen free radicals is, therefore, an additional therapeutic opportunity in IBD patients. Since deferiprone is already used in humans for other indications, it should also be evaluated in patients with Crohn's disease and ulcerative colitis.

Amelioration of colitis by hyperbaric oxygen

Hyperbaric oxygen (HBO) has been suggested to be beneficial in inflammatory bowel disease. HBO was reported, though never in a controlled trial, to be beneficial in patients with perianal Crohn's disease. The mechanisms responsible for its therapeutic effect have not been elucidated. HBO, which is 100% O_2 at 2–3 times the atmospheric pressure at sea level, may result in increased PaO_2 of almost 400 mmHg. Alleviation of tissue hypoxia and restoration of tissue defence against bacterial infection are among its possible beneficial biochemical, physiological and cellular effects. When used with pressures of 3 atm or less in sessions of 120 min or less, HBO treatment is safe. If these limits are exceeded, it may cause generalized seizures and impairment of inner ear function. The positive anti-inflammatory effects of HBO were substantiated in models of experimental colitis. A significant decrease in the extent of tissue damage was already observed 24 h after induction of injury with acetic acid or TNB and, in the TNB model, also after 7 days[10]. The decrease in tissue injury was accompanied, as in other pharmacological manipulations, by a decrease in MPO activity. Amelioration of tissue injury was also accompanied by a significant decrease in NOS activity. The possibility that the decrease in colonic NOS activity may be a primary event whereby HBO exerts its beneficial effects is supported by the observation that 7 days of exposure of control untreated rats to HBO also resulted in significant suppression of this enzyme activity. HBO treatment is definitely not advised for uncomplicated IBD patients. However, it is highly recommended that a controlled therapeutic trial be conducted, especially in complicated patients such as Crohn's disease patients with severe perianal involvement.

THERAPEUTIC POSSIBILITIES WITH PROBIOTICS

For several years, the possible role of the intestinal microflora in the pathogenesis of IBD has been evaluated. With few exceptions, so far, most attempts to correlate the presence of bacteria with IBD has not provided convincing evidence. Among the exceptions is the somewhat positive effect of antibiotics on Crohn's disease activity and in patients with pouchitis. In experimental animals, it was clearly shown that spontaneous colitis, that develops in transgenic knockout mutant murine models of colitis, may not occur in germ-free conditions.

Concomitantly, it was suggested that ingestion of living organisms might be beneficial due to changes in the microbial balance and also because of their function as immune modulators[11]. Recently, probiotics have been shown to modulate the extent of experimental colitis[12]. Intragastric administration of four strains of lactobacilli, three strains of bifidobacteria and one strain of streptococci for 7 days prior to induction of colitis by iodoacetamide was found to reduce the lesion area by 69%. However, this treatment had no effect on the severity of damage in the DNB model. It is of interest that intragastric administration of another bacterial preparation, LGG, was also found to be beneficial in decreasing damage in the iodoacetamide model. The observations in experimental models of colitis support the positive trials conducted in human IBD and encourage further controlled trials especially in ulcerative colitis patients.

MODULATION OF IBD BY NICOTINE

The search for the elucidation of the aetiology of IBD led to the epidemiological observation that cigarette smoking has diverse effects on IBD since it is beneficial in ulcerative colitis and deleterious in Crohn's disease. The ingredient in tobacco which is responsible for its effect on IBD is most probably nicotine. However, the mechanisms whereby smoking or nicotine affect the course of IBD are not clear.

Recently, both active and passive exposure to cigarette smoke was found, as in human Crohn's disease, to potentiate the severity of the inflammatory response in DNB-induced colitis in rats. On the other hand, nicotine administration was found to have a bivalent effect on the severity of experimental colitis. Whereas small quantities were found to reduce the severity of the damage, higher doses had an opposite effect. In ulcerative colitis patients, nicotine therapy was found to have a positive effect, both when administered in patches or as an enema[13]. It is therefore suggested that nicotine may be regarded as a complementary therapeutic modality in non-smokers with ulcerative colitis, whereas smokers with Crohn's disease should be advised to stop smoking.

PREVENTION AND TREATMENT WITH IMMUNOSTIMULATORY DNA SEQUENCES

Immunostimulatory DNA sequences (ISS) and their synthetic oligonucleotides (ODN) analogues (ISS–ODNs), also known as CpG motifs, are unmethylated CpG dinucleotides within a consensus sequence of 5′-purine-purine-CG-pyrimidine-pyrimidine-3′ or 5′-purine-TCG-pyrimidine-pyrimidine-3′, which are common in certain bacterial and viral genomes[14]. Immunostimulatory DNA induces the secretion of Th1-like cytokines; up-regulates cell-surface molecules involved in T-cell activation on macrophages and dendritic cells; and possesses anti-apoptotic and anti-inflammatory properties. We recently found[15] that systemic and intragastric administrations of ISS ameliorate and prevent colonic inflammation in four models of experimental colitis: DSS colitis in mice (Th-1/Th-2 biased), TNB/DNB-induced colitis in mice (Th-2 biased), spontaneous colitis in IL-10 KO mice (Th-1 biased), and DSS colitis in IL-10 KO mice. ISS was also found to inhibit pro-inflammatory cytokine generation (TNF-α and IL-1β) by colonic mucosa of patients with active IBD. These findings suggest a role for ISS in amelioration of colitis regardless of the underlying T-cell response and may explain the mechanism responsible for the therapeutic efficacy of probiotics.

References

1. Karmeli F, Cohn P, Rachmilewitz D. Cyclooxygenase-2 inhibitors ameliorate the severity of experimental colitis in rats. Eur J Gastroenterol Hepatol. 2000;12:223–31.
2. Belluzi A, Brignola C, Campieri M *et al.* Effects of an enteric coated fish oil preparation on relapses in Crohn's disease. N Engl J Med. 1996;334:1557–61.
3. Stenson WF, Cort D, Rodgers J. Dietary supplementation with fish oil in ulcerative colitis. Ann Intern Med. 1992;116:609–14.
4. Eliakim R, Karmeli F, Okon E, Rachmilewitz D. Ketotifen ameliorates capsaicin-augmented acetic acid-induced colitis. Dig Dis Sci. 1995;40:503–9.
5. Dotan I, Herskoviz R, Karmeli F, Rachmilewitz D, Peled Y, Halperin Z. Low molecular weight heparin (clexane) significantly ameliorates experimental colitis. Gastroenterology. 1999;116: A372.
6. Karmeli F, Eliakim R, Okon E, Samuni A, Rachmilewitz D. A stable nitroxide radical effectively decreases mucosal damage in experimental colitis. Gut. 1995;37:386–93.
7. Hershkovitz R, Karmeli F, Dotan I, Halperin Z, Rachmilewitz D. Allicin: A novel modality to ameliorate experimental colitis. Gastroenterology. 1999;116:A736.
8. Rachmilewitz D, Karmeli F, Okon E, Bursztyn M. Experimental colitis is ameliorated by inhibition of nitric oxide synthase activity. Gut. 1995;37:247–55.

9. Ablin J, Shalev O, Okon E, Karmeli F, Rachmilewitz D. Deferiprone, an oral iron chelator, ameliorates experimental colitis and gastric ulceration in rats. Inflamm Bowel Dis. 1999;5:253–61.
10. Rachmilewitz D, Karmeli F, Okon E, Rubenstein I, Better OS. Hyperbaric oxygen – A novel modality to ameliorate experimental colitis. Gut. 1998;43:512–18.
11. Campieri M, Gionchetti P. Probiotics in inflammatory bowel disease: New insight to pathogenesis or a possible therapeutic alternative? Gastroenterology. 1999;116:1246–60.
12. Shibolet O, Karmeli F, Eliakim R, Campieri M, Giochetti P, Rachmilewitz D. Probiotics ameliorate iodoacetamide-induced colitis. Gastroenterology. 1999;116:A818.
13. Rachmilewitz D. On smoking rats and inflammatory bowel disease. Gastroenterology. 1999; 117:1008–11.
14. Van Uden J, Raz E. Immunostimulatory DNA and applications to allergic disease. J Allergy Clin Immunol. 1999;104:902–10.
15. Rachmilewitz D, Karmeli F, Raz E. Immunostimulatory DNA sequences ameliorate the extent of experimental colitis in mice and rats. Gastroenterology. 2000;118;A576–7.

Section VII
Miscellaneous topics

34
Diagnostic and therapeutic challenges in indeterminate refractory colitis

M. DAPERNO, R. SOSTEGNI, S. TARAGLIO, R. ROCCA, B. TORCHIO and A. PERA

CASE HISTORY

A 45-year-old male presented in November 1994 with bloody diarrhoea. A total colonoscopy showed endoscopic features of ulcerative colitis (UC) with involvement up to the splenic flexure. Ileoscopy was normal. Histology confirmed the diagnosis of inflammatory bowel disease (IBD) with findings suggestive for ulcerative colitis.

Prednisone 1 mg/kg body weight (bw) oral treatment was given, with a good clinical response and gradual tapering of steroids. Subsequently, the patient relapsed in August 1996, March 1997 and June 1997; oral steroids were given with a good clinical response but with steroid-dependency. In May 1997, a total colonoscopy showed left-side colitis with continuous lesions and mild endoscopic activity. Isolated pseudopolyps were found. In August 1997, the patient was admitted to the Gastroenterology Unit because of a flare-up and steroid-dependent refractory disease.

Because of the lack of response to parenteral steroids, oral cyclosporine 5 mg/kg bw/day was administered. After clinical improvement, azathioprine 2 mg/kg bw/day was given and steroids were tapered. Cyclosporine was stopped 3 months later. A radiological examination of the small bowel was normal.

In July 1998, there was a new relapse during azathioprine therapy 2 mg/kg bw/day. Surgery was suggested but the patient did not follow the indication. Topical budesonide was added. During the subsequent year, the disease was cronically active despite immunosuppressive and topical steroid therapy.

In June 1999, the patient was admitted to the Gastroenterology Department in order to evaluate the indications for surgery. A total colonoscopy was performed and showed moderate to severe disease activity in the left colon, with linear and large ulcers, with an overall endoscopic diagnosis of Crohn's (CD) colitis (Figure 1).

Histology confirmed a diagnosis of IBD but with signs suggestive of ulcerative colitis. No sign of cytomegalovirus (CMV) disease was present at histology.

Anorectal manometry was also performed and demonstrated a pattern suggestive of microrectum. Topical 2% lidocaine was started but no relevant effect on tenesmus or on bowel movements was noted. ASCA and p-ANCA evaluation was carried out: both tests were negative. An indication for surgery was given. A subtotal colectomy was carried out in August 1999 with temporary ileostomy. Histology of the surgical specimen showed features commonly found both in ulcerative colitis and Crohn's disease, with a final diagnosis of indeterminate colitis (Figure 2).

On the basis of the diagnosis, the patient underwent ileal pouch anal anastomosis (IPAA) with a 3-step procedure. At present the patient is in good clinical condition with 4–5 stools/day. No clinical or endoscopic sign of pouchitis and no complication related to the surgical procedure has appeared.

COMMENTS:

Two main problems were met in managing this patient:

- Diagnostic uncertainty (indeterminate colitis)
- Therapeutic options for refractory colitis

Indeterminate colitis

The differential diagnosis between Crohn's disease (CD) and ulcerative colitis (UC) is possible in about 80–90% of patients with inflammation confined to the colon, while in the remaining 10–20%, differentiation is not possible[1,2].

According to Hodgson's proposals[3], the definition of **indeterminate colitis** (IC) should be reserved for cases in whom a definite diagnosis is not possible from the surgical specimen. For patients in whom colectomy has not been performed and the diagnosis is not sure, a definition of **IBD type uncertain** should be used (Table 1). It has been demonstrated that follow-up may lead to a diagnostic definition of Crohn's disease or ulcerative colitis in a large proportion of patients initially diagnosed as having indeterminate colitis[4].

To summarize the diagnostic difficulties encountered in IBD, we must keep in mind that no sign is absolutely specific; granulomas and perianal disease can rarely be found in patients with all other findings typical of ulcerative colitis, while bloody diarrhoea and a UC-like pattern of disease can be present in Crohn's disease.

Indeterminate colitis and IBD type uncertain show endoscopic and histological features commonly found in both Crohn's disease and ulcerative colitis (Figures 1 and 2).

Table 1 Uncertain or indeterminate colitis

IBD type uncertain	Typical features of IBD, but not enough data to establish a definite diagnosis of Crohn's disease or ulcerative colitis. Follow-up may allow a classification of these patients into Crohn's disease or ulcerative colitis.
Indeterminate colitis (IC)	Presence of features commonly found in ulcerative colitis and Crohn's disease on the surgical specimen.

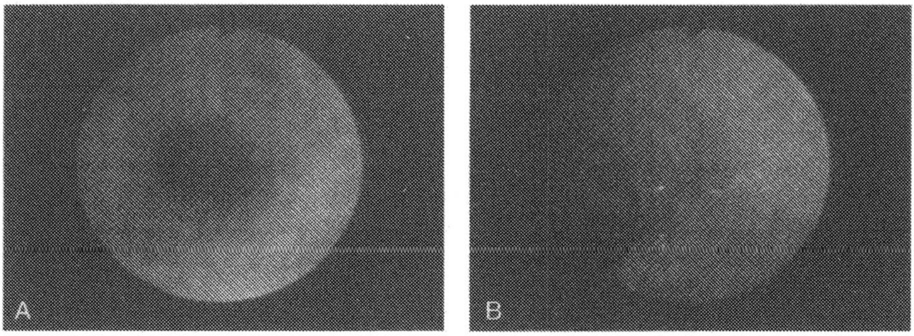

Figure 1 Overlapping endoscopic patterns in IBD, type uncertain. (**A**) Large superficial ulcers with almost normal mucosa interposed. Marked haustral reduction. (**B**) Granularity and continuous involvement of the mucosa

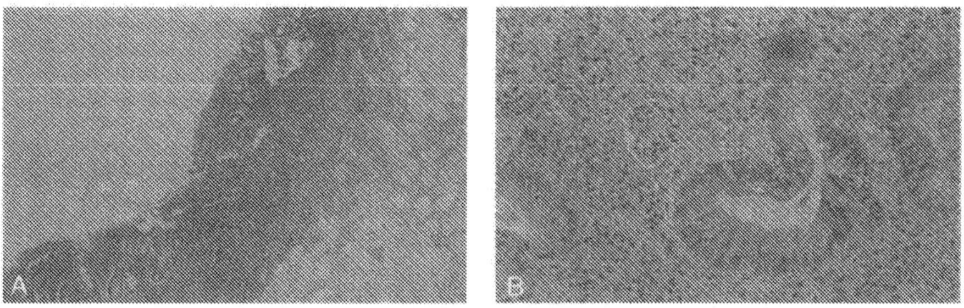

Figure 2 Histopathological patterns of indeterminate colitis. (**A**) Large superficial ulcer with a tendency to intramucosal fissure. Heavy lymphocytic infiltrate of the mucosa. Fibrolipomatosis of the submucosa × 80. (**B**) Crypt abscess, cryptitis and mucus depletion of the glands × 250

It is not clear whether we should consider indeterminate colitis a disease different from ulcerative colitis and Crohn's disease or whether the three patterns are part of a whole spectrum of patients with IBD.

Medical therapy and surgical management of indeterminate colitis represent a challenge for clinicians. Medical treatment[5] is based on 5-aminosalicylic acid (5-ASA) and glucocorticosteroids for mild to moderately active disease. If steroid refractoriness or steroid dependency develops, 6-mercaptopurine (6-MP) or azathioprine (AZA) could be considered, while infliximab, being effective for active Crohn's disease, could be of some interest.

However, no trial (to our knowledge) has proved the efficacy of infliximab in indeterminate colitis; furthermore, the drug was not available in Italy before our patient was operated on.

Refractoriness to medical treatment is an indication for colectomy. Data on outcome after surgery in indeterminate colitis are controversial and probably confused by differences in definitions, but the possibility of performing an IPAA in a patient with Crohn's disease can increase the risk of postoperative morbidity. In fact, clinical trials showed no differences between indeterminate colitis and ulcerative colitis[6], or a slight increase in minor adverse events without an increased rate of pouch removal in indeterminate colitis[7,8].

Mortensen and colleagues[9] proposed a management algorithm for surgery of patients with indeterminate colitis based on delayed reconstruction after colectomy, when the diagnosis is confirmed in the surgical specimen. Biopsies of rectal stump during a 12-month period are suggested in order to clarify the diagnosis. If Crohn's disease becomes more likely, Mortensen prefers to perform an ileorectal anastomosis if the rectum is spared, while, if a diagnosis of ulcerative colitis becomes more likely during follow-up, an IPAA is suggested.

Medical treatment of refractory colitis

Before assigning to a patient the label of 'refractory disease', we must rule out the possible causes of the lack of response to medical therapy (e.g. irritable bowel syndrome or other causes of diarrhoea not due to IBD).

True refractory disease can be associated with both endogenous (e.g. disease activity) and exogenous (e.g. superinfections, compliance with treatment, drug dosing) factors.

As an example, CMV infection has been reported as a common cause of steroid-refractory IBD[10]. Recently, Cottone and colleagues[11] found a positivity for CMV in 36% of severe acute refractory IBD patients, and over 70% of these achieved clinical remission after specific antiviral chemotherapy. These data suggest that testing for serum CMV antigens and antibodies and examination of rectal biopsies for CMV have a key role in the management of refractory IBD.

Endoscopic examination (distal or extensive) may play an important role in evaluating activity, in the differential diagnosis and it allows biopsy sampling.

Refractory distal colitis

Refractory proctosigmoiditis seems to represent a specific subgroup of the disease, with resistance to standard therapies[12,13]. Topical mesalamine has been shown to be an effective treatment for distal ulcerative colitis[14].

Intolerance to topical 5-ASA with diarrhoea is a cause of pseudo-refractoriness. If topical 5-ASA does not lead to remission, a combination therapy with topical steroids may be employed. An alternative to classical topical steroids is budesonide, a steroidal drug with high first-passage liver metabolism and fewer steroidal side effects (e.g. less hypothalamo–pituitary–adrenal axis suppression).

When topical treatments are not effective, an intensive steroid regimen can be used. Alternative proposed treatments are: nicotine enemas, nicotine patches, resumption of smoking, short chain fatty acids (butyrate), and topical lidocaine[15].

Refractory ulcerative pancolitis

In patients with extensive ulcerative colitis, when therapy with full-dosage 5-ASA and steroids fails to induce remission and exogenous factors of refractoriness have been ruled out, parenteral steroids (methylprednisolone 1 mg/kg bw/day or equivalent) alone should be tried in order to exclude 5-ASA intolerance.

AZA and 6-MP are beneficial in chronic active ulcerative colitis but they require one to three months in order to be efficacious and a key question is whether the patient can tolerate an additional 3 months of ulcerative colitis symptoms and potential steroid toxicity while awaiting the therapeutic effects of the drugs. In the subgroups steroid-dependent and chronic active patients, AZA and 6-MP are the drugs of choice.

Understanding **azathioprine** metabolism in IBD has led to a better knowledge of metabolic pathways of toxicity and to the possibility of preventing it.

In recent years, the metabolism of AZA and its non-enzymatic metabolite 6-MP has been clarified. Two rate-limiting steps are represented by activity of thiopurine methyl transferase (TPMT) and of hypoxanthine phosphoribosyl transferase (HPRT). Enzymatic metabolites of the previous mentioned metabolic pathways are 6-methyl-mercaptopurine (6-MMP) and 6-thioguanosine nucleotides (6-TG), respectively. The therapeutic effect is linked to 6-TG, with its incorporation into RNA and DNA and consequent immunosuppressive effect. 6-MMP is the main factor responsible for toxic effects of AZA and 6-MP, specifically for pancreatitis, bone marrow suppression and hepatitis. Figure 3 summarizes AZA metabolism.

In a previous study, Cuffari *et al.*[16] showed that intra-erythrocyte 6-TG levels correlate with therapeutic efficacy, while high levels of 6-MMP seem to be associated with more frequent toxic effects. In a recent paper, Cuffari *et al.*[17] suggested that a tailored therapy with dosages of AZA/6-MP based on TPMT activity and on reaching therapeutic levels of 6-TG ($>$250 pmol/8 $\times$ 10^8 red blood cells) achieves better results and fewer adverse events.

In severe extensive steroid-refractory ulcerative colitis, there is a therapeutic role for **cyclosporine** (Cy-A). Cy-A is a lipophilic hydrophobic drug that inhibits T-helper lymphocyte production of interleukin-2 (IL-2) and interferon-γ (IFN-γ). Downstream effects of this action on cytokine balance lead to impairment of humoral and T-cellular immunity. Prior to initiating Cy-A treatment, cholesterol and Mg^{2+} levels should be investigated: low levels are associated with higher risk of seizure.

Blood-levels of Cy-A, tested either by high-performance liquid chromatography (HPLC) or by a monoclonal radioimmunoassay (RIA), should be monitored to adjust dosing of the drug in order to maintain levels within the therapeutic

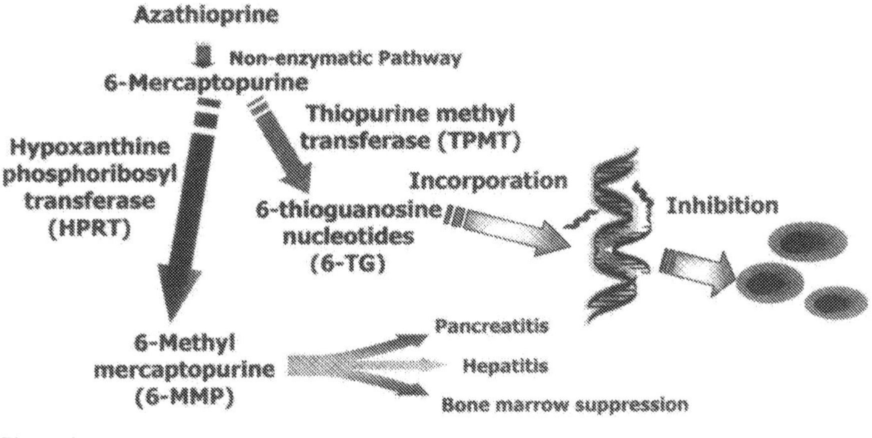

Figure 3 Metabolism of azathioprine and 6-mercaptopurine

range (100–300 ng/ml) and to reduce the risk of adverse events. Earlier data showed the efficacy of an intravenous 4 mg/kg bw/day regimen, with continuous infusion[18], in reducing the need for colectomy, but long-term results were disappointing. An earlier start of a maintenance treatment with AZA/6-MP led to considerably fewer relapses and reduced the rate of late colectomy[19]. Oral administration of a microemulsified formulation of Cy-A (Neoral, 5 mg/kg bw/day) seemed to be as effective as iv administration[20].

In a recent trial by D'Haens *et al.*[21], intravenous Cy-A monotherapy showed similar results when compared with steroids in patients with acute severe ulcerative colitis.

Among new drugs for acute severe ulcerative colitis, **tacrolimus** showed a short-term efficacy similar to that reported for Cy-A, with poor results in the long term when administered as monotherapy; it could represent an alternative to Cy-A when adverse events arise[22].

Data on the use of **infliximab** in refractory ulcerative colitis are limited to a pilot study by Chey[23] on 16 patients, with an efficacy of over 85% in the short term, and of about 25% at a 7–10 months follow-up. A randomized controlled study of infliximab in severe acute refractory ulcerative colitis[24] was stopped because of slow enrollment; it showed that 4/8 (50%) of treated patients responded to the active drug, while no responder was observed among controls.

Use of infliximab as a *bridge treatment* until AZA reaches therapeutic effects seems to be promising but needs to be demonstrated.

CONCLUSIONS

- The patient discussed here can be defined as having indeterminate colitis since this diagnosis was made on the surgical specimen.
- Indeterminate colitis is usually managed, from the medical point of view, as ulcerative colitis.
- Distal colitis refractory to standard treatments is a challenging problem and it is not uncommon to try different medical options (in this case topical and systemic 5-ASA, topical and systemic steroids, cyclosporine, azathioprine, budesonide enemas and topical lidocaine) before choosing surgery.
- Infliximab could represent an alternative treatment for refractory colitis (either ulcerative colitis or 'IBD, type uncertain') but its use in this clinical condition needs to be further evaluated.
- In **true** indeterminate colitis, colectomy with ileal pouch–anal anastomosis should represent the treatment of choice, although some authors recommend a delayed reconstruction to allow a possible better definition of the disease.

References

1. Price AB. Overlap in the spectrum of non-specific inflammatory bowel disease – "colitis indeterminate". J Clin Pathol. 1978;31:567–77.
2. Wells AD, McMillan I, Price AB, Ritchie JK, Nicholls RJ. Natural history of indeterminate colitis. Br J Surg. 1991;78(2):179–81.
3. Hodgson HJF. Ulcerative colitis versus Crohn's disease – one disease or two? In: Allan RN, Rhodes JM, Hanauer SB, Keighley MRB, Alexander-Williams J, Fazio VW, editors, Inflammatory Bowel Diseases, Third edition, Edinburgh: Churchill Livingstone, 1997:343–7.

4. Meucci G, Bortoli A, Riccioli FA *et al.* Frequency and clinical evolution of indeterminate colitis: a retrospective multi-centre study in northern Italy. GSMII (Gruppo di Studio per le Malattie Infiammatorie Intestinali). Eur J Gastroenterol Hepatol. 1999;11(8):909–13.
5. MacDermott RP. Indeterminate colitis. In: Bayless TM, Hanauer SB, editors, Advanced Therapy of Inflammatory Bowel Disease. Hamilton, Ontario: BC Decker Inc., 2001:157–60.
6. Poggioli G, Laureti S, Stocchi L *et al.* Immediate and long-term results in ileoanastomosis with reservoir in 335 consecutive cases. Chir Ital. 2000;52(3):215–22.
7. Breen EM, Schoetz DJ Jr, Marcello PW *et al.* Functional results after perineal complications of ileal pouch–anal anastomosis. Dis Colon Rectum. 1998;41(6):691–5.
8. McIntyre PB, Pemberton JH, Wolff BG, Dozois RR, Beart RW Jr. Indeterminate colitis. Long-term outcome in patients after ileal pouch–anal anastomosis. Dis Colon Rectum. 1995;38(1):51–4.
9. Lindsey I, Warren BF, Mortensen NJ. Indeterminate colitis: Surgical approaches. In: Bayless TM, Hanauer SB, editors, Advanced Therapy of Inflammatory Bowel Disease. Hamilton, Ontario: BC Decker Inc., 2001:241–4.
10. Vega R, Bertran X, Menacho M *et al.* Cytomegalovirus infection in patients with inflammatory bowel disease. Am J Gastroenterol. 1999;94(4):1053–6.
11. Cottone M, Pietrosi G, Martorana G *et al.* Prevalence of cytomegalovirus infection in severe refractory ulcerative and Crohn's colitis. Am J Gastroenterol. 2001;96(3):773–5.
12. Samuelsson SM, Ekbom A, Zack M, Helmick CG, Adami HO. Risk factors for extensive ulcerative colitis and ulcerative proctitis: a population based case-control study. Gut. 1991;32(12):1526–30.
13. Griffin MG, Miner PB. Review article: refractory distal colitis – explanations and options. Aliment Pharmacol Ther. 1996;10(1):39–48.
14. Campieri M, Gionchetti P, Belluzzi A *et al.* Optimum dosage of 5-aminosalicylic acid as rectal enemas in patients with active ulcerative colitis. Gut. 1991;32:929–31.
15. Hanauer SB. Treatment of active, severe and refractory ulcerative colitis: state of the art. In: IBD at the End of its First Century, Falk symposium no. 111. Dordrecht: Kluwer Academic Publisher, 2000:178–87.
16. Cuffari C, Theoret Y, Latour S, Seidman G. 6-Mercaptopurine metabolism in Crohn's disease: correlation with efficacy and toxicity. Gut. 1996;39(3):401–6.
17. Cuffari C, Hunt S, Bayless T. Utilisation of erythrocyte 6-thioguanine metabolite levels to optimise azathioprine therapy in patients with inflammatory bowel disease. Gut. 2001;48:642–6.
18. Lichtiger S, Present DH, Kornbluth A *et al.* Cyclosporine in severe ulcerative colitis refractory to steroid therapy. N Engl J Med. 1994;330:1841–5.
19. Fernandez-Banares F, Bertran X, Esteve-Comas M *et al.* Azathioprine is useful in maintaining long-term remission induced by intravenous cyclosporine in steroid-refractory severe ulcerative colitis. Am J Gastroenterol. 1996;91:2498–9.
20. Actis GC, Aimo G, Priolo G, Moscato D, Rizzetto M, Pagni R. Efficacy and efficiency of oral microemulsion cyclosporin versus intravenous and soft gelatin capsule cyclosporin in the treatment of severe steroid-refractory ulcerative colitis: an open-label retrospective trial. Inflamm Bowel Dis. 1998;4(4):276–9.
21. D'Haens G, Lemmens L, Geboes K *et al.* Intravenous cyclosporine versus intravenous corticosteroids as single therapy for severe attacks of ulcerative colitis. Gastroenterology. 2001; 120(6):1323–9.
22. Bousvaros A, Kirschner BS, Werlin SL *et al.* Oral tacrolimus treatment of severe colitis in children. J Pediatr. 2000;137(6):794–9.
23. Chey WY. Infliximab for patients with refractory ulcerative colitis. Inflamm Bowel Dis. 2001;7(Suppl 1):S30–3.
24. Sands BE, Tremaine WJ, Sandborn WJ *et al.* Infliximab in the treatment of severe, steroid-refractory ulcerative colitis: a pilot study. Inflamm Bowel Dis. 2001;7(2):83–8.

35
Indeterminate colitis

G. C. STURNIOLO, V. MEDICI, L. BENAZZATO and R. D'INCÀ

INTRODUCTION

Indeterminate colitis (IC) is defined as colitis with overlapping histological features of both ulcerative colitis (UC) and Crohn's disease (CD). IC occurs as an initial diagnosis in 5–13% of IBD patients. Most of the patients present with acute colitis (bloody diarrhoea, abdominal pain); about 25% of the patients have initial symptoms indicative of CD (diarrhoea without haematochezia, fever or weight loss). Diagnosis is based on endoscopic and histological features but ANCA and ASCA evaluation may be helpful. Follow-up is useful to classify about 70% of cases as either CD or UC. Patients with a diagnosis of IC in spite of accurate pre- and post-operative assessment are unlikely to show features of CD in the long term.

Medical treatment could be the same as for UC. Immunomodulatory agents are often used because of steroid dependency.

Restorative proctocolectomy seems to be the preferred treatment since the risk of pouch dysfunction is around 20% and the overall removal rate of the pouch does not exceed 10%. A recent 10-year follow-up of 82 IC patients who underwent an ileal pouch–anal anastomosis demonstrated more episodes of pelvic sepsis and fistulas. However, new biological therapies may offer another opportunity to help patients with ileal pouch–anal anastomosis (IPAA) complications.

CASE REPORT

This case shows the clinical features of a 45-year-old male complaining of bloody diarrhoea: at presentation, this case was suggestive of UC, due to the clinical, endoscopic and histological findings. Steroid treatment was rapidly effective but frequent episodes of flare-up followed, with the development of a steroid-dependent/refractory condition. A further episode of acute relapse was therefore treated with cyclosporine (CyA) and then azathioprine.

Recently, the efficacy of CyA followed by a combination of CyA and azathioprine has been demonstrated in active severe UC: patients treated with this drug combination have an increased probability of avoiding colectomy[1].

Fifty-four patients with severe colitis were observed over a 4-year period (age = 45 ± 17 years; 35 males) at the Gastroenterology Unit of the University of Padua: 11 (20%) were operated within 1 month of admission, 26 (48%) went into remission with steroids (dose 1 mg kg^{-1} day^{-1} oral or i.v.) and 17 (31%) with CyA i.v. (dose 2–4 mg kg^{-1} day^{-1}); 11 of them had a long-term remission period (mean follow up: 46 months). Travis *et al.*[2] demonstrated that bowel frequency (more than 8 bowel movements/day at day 3) and CRP (more than 80 Units at day 3) are factors predictive of a negative outcome (colectomy). In our experience, an increased risk of colectomy was identified, by means of logistic regression analysis, for patients having fever (>37°C) and ESR exceeding 54 at day 5 after admission.

The patient presented here benefited from azathioprine: azathioprine allows reduction of steroids and is effective in maintaining long-term remission. In spite of the encouraging results, the patient experienced a new flare-up and total colonoscopy outlined moderate to severe disease activity in the left colon.

Recently, a new therapeutic option with infliximab has been proposed for refractory UC[3]. Seventeen patients with refractory UC were treated with infliximab infusions at the dosage of 5 mg/kg: 16 improved, one underwent surgery.

Surgery was suggested for our patient. Subtotal colectomy with temporary ileostomy was carried out: the pathological features of the resected colon were compatible with either UC or CD, leading to a final diagnosis of IC.

IC could be defined in different ways: chronic colitis with divergent endoscopic or histological patterns and clinical features; or colitis with overlapping histological features of both UC and CD[4]: it has been estimated that about 10–15% of all surgical specimens fall into this category for both macroscopic and microscopic features. The pathological differential diagnosis between CD and UC is often more difficult in acutely inflamed specimens, when the appearances of these two conditions approximate to one another and several of the discriminating diagnostic attributes present in the chronic state become common to both conditions. Monocytolysis, capillary engorgement and acute V-shaped clefts were frequently described in Price's series[5]. Moreover, 'indeterminate colitis' is not even mentioned in some well-known diagnostic criteria for IBD, nor in the International Classification of Diseases.

The incidence of IC may vary if we consider the different definitions of the disease. Moum[6] studied retrospectively the IC incidence in four regions in south-eastern Norway: 93 cases of IC yielded a mean annual incidence of 2.4/100 000. The median age at diagnosis was 35 years. IC occurs as an initial diagnosis in 5–13% of IBD patients, although rates as high as 23% have been reported in children. Most of the patients show the clinical picture of an acute colitis (bloody diarrhoea, abdominal pain); about 25% of the patients have initial symptoms indicative of CD, such as diarrhoea without haematochezia, fever or weight loss.

A co-operative yet retrospective Italian study[7] involving 1113 IBD patients found 50 patients with a diagnosis of IC. Seventy-two per cent of these IC cases had a definite diagnosis of either CD or UC during the follow up. Wells[8], observing 16 patients with an IC diagnosis who underwent colectomy, found that patients who continue to have a diagnosis of IC after surgery in spite of careful assessment are unlikely to show features of CD in the long term.

ANCA and ASCA evaluation could be helpful for the diagnosis of IBD, p-ANCA being more specific for UC (>60% positivity in UC patients), and ASCA for CD. Quinton *et al.*[9] demonstrated that simultaneous ANCA and ASCA testing can improve the positive predictive value of these antibodies. In particular, the combination of ANCA+/ASCA− is strongly suggestive for ulcerative colitis (with a sensitivity of 57%, specificity of 97% and positive predictive value of 92.5%), while ANCA−/ASCA+ suggests Crohn's disease (sensitivity, specificity and positive predictive value of 49%, 97% and 96%, respectively). Unfortunately, as pointed out in a recent study[10], there is still no complete agreement among the different ASCA assays on the market.

Although medical management of UC and CD is often similar, the need for a differential diagnosis is expecially needed when surgery is under consideration; poor results occur more frequently in patients with a clinical diagnosis of Crohn's disease after IPAA. McIntyre *et al.*[11] compared functional outcomes of IPAA in patients with typical UC (1232 patients) and IC (71 patients). He observed that, five years after surgery, pouch failure occurred significantly more frequently in patients with an IC diagnosis than in those with UC (19% vs. 8%); however, more than 80% of IC patients had satisfactory pouch function follow up in the long term.

Yu *et al.*[12] demonstrated that IC and UC patients who underwent IPAA had the same rate of complications (pelvic sepsis, fistula, pouch failure) in a median follow up of 83 months. Interestingly, after ten years, patients with IC had significantly more episodes of complications if a final diagnosis of CD was made during follow up. Restorative proctocolectomy seems to be the preferred form of treatment since the risk of pouch dysfunction is about 20% and the overall removal rate of the pouch is 6–10%: the presented case had a positive outcome after IPAA.

New biological therapies could represent an important and useful alternative in cases of pouchitis: a recent study by Ricart[13] reported on the use of infliximab in pouchitis of patients with an initial UC diagnosis who turned out to have CD, showing a complete response in 6 of the 7 patients.

IC still represents a challenge for the clinician but new frontiers in diagnosis and therapy will reduce its frequency.

References

1. Cohen RD, Stein R, Hanauer SB. Intravenous cyclosporin in Ulcerative Colitis: a five year experience. Am J Gastroenterol. 1999;94:1587–92.
2. Travis DP, Farrant JM, Ricketts C *et al.* Predicting outcome in severe ulcerative colitis. Gut. 1996;38:905–10.
3. Chey WY. Infliximab for patients with refractory ulcerative colitis. Inflamm Bowel Dis. 2001;7 Suppl 1:S30–3.
4. Nicholls RJ, Wells AD. Indeterminate colitis. Bailliere's Clin Gastroenterol. 1992;6:105–12.
5. Price AB. Overlap in the spectrum of non-specific inflammatory bowel disease-"colitis indeterminate". J Clin Pathol. 1978;31:567–77.
6. Moum B, Vatn MH, Ekbom A *et al.* Incidence of ulcerative colitis and indeterminate colitis in four countries of Southeastern Norway, 1990–93. Scand J Gastroenterol. 1996;31:362–6.
7. Meucci G, Bortoli A, Albini Riccioli F *et al.* Frequency and clinical evolution of indeterminate colitis: a retrospective multi-centre study in Northern Italy. Eur J Gastroenterol Hepatol. 1999;11:909–13.

8. Wells AD, McMillian I, Price AB, Ritchie JK, Nicholls RJ. Natural history of indeterminate colitis. Br J Surg. 1991;78:179–81.
9. Quinton JF, Sendid B, Reumaux D *et al.* Anti-*Saccharomyces cerevisiae* mannan antibodies combined with antineutrophil cytoplasmic autoantibodies in inflammatory bowel disease: prevalence and diagnostic role. Gut. 1998;42:788–91.
10. Vermiere S, Joossens S, Peeters M *et al.* Comparative study of ASCA assays in Inflammatory Bowel Disease. Gastroenterology. 2001;120:827–33.
11. McIntyre PB, Pemberton JH, Wolff BG, Dozois RR, Beart RW. Indeterminate colitis. Long term outcome in patients after ileal pouch-anal anastomosis. Dis Colon Rectum. 1995;38:51–4.
12. Yu CS, Pemberton JH, Larson D. Ileal pouch-anal anastomosis in patients with indeterminate colitis: long term results. Dis Colon Rectum. 2000;43(11):1487–96.
13. Ricart E, Sandborn WJ. Infliximab for the treatment of fistulas in patients of Crohn's disease. Gastroenterology. 1999;117(5):1247–8.

36
IBD: UC or CD

K. GEBOES, I. DALLE and K. P. GEBOES

INTRODUCTION

Colorectal biopsy is widely used for the diagnosis of patients with colitis and is especially important for the diagnosis of ulcerative colitis (UC) or Crohn's disease (CD), the two major forms of idiopathic inflammatory bowel diseases (IBD). A variety of colitides may, however, be clinically confused with UC or CD. The differential diagnosis between IBD and other forms of colitis (non-IBD) is thus an important but often controversial issue. Diagnostic problems can arise in different clinical situations such as acute (prolonged) colitis, acute fulminant colitis, chronic relapsing disease and relapse of established IBD. The differential diagnosis between Crohn's disease involving the colon and UC is another differential diagnostic problem which can be difficult. Established biopsy criteria distinguishing between the two conditions do not exceed a sensitivity or specificity of 75%[1]. Analysis of multiple biopsies from different sites of the colon and the ileum can increase diagnostic accuracy. An increase from 5% to 40% was reached in a workshop organized in 2000 by the IBD Morphology Study Group and involving 24 pathologists, experts and non-experts, from different countries from Europe, North America and Asia. When it is impossible to solve the distinction between UC and CD, a diagnosis of 'indeterminate colitis' can be proposed. Originally, the term 'colitis indeterminate' was introduced for the small group of unclassified cases in which there was difficulty in distinguishing CD from UC or infections in the excised specimen[2]. Most of the cases were in fulminant disease and the classification was essentially temporary before a final diagnosis was established. More recently, 'indeterminate colitis' has also been applied as a temporary classification to cases where a definite diagnosis was not possible with endoscopic samples. In these cases, it was also not only a problem of distinguishing between CD and UC but also of discrimination between non-IBD colitis and IBD. It might, however, have been more appropriate to use the term 'indeterminate colitis' only for surgical specimens and the term 'unclassifiable' for endoscopic samples, especially for those obtained early after onset.

For the solution of differential diagnostic problems, a proper knowledge of the clinical history is essential. It is for instance important to know if the colitis occurs in an immunocompetent or an immunocompromised patient and it is essential to know if the patient is taking or has been taking drugs.

The present review is divided into three parts. The first part discusses acute or acute prolonged conditions which can mimic IBD but for which a definite diagnosis should be possible on the basis of clinical data, routine investigations and microscopy. In the second part, the diagnosis of IBD and the differential diagnosis between CD and UC are discussed. In the third part, situations where the differential diagnosis between CD and UC cannot be solved easily are discussed.

PATHOLOGICAL MIMICS OF IBD

Infectious diseases

The differential diagnosis with infectious or drug-related diseases is important both in fulminant colitis and in acute colitis because treatment and outcome are entirely different and proper treatment is essential. In these clinical circumstances, the differential diagnosis includes diffuse forms of colitis similar to ulcerative colitis which can occur as fulminant diseases due to *C. difficile* or antibiotic-associated colitis and a variety of infectious diseases, such as salmonellosis, shigellosis, *Escherichia coli* colitis, *Campylobacter* colitis, amoebiasis and schistosomiasis and toxic colitis due to potent antineoplastic agents[3,4]. Histopathology can help to solve many diagnostic problems, especially in non-fulminant cases (Figure 1). The microscopic features which can be used for the diagnosis of IBD are, however, often not present in the early stages of these diseases[5].

Some infectious or drug-related diseases have a more indolent course and may mimic CD or UC. In some of these cases, histopathology may even lead to confusion. *Entamoeba histolytica* may present as an indolent illness with apparent relapses and remissions over the course of weeks or months. It is thus essential to distinguish rapidly these conditions since inappropriate use of corticosteroids or other drugs or delay in administering an antibiotic is highly undesirable. Misdiagnosis of amoebiasis or tuberculosis with inappropriate use of corticosteroids can lead to serious complications.

Drug-related diseases

A medication history is indispensable in the investigation of patients with diarrhoea. A variety of drugs given either topically or systemically can cause colitis, ileocolitis or proctitis. Some of these drugs may mimic IBD more than others.

Non-steroidal anti-inflammatory drug (NSAID)-induced colitis is a significant clinical problem. Usually the patients are elderly. Symptoms can develop after 2 months to 5 years. They include abdominal complaints and blood in the stool. Night sweats and weight loss are not uncommon. Anaemia and elevated ESR can be present. NSAIDs can induce small bowel and colonic lesions. In the small bowel, discrete ulcers, perforation and diaphragm-like strictures have been reported[6]. In the colon, ulcers, perforation, or fistulas related to diverticulosis and exacerbations of colitis can appear (Figure 2).

The proposed mechanism for the small bowel is direct topical irritation facilitated by enterohepatic circulation of active NSAID metabolites. For the colon,

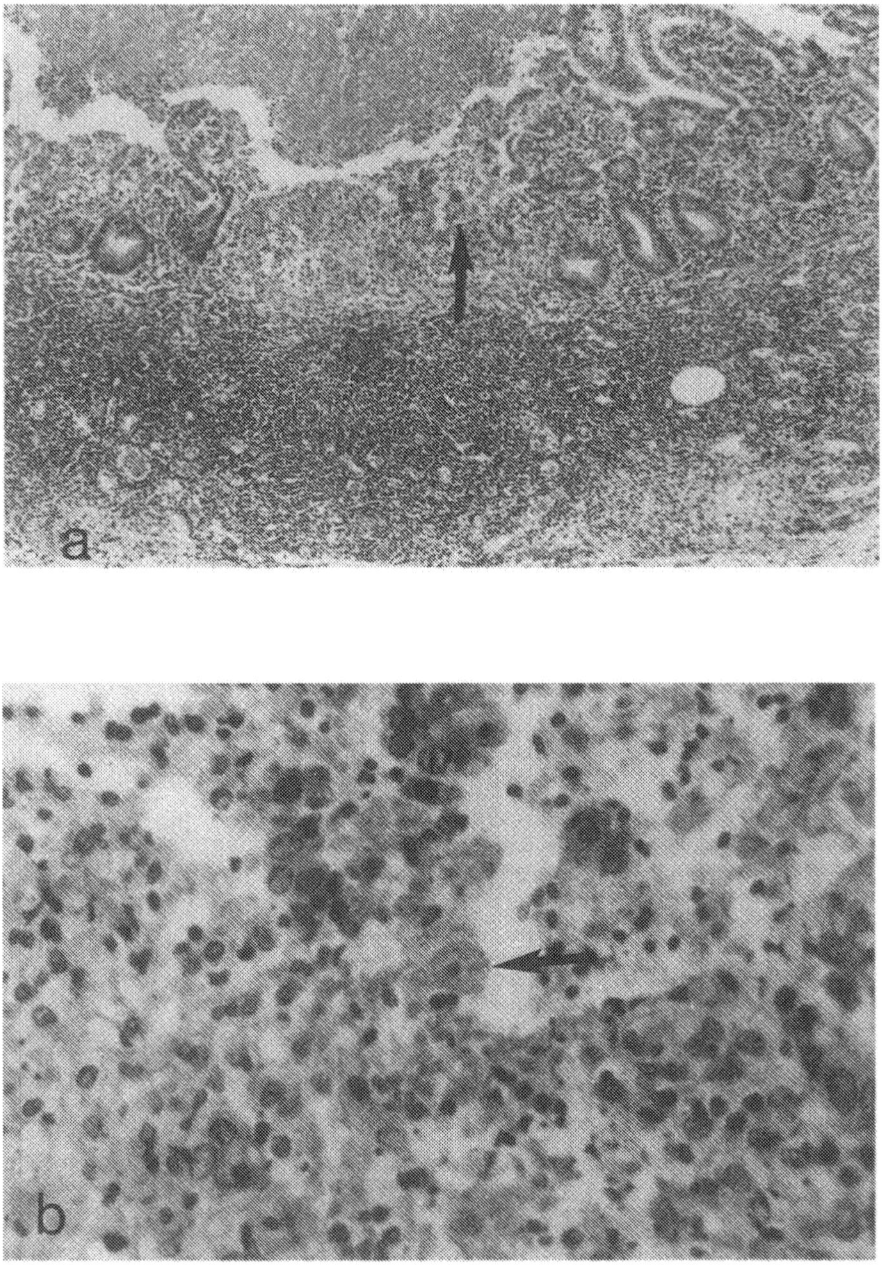

Figure 1 Ileal biopsy from a patient presenting with fulminant enterocolitis involving the colon and distal small intestine. The microphotograph (**a**) shows a superficial erosion overlying a lymphoid follicle in the centre. The villi in the mucosa at the edge of the ulcer can still be recognized and appear regular (haematoxylin and eosin (H&E); ×325). In the exudate, overlying the mucosal defect, amoebae can be identified (arrow) as shown at higher magnification in (**b**) (H&E; ×500)

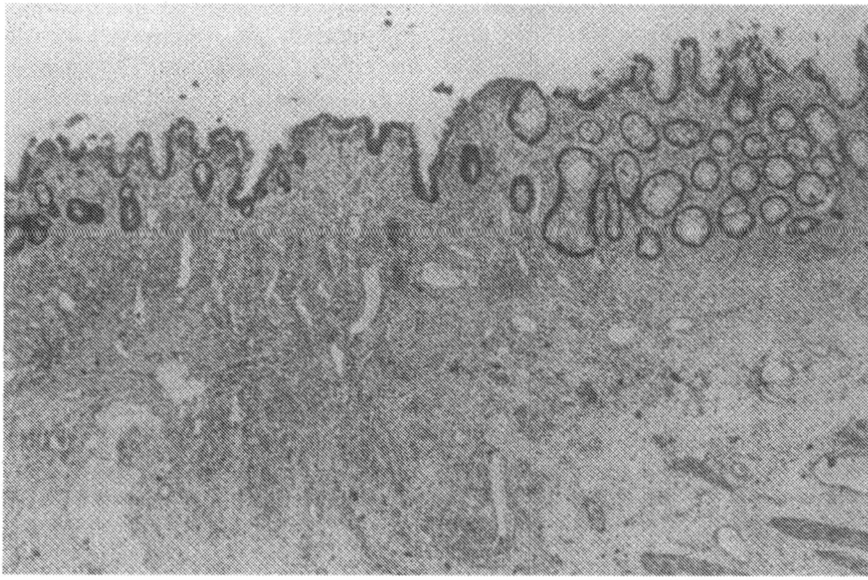

Figure 2 Colonic biopsy showing crypt architectural distortion in the mucosa, limited inflammation and loss of muscularis mucosae. The patient presented with multiple ulcers in the terminal ileum and proximal colon caused by NSAIDs (H&E; ×325)

the mechanism relates probably to decreased mucosal prostaglandins and a decreased production of COX-2 in underlying colitis[7].

Diclofenac, mefenamic acid and indomethacin are frequent offenders, especially the sustained-release preparations. Patients present with abdominal cramps, diarrhoea or constipation and laboratory tests reveal iron deficiency and positive faecal occult blood test. Colitis induced by NSAIDs can present as: non-specific colitis; *de novo* colitis; reactivation of quiescent inflammatory bowel disease; hypersensitivity reaction; allergic colitis (with eosinophils)[8]; constipation with perforation (stercoral ulcer)[9,10]; non-specific caecal or ileocaecal ulceration following the administration of oxyphenbutazone, slow-release diclofenac and ibuprofen; or more distal ulcers (naproxen in association with acetylsalicylic acid).

The differential diagnosis may be difficult, especially because rheumatic diseases may be associated with genuine IBD or with a Crohn-like non-specific form of chronic intestinal inflammation. Other drugs that can cause colitis are penicillamine and gold salts. Oral contraceptives and cocaine rather mimic ischaemic colitis[11,12].

Diverticular disease-associated colitis

A clinical syndrome of chronic colitis, localized to the sigmoid colon and occurring in association with diverticular disease, has been recognized repeatedly. Mucosal biopsies of this condition show features of idiopathic inflammatory bowel disease, including a distorted crypt architecture and basal plasmacytosis.

Colonic mucosa proximal and distal is usually normal. Overall, the inflammatory features can mimic either UC or CD. Crohn's disease-like features can include fat wrapping, fissures or sinuses and the presence of granulomas. The relationship between the inflammatory reaction and genuine IBD is unclear. Diverticular disease-associated chronic colitis may precede the onset of conventional ulcerative proctitis and colitis (3 out of a series of 23) or Crohn's disease (2 out of a series of 25) in a minority of the cases[13,14].

Endometriosis

The prevalence of intestinal endometriosis varies between 3% and 37% of all endometriosis. The anatomic distribution within the gastrointestinal tract is as follows: rectosigmoid in 50–90%, rectovaginal septum in 10–20%, caecum in 2–5%, appendix in 3–18% and small intestine in 2–16%. Small intestinal involvement is nearly always confined to the terminal ileum. Most commonly, intestinal endometriosis is asymptomatic. Ileal endometriosis, however, may present with acute, chronic or recurrent distal small bowel obstruction, in the same way as Crohn's ileitis. These symptoms occur mostly only when the endometriosis is deep and invasive. The most common complaint is midabdominal, rather than right lower quadrant, crampy pain. Diarrhoea or constipation, nausea and vomiting, fever, anorexia, weight loss and even haematochezia may be present. A relationship with the menstrual cycle is not always apparent[15–17].

Miscellaneous

A variety of other conditions can mimic IBD. Lesions similar to CD have been reported in ileal and colonic biopsies from patients with reactive arthritis and ankylosing spondylitis[18]. Less common pathological mimics include different forms of vasculitis, Behçet's disease, iatrogenic conditions such as graft-versus-host disease and radiation colitis and cancer.

BIOPSY DIAGNOSIS OF CHRONIC IDIOPATHIC INFLAMMATORY BOWEL DISEASES

The histological features which allow a reliable distinction between IBD and other causes of colorectal inflammation can be subdivided in two major categories: architectural abnormalities and inflammatory features. Abnormalities of the mucosal architecture include crypt architectural distortion (non-parallel, variable diameter or cystically dilated crypts), crypt branching, crypt shortening, decreased crypt density (increased spacing between crypts) and irregular (pseudovillous) mucosal surface (Figure 3). Diagnostic inflammatory features are transmucosal increased lamina propria cells, epithelioid granulomas and large numbers of neutrophils, especially in crypt abscesses[1,5,19] (Figure 4). The diagnostic value (specificity, sensitivity, inter- and intraobserver variability and predictive value) of these features have been studied extensively. Increased basal lamina propria cellularity and basal plasmacytosis for instance are common in UC (frequency of detection 76–92%) and in CD (frequency of detection 72–81%)[19]. Basal plasmacytosis occurs in approximately 38% of cases within

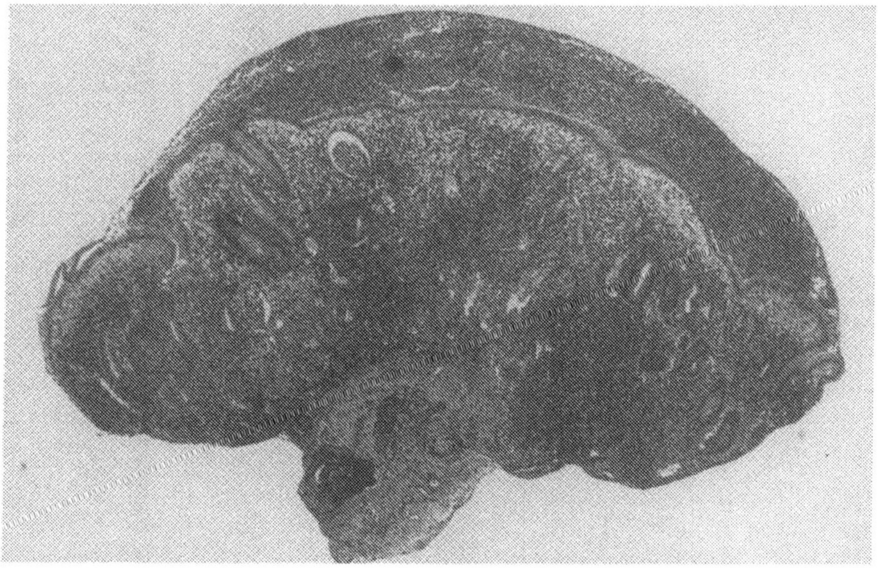

Figure 3 Colonic biopsy showing widespread crypt architectural distortion of the mucosa with shortening of crypts. The inflammation is transmucosal and diffuse. These features incline towards a diagnosis of ulcerative colitis. The presence of crypt abscesses indicates disease activity (H&E; ×325)

two weeks following onset of colitis and has a high predictive diagnostic value for IBD[5]. Granulomas are characteristic for CD being present in 21–37% of the endoscopic biopsies[19,20]. Histiocytic inflammation can occur in both CD and UC although, in some studies, it is considered as an argument in favour of CD[5,21,22]. Discontinuous inflammation and discontinuous crypt distortion favour a diagnosis of CD, while severe crypt architectural distortion and heavy diffuse transmucosal lamina propria cell increase favour UC (Table 1). Some of these features, like the presence of crypt abscesses, are not only used for diagnosis but also for the assessment of disease activity[23].

DIFFERENTIAL DIAGNOSIS BETWEEN CROHN'S DISEASE AND ULCERATIVE COLITIS

General pathological features

Crohn's disease can affect any part of the alimentary tract while ulcerative colitis is a colonic disease. Biopsies from the oesophagus, the stomach and the small intestine (ileum) can thus be helpful for the differential diagnosis. There are, however, some pitfalls. Severe duodenitis can occur in ulcerative colitis[24].

CD is characterized by segmental involvement of the colon and small intestine with deeper (fissuring) ulceration and prominent transmural inflammation and is often associated with strictures, fistula and anal lesions[25,26]. In UC, the rectum is nearly always involved. The disease may extend more proximal to any part of

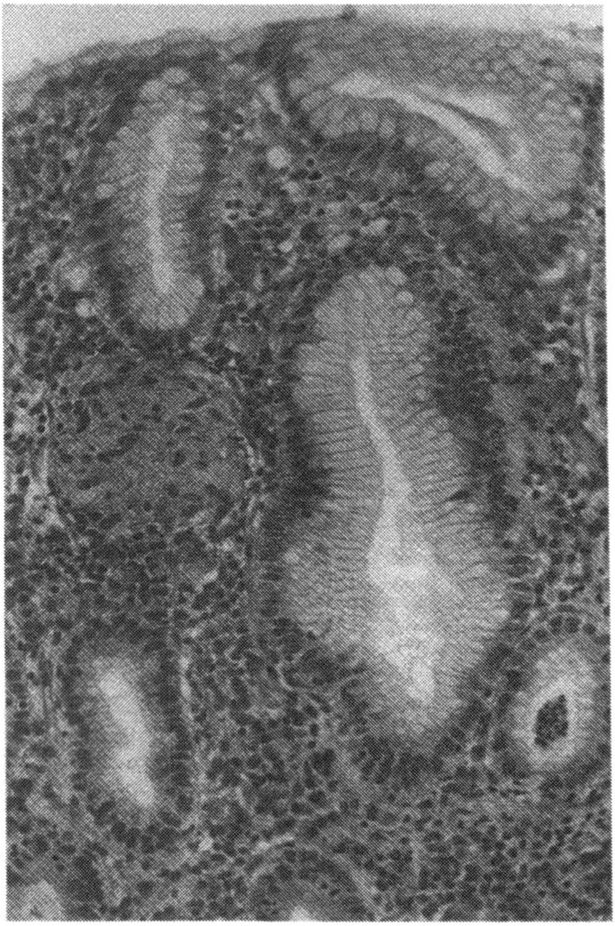

Figure 4 The presence of granulomas incline towards a diagnosis of Crohn's disease (H&E; ×500)

the colon from the left side to the entire large intestine. The anal canal can be spared but the transitional epithelium of the anal zone is often involved[27]. There are no skip lesions (although gross and microscopic caecal lesions can occur in predominantly left-sided colitis) and the disease does not affect the small intestine or other parts of the gut[28]. However, back-wash ileitis may be present. It is characterized by diffusely inflamed ileal mucosa in continuity with colonic lesions.

The gross appearance of the colon is extremely varied. It is determined by the fact that the disease may be continuous despite treatment or follow a pattern of remission and exacerbation. The disease intensity also may vary markedly from mild mucosal inflammation to severe inflammation with deep and/or widespread ulceration or a resolving quiescent colitis. Several features, such as the diffuse nature of the lesions, can be better evaluated on resection specimens although

Table 1 Frequency of detection in percentages of diagnostic microscopic features

	Normal	*Infective*	*IBD*	*UC*	*CD*
Architecture					
Irregular surface	0–5	0–7	39	63	24
Branched crypts	0–5		75	63–83	39–67
Crypt shortening	0–5	0		29–78	12–37
Chronic inflammation					
Increased basal cellularity	0	0		63	62
Increased lamina propria cellularity	0–19	30	89–93	76–92	72–81
Granulomas	0	0–2	25–27	0–5	21–100
Discontinuous inflammation	7			10	26
Epithelial alterations					
Mucin depletion	17			35–69	5–57
Mucin preservation at ulcer edge					+++
Neuronal changes				+	++

+indicates frequency of presence assessed on a subjective approach.

multiple stepwise endoscopic colonic biopsies with reliable identification of the site of the biopsies might help the pathologist in the differential diagnosis. The distribution of the lesions may, however, be modified seriously by medical treatment and hence it is not always a reliable feature for diagnostic purposes[29]. Features such as the transmural nature of the inflammation, the occurrence of lesions of the intrinsic innervation and the presence of granulomatous vasculitis or lymphangitis in CD can only reliably be assessed in surgical samples[30–32].

Macroscopy

Classical UC is a mucosal disease. It begins in the rectum and spreads proximal and in continuity involving a variable length of the colon. Ulcerative colitis is characteristically a left-sided disease. Rectitis (9%), rectosigmoiditis (23%) and left colonic involvement (24%) are the most common forms. Pancolitis is observed in 11–30% of cases[33]. UC is clinically characterized by acute exacerbations of symptoms and periods of remission. The gross appearance of the mucosal lesions varies with the stage of the disease. In the acute or early form, the mucosal surface is wet and glaring from blood and mucus and shows numerous petechial haemorrhages. Various-sized ulcers can appear. They can become extensive and undermine the mucosa. Multiple confluent ulcerations provoke denudation of the mucosa. The serosal side may appear congestive. Mesenteric fat hyperplasia is absent, in contrast to what is commonly seen in CD. Following healing of mucosal ulcers, elevated sessile reddish nodules, known as pseudopolyps, are often seen in an otherwise flat surface. They are typically small and multiple. Rarely, they may have a filiform configuration. In the more advanced stages the entire bowel becomes fibrotic, narrowed and shortened. In severe and active forms the entire colon or a segment may become dilated (toxic megacolon). In such cases the wall is usually thin and perforation can occur. There is some variability in the prevalence of the lesions depending upon the colonic segment involved. Pseudopolyps are rare in the rectum where mucosal congestion and friability predominate. During remission the mucosa may become normal again.

Healing, however, often occurs in an irregular way leading to a discontinuous, heterogeneous aspect of the mucosa which can be confused with CD. Treatment may increase the heterogeneous nature of the lesions. Topical treatment of the rectum with steroid or 5-ASA enemas may induce complete rectal healing while the lesions in the other segments of the colon may persist. Cases of UC with rectal sparing, although rare, must therefore not be confused with CD[34]. Palnaes-Hanson *et al.*, reviewing a series of surgical specimens of CD and UC, demonstrated the difficulty of making a reliable diagnosis of UC or CD on macroscopic examination alone[35].

The macroscopic lesions of CD are apparent both on the mucosal and serosal side of the bowel wall. Lesions are visible in the colon and/or small intestine often in association with the ascending colon but separated by uninvolved 'skip areas'. The length of the segments involved is variable. The mucosal appearance is heterogeneous. Lesions of different size (and probably of variable duration) are simultaneously present in the same surgical specimen. The ileal or colonic mucosa may appear normal or may show small, punctiform, rounded superficial erosions, often in the proximity of the section margin. Commonly larger, serpiginous ulcerations separated by normal-appearing mucosa are present. The combination of longitudinal and transverse ulceration in an oedematous mucosa is responsible for the characteristic cobblestone aspect. Ulcerations are more common on the mesenteric border of the small intestine. More severe ulcerations with complete circumferential loss of the mucosa are seen in stenosing areas. In rare cases CD can present a macroscopic picture of the left colon with continuous involvement, reminiscent of UC, in association with ileal disease[36].

Pseudopolyps of the colon and small intestine (in approximately 20% of the cases) are identical to those described in UC[37]. They are usually tall mucosal outgrowths, most commonly measuring a few millimetres in length but giant forms have been described. These are more common in CD[38]. Early mucosal lesions in CD are usually small, 1–2 mm in size and often multiple[39]. They appear as reddish plaques or as small nodules which may be eroded at the surface. When found overlying lymphoid nodules they correspond to aphthoid lesions. Erosions can become confluent and give rise to larger longitudinal ulcers known as serpiginous ulcers. Endoscopic studies have documented the progress from small to typical linear ulceration over 2–3 years[40]. They can also produce deeply situated fissuring ulcers and give rise to abscesses or fistulas between the involved segments and adjacent organs or nearby uninvolved loops. The bowel wall is usually thickened with involvement of the serosa and fat. The serosal side is characterized by overgrowth of mesenteric fats, called fat wrapping in the involved segments. This phenomenon is specific for CD. It is observed in 75% of the surgical specimens[41,42]. The mesenteric lymph nodes are commonly swollen but the number and size of the swollen lymph nodes in CD is not different from that observed in UC[43].

Microscopy

Several histological features are common to both UC and CD differing only in relative amounts[44,45]. These include mucosal distortion, cryptitis and crypt abscesses. Crypt architectural abnormalities in the colon are more common in UC (57–100% of cases) than in CD (27–71% of cases)[19]. Crypt abscesses are also more common in UC (frequency of detection = 41%) than in CD (frequency of detection = 19%)[19]. Paneth cell metaplasia (distal to the hepatic flexure) is common in long-standing IBD and more often seen in UC. Lymphoid nodules and lymphatic dilation are usually more common in CD. Differences have been noted between the results obtained with biopsies from children and adolescents compared with those of adults. Deformation of crypts, fibrosis and number of eosinophils were the most efficient variables for separating UC and CD in adults. In children the variables, granuloma and density of infiltration, were most separating. This outcome corresponds rather to the actual duration of the illness than to basic differences[45].

The distribution of inflammation may help in the distinction between UC and CD[43]. The possible inflammatory patterns available in a single mucosal colonic biopsy or in a set of biopsies are: normal mucosa; diffuse inflammation which may be *active* (neutrophils), *inactive* (increased number of lymphocytes and plasma cells) or *quiescent* (normal number of leukocytes within a mucosa showing disturbed crypt architecture); segmentary or patchy inflammation (background of inflammation with variable intensity); focal inflammation (normal background) and the presence of granulomas[44–46]. It is traditionally accepted that diffuse mucosal inflammation is common in UC and focal or patchy inflammation more common in CD. Discontinuous inflammation is therefore often considered to be a good criterion of Crohn's disease in stepwise endoscopic biopsies of the large bowel in both children and adults although it can be found in biopsies of resolving ulcerative colitis too[47]. When evaluating endoscopic biopsies for the differential diagnosis between UC and CD, the pathologist must be aware of the possibility of changes in time of various microscopic features[5,29]. The diagnostic criteria which can be applied on an initial set of biopsies obtained in an untreated patient may not be the same as those which can be used in follow-up biopsies[29]. When only colonic or rectal biopsies are available, a diagnosis of CD is thus supported by the finding of a focal active colitis or a normal mucosa within a set of otherwise inflamed biopsies (which is indicative of skip areas). Confirmation is obtained by the presence of granulomas or of a combination of features[48]. The diagnosis of UC is supported by the presence of severe mucosal architectural distortion and a diffuse transmucosal inflammation (with numerous crypt abscesses or extensive cryptitis).

Granulomas and microgranulomas are characteristic for CD. Granulomas in Crohn's disease are found in about 25% of colorectal biopsies[20]. Multiple serial sections and *en face* orientation of biopsies may increase the yield of granulomas. Aphthous ulcerations (histologically, ulcerations overlying lymphoid follicles – ulcer at a crypt base later becoming a 'mountain peak ulcer') in a seemingly normal mucosa are characteristic endoscopic features of Crohn's disease and are believed to represent early lesions[46]. Biopsies of these aphthous lesions often reveal diagnostic histological findings[48,49]. 'Cryptolytic lesions' and pericryptal granulomas present a special diagnostic problem. According to most authors, these granulomas can also be found in UC and are not reliable for a diagnosis of CD[50]. Yet, in a series of 22 patients with suspected inflammatory bowel disease, this type of lesion was present in 14 cases in the colorectal biopsies.

Ten of these patients were subsequently found to have CD[51]. Granulomas on their own are, however, not diagnostic of CD since they may be found in other conditions such as tuberculosis, schistosomiasis and *Yersinia* pseudotuberculosis. The simultaneous presence of a granuloma and other histopathological features, such as a disproportionate infiltrate (higher intensity in the submucosa than in the mucosa) with patchy distribution and relative preservation of the mucosal crypts, can be regarded as reliably diagnostic provided that specific infections are ruled out. Most of these features have been established some time ago, on surgical samples or biopsies from patients without important medical treatment.

Some studies have suggested that immunohistological methods may help in differentiating UC and CD. In CD, a partial replacement of interdigitating cells by scavenger macrophages has been reported. In acute infectious colitis, immunoglobulin A-and-IgM- or IgA-and-IgE-containing plasma cells are increased while, in IBD, most authors find an increase of all three major classes of IgG-containing cells or of IgG-containing cells in ulcerative colitis, of IgG and IgM in active Crohn's disease and a relative increase of IgM-containing cells in quiescent Crohn's disease[52]. A more recent finding was that epithelial cells in UC express CD44 isoform variants, v6 and v3, but, in patients with CD, CD44 v9. Additional studies have not however confirmed the initial hope that these markers could distinguish between CD and UC. Their appearance is more likely linked to increased proliferation of epithelial cells in severely inflamed tissue and not specific for a certain disease[53,54].

THE DIFFERENTIAL DIAGNOSIS BETWEEN UC AND CD: INDETERMINATE COLITIS (IC)

Terminology

Difficulties in diagnosis due to overlapping in the pathological features of Crohn's disease and ulcerative colitis have first been studied in surgical specimens. The term 'colitis indeterminate' was proposed for the small group of unclassified cases in which there was difficulty in distinguishing Crohn's disease from ulcerative colitis (and even infectious diseases) in the excised specimen. The difficulty was due to the fact that features of both conditions were present in the same specimen. Most of the cases were in fulminant disease and the classification was essentially temporary before a final diagnosis was established[2]. Later 'indeterminate colitis' has also been applied as a temporary classification to cases where a definite diagnosis was not possible with endoscopic samples because of absence of diagnostic features discriminating between CD and UC.

The morphological features of indeterminate colitis diagnosed on endoscopic samples include: (1) lesions which are suggestive or diagnostic for IBD such as (minimal) architectural distortion; (2) inflammatory features (usually transmucosal inflammation) which do not allow a firm distinction between ulcerative colitis and Crohn's disease because of their patchy nature; and (3) absence of small bowel involvement.

Diagnostic problems

The differential diagnosis between CD and UC can be made in most cases on the cumulative clinical, radiological, endoscopic, biochemical and pathological evidence. However, owing to the variable occurrence of even the most reliable features, diagnostic difficulties still occur. A confident diagnosis could not be reached in 10–20% of cases in older series. Colonoscopy and an improved knowledge of the evolution of the histopathological features in time have increased the diagnostic yield but diagnostic difficulties have not disappeared completely. In a prospective study of IBD from 20 European centres, 5% of all patients with IBD were classified as having indeterminate colitis[55]. Diagnostic difficulties occur in different clinical situations including early onset disease, atypical clinical presentations, and following medical or surgical therapy.

In the initial period shortly after onset of the disease, it may be difficult to reach a definite diagnosis because biopsies are less characteristic due to the absence of pathognomonic features. While one or more of the characteristic features of IBD are present in about 80% of the biopsies after 3–8 weeks, they are absent in about 20% of the cases and in an even larger group of patients in the first 3 weeks after clinical onset[5].

Patients with CD may present with an ulcerative colitis-like pattern both on endoscopy and on biopsy[37]. The presence of ileal lesions can be of major importance for this differential diagnostic problem[56].

Microscopic colitis is clinically and morphologically different from IBD. Yet in some cases, collagenous or lymphocytic colitis can precede (or follow) genuine UC (or CD)[57].

Diagnostic difficulties may appear or reappear in patients with long-standing disease presenting with a relapse. Histopathological and endoscopic features may change or even disappear because of the relapsing nature of IBD and variability with time and treatment[29,47]. Discontinuous inflammation, which has long been considered a good criterion for CD, has been shown to be common in resolving and long-standing UC. The proximal to distal gradient of inflammation, which means that inflammation is more pronounced in the proximal colon and terminal ileum in CD, can also change[58]. Review of previous biopsies is essential in such a situation.

Cytomegalovirus can be associated with an initial attack of IBD, usually UC. The patient can present with fulminant colitis. CMV infection can also be responsible for a clinical relapse of UC or for therapy refractory disease. It was found in 36% of refractory patients[59]. It may further complicate pouchitis and immunomodulatory treatment[60,61].

Major diagnostic problems can be observed also in operated patients presenting with severe pouchitis or perianal disease. Granulomas and transmural inflammation, which are considered to be diagnostic for CD, can be observed in pouchitis, following surgery for ulcerative colitis. Review of the original surgical specimen and of any other material available is essential before considering changing a diagnosis of ulcerative colitis to Crohn's disease[62].

Evolution

While only a minority of patients have a diagnosis of indeterminate colitis (IC), it is important to realize that such a diagnosis has certain consequences.

A diagnosis of indeterminate colitis means that the patient has IBD and that other conditions, especially infections, are less likely or indeed excluded. Relapse of symptoms due to complications such as CMV infection is equally excluded. A diagnosis of IC means also that the patient needs to be followed carefully in order to reach a more definite diagnosis. The latter can be obtained during follow-up (development of small intestinal involvement), by examination of gastric biopsies and the identification of focal gastritis, by using serological markers such as pANCA (perinuclear antineutrophil cytoplasmic antibodies) and ASCA (anti-*Saccharomyces cerevisiae* antibodies)[63]. In a prospective multicentre study involving 83 patients, a final diagnosis was reached in 22 patients after a mean follow-up of 7.5 months. Thirteen of 22 patients had Crohn's disease and 9 had ulcerative colitis.

The clinical course of patients with IC is at least as severe as that of patients with UC. Studies of clinical characteristics of IC, when compared with UC, revealed that patients with IC have younger age at onset, more extensive disease and a more severe clinical course (severity of first attack, frequency of clinical remissions and surgery). The risk of colorectal cancer is similar to that for UC or even somewhat enhanced[55]. Immunomodulatory agents are used more frequently because of steroid dependency, resistance or toxicity[64]. When surgery is needed, different options have to be considered. It might, for instance, be considered to postpone the construction of an ileoanal anastomosis. The course of IC is indeed more refractory than UC with regard to relapse, incidence of colectomy and pouch failure after ileal pouch–anal anastomosis.

CONCLUSIONS

Colorectal biopsy is widely used for the differential diagnosis of various colitides. Several histological features are discriminative in the diagnosis of IBD and non-IBD. These include, in general, mucosal distortion and basal plasmacytosis. The distinction between UC and CD relies on the extent of mucosal distortion, mucin depletion and mucin preservation at the edge of an ulcer[1], the distribution of the inflammatory infiltrate and the presence of granulomas. Indeterminate colitis is a temporary diagnosis for a patient presenting with symptoms which are suggestive of genuine IBD. The biopsy contains features which indicate IBD, such as architectural distortion, but the differential diagnosis between UC and CD cannot be solved. In acute cases, infections must be ruled out. A diagnosis of IC must not be a substitute diagnosis for lack of knowledge or fear of decision. The clinical course of patients with indeterminate colitis is usually more severe when compared with classical UC. Medical and surgical treatment must be considered carefully because of possible complications and uncertain natural evolution, although basically, treatment is comparable with routine treatment for IBD.

References

1. Tanaka M, Riddell RH, Saito H, Soma Y, Hidaka H, Kudo H. Morphologic criteria applicable to biopsy specimens for effective distinction of inflammatory bowel disease from other forms of colitis and Crohn's disease from ulcerative colitis. Scand J Gastroenterol. 1999;34:55–67.

2. Price A. Overlap in the spectrum of non-specific inflammatory bowel disease – 'colitis indeterminate'. J Clin Pathol. 1978;31:567–77.
3. Meuwissen SGM, Vandenbroucke-Grauls C, Geboes K. Spectrum of acute self-limiting colitis: role of the clinician and pathologist. Ital J Gastroenterol Hepatol. 1999;31:807–16.
4. Floch MH, Hellman L. The effect of 5-fluorouracil on rectal mucosa. Gastroenterology. 1965;48:430–7.
5. Schumacher G, Kollberg B, Sandstedt B. A prospective study of first attacks of inflammatory bowel disease and infectious colitis. Histologic course during the 1st year after presentation. Scand J Gastroenterol. 1994;29:318–32.
6. Lang J, Price AB, Levi AJ, Burke M, Gumpel JM, Bjarnason I. Diaphragm disease: pathology of disease of the small intestine induced by non-steroidal anti-inflammatory drugs. J Clin Pathol. 1988;41:516–26.
7. Eaker EY. Gastrointestinal injury related to use of nonsteroidal anti-inflammatory drugs. Gastrointest Dis Today. 1997;6:1–8.
8. Goere D, Brocheriou-Spelle I, Baron-Josselin V, Salmeron M, Houdart R. Colite aiguë grave secondaire à la prise d'aspirine. Gastroenterol Clin Biol. 1999;23:586–7.
9. Gibson GR, Whitacre EB, Ricotti CA. Colitis induced by nonsteroidal anti-inflammatory drugs. Report of four cases and review of the literature. Arch Intern Med. 1992;152:625–32.
10. Hollingworth J, Alexander-Williams J. Non-steroidal anti-inflammatory drugs and stercoral perforation. Ann Roy Coll Surg. 1991;73:337–40.
11. Lewis JH. Gastrointestinal injury due to medicinal agents. Am J Gastroenterol. 1986;81:819–34.
12. Nalbandian H, Sheth N, Dietrich R, Georgiou J. Intestinal ischemia caused by cocaine ingestion: report of two cases. Surgery. 1985;97:374–6.
13. Makapugay LM, Dean PJ. Diverticular-disease-associated chronic colitis. Am J Surg Pathol. 1996;20:94–102.
14. Goldstein N, Leon-Armin C, Mani A. Crohn's colitis-like changes in sigmoid diverticulitis specimens is usually an idiosyncratic inflammatory response to the diverticulosis rather than Crohn's colitis. Am J Surg Pathol. 2000;24:668–75.
15. Boulton R, Chawla MH, Poole S, Hodgson HJF, Barrison IG. Ileal endometriosis masquerading as Crohn's ileïtis. J Clin Gastroenterol. 1997;25:338–42.
16. Langlois NEI, Park MKG, Keenan RA. Mucosal changes in the large bowel with endometriosis: a possible cause of misdiagnosis of colitis? Hum Pathol. 1994;25:1030–4.
17. Craninx M, D'Haens G, Cokelaere K *et al.* Crohn's disease and intestinal endometriosis: an intriguing co-existence. Eur J Gastroenterol Hepatol. 2000;12:217–21.
18. Cuvelier C, Barbatis C, Mielants H, De Vos M, Roels H, Veys E. Histopathology of intestinal inflammation related to reactive arthritis. Gut. 1987;28:394–401.
19. Jenkins D, Balsitis M, Gallivan S *et al.* Guidelines for the initial biopsy diagnosis of suspected chronic idiopathic inflammatory bowel disease. The British Society of Gastroenterology Initiative. J Clin Pathol. 1997;50:93–105.
20. Heresbach D, Heresbach-Le Berre N, Ramée MP, Séman G, Gosselin M, Bretagne JF. Fréquence et valeur pronostique du granulome épithélioïde au cours des maladies inflammatoires chroniques de l'intestin. Gastroentérol Biol Clin. 1999;23:1376–87.
21. Tsang P, Rotterdam H. Biopsy diagnosis of colitis. Possibilities and pitfalls. Am J Surg Pathol. 1999;23:423–30.
22. Seldenrijk CA, Morson BC, Meuwissen SGM, Schipper NW, Lindeman J, Meijer CJLM. Histopathological evaluation of colonic mucosal biopsy specimens in chronic inflammatory bowel disease: diagnostic implications. Gut. 1991;32:1514–20.
23. Geboes K, Riddell R, Öst Ä, Jensfelt B, Persson T, Löfberg R. A reproducible grading scale for histological assessment of inflammation in ulcerative colitis. Gut. 2000;47:404–9.
24. Valdez R, Appelman HD, Bronner MP, Greenson JK. Diffuse duodenitis associated with ulcerative colitis. Am J Surg Pathol. 2000;24:1407–13.
25. Oberhuber G, Stangl PC, Vogelsang H, Schober E, Herbst F, Gasche C. Significant association of strictures and internal fistula formation in Crohn's disease. Virchows Arch. 2000;437:293–7.
26. Graham MF, Diegelmann RF, Elson CO *et al.* Collagen content and types in the intestinal strictures of Crohn's disease. Gastroenterology. 1988;94:257–65.
27. Ambroze WL, Pemberton JH, Dozois RR, Carpenter HA, O'Rourke JS, Ilstrup DM. The histological pattern and pathological involvement of the anal transition zone in patients with ulcerative colitis. Gastroenterology. 1993;104:514–18.

28. D'Haens G, Geboes K, Peeters M, Baert F, Ectors N, Rutgeerts P. Patchy cecal inflammation associated with distal ulcerative colitis: a prospective endoscopic study. Am J Gastroenterol. 1997;92:1275–9.
29. Geboes K. Pathology of inflammatory bowel diseases (IBD): variability with time and treatment. Colorectal Dis. 2001;3:2–12.
30. Geller SA, Cohen A. Arterial inflammatory-cell infiltration in Crohn's disease. Arch Pathol Lab Med. 1983;107:473–5.
31. Wakefield AJ, Dhillon AP, Rowles PM, Sawyerr AM, Pittilo RM, Lewis AAM. Pathogenesis of Crohn's disease: multifocal gastrointestinal infarction. Lancet. 1989;2:1057–62.
32. Wakefield AJ, Sankey EA, Dhillon AP *et al.* Granulomatous vasculitis in Crohn's disease. Gastroenterology. 1991;100:1279–87.
33. Both H, Torp-Pedersen S, Kreiner S, Hendriksen C, Binder V. Clinical appearance at diagnosis of ulcerative colitis and Crohn's disease in a regional patient group. Scand J Gastroenterol. 1983;18:987–91.
34. Bernstein CN, Shanahan F, Anton PA, Weinstein WM. Patchiness of mucosal inflammation in treated ulcerative colitis: a prospective study. Gastrointest Endosc. 1995;42:232–7.
35. Palnaes-Hanson C, Hegnhoj J, Moller A, Brauer C. Ulcerative colitis and Crohn's disease of the colon: is there a macroscopic difference? Ann Chir Gynaecol. 1990;79:78–81.
36. Vasiliauskas EA, Plevy SE, Landers CJ *et al.* Perinuclear antineutrophil cytoplasmic antibodies in patients with Crohn's disease define a clinical subgroup. Gastroenterology. 1996;110:1810–19.
37. Kahn E, Daum F. Pseudopolyps of the small intestine in Crohn's disease. Hum Pathol. 1984;15:84–6.
38. Kelly JK, Langevin JM, Price LM, Hershfield NB, Share S, Blustein P. Giant and symptomatic inflammatory polyps of the colon in idiopathic inflammatory bowel disease. Am J Surg Pathol. 1986;10:420–8.
39. Watier A, Devroede G, Perey B, Haddad P, Madarnas P, Grand-Maison P. Small erythematous mucosal plaques: an endoscopic sign of Crohn's disease. Gut. 1980;21:835–9.
40. Rutgeerts P, Geboes K, Vantrappen G, Kerremans R, Coenegrachts JL, Coremans G. Natural history of recurrent Crohn's disease at the ileocolonic anastomosis after curative surgery. Gut. 1984;25:665–72.
41. Sheehan AL, Warren BF, Gear MWL, Shepherd NA. Fat-wrapping in Crohn's disease: pathological basis and relevance to surgical practice. Br J Surg. 1992;79:955–9.
42. Desreumaux P, Ernst O, Geboes K *et al.* Inflammatory alterations in mesenteric adipose tissue in Crohn's disease. Gastroenterology. 1999;117:73–81.
43. Cook MG. The size and histological appearances of mesenteric lymph nodes in Crohn's disease. Gut. 1972;13:970–2.
44. Goldman H. Colonic mucosal biopsy in inflammatory bowel disease. Surg Pathol. 1991;4:3–24.
45. Schmitz-Moormann P, Himmelman GW. Does quantitative histology of rectal biopsy improve the differential diagnosis of Crohn's disease and ulcerative colitis. Path Res Pract. 1988; 183:481–8.
46. Tanaka M, Riddell RH. The pathological diagnosis and differential diagnosis of Crohn's disease. Hepato-gastroenterology. 1990;37:18–31.
47. Kleer CG, Appelman HD. Ulcerative colitis: patterns of involvement in colorectal biopsies and changes with time. Am J Surg Pathol. 1998;22:983–9.
48. Geboes K, Vantrappen G. The value of colonoscopy in the diagnosis of Crohn's disease. Gastrointest Endosc. 1975;22:18–23.
49. Jouret A, Mainguet P. Diagnostic value of systematic endoscopic biopsies in ileocolonic Crohn's disease. Acta Gastroenterolog Belg. 1993;56:C71.
50. Dundas SAC, Dutton J, Skipworth P. Reliability of rectal biopsy in distinguishing between chronic inflammatory bowel disease and acute self-limiting colitis. Histopathology. 1997;31:60–6.
51. Lee FD, Maguire C, Obeidat W, Russell RI. Importance of cryptolytic lesions and pericryptal granulomas in inflammatory bowel disease. J Clin Pathol. 1997;50:148–52.
52. Oshitani N, Campbell A, Kitano A, Kobayashi K, Jewell DP. *In situ* comparison of phenotypical and functional activity of infiltrating cells in ulcerative colitis mucosa. J Pathol. 1996;178:95–9.
53. Fromont-Hankard G, Cezard JP, Aigrain Y, Navarro J, Peuchmaur M. CD44 variant expression in inflammatory colonic mucosa is not disease specific but associated with increased crypt cell proliferation. Histopathology. 1998;32:317–21.

54. Reinisch W, Heider KH, Oberhuber G *et al.* Poor diagnostic value of colonic CD44v6 expression and serum concentrations of its soluble form in the differentiation of ulcerative colitis from Crohn's disease. Gut. 1998;43:375–82.
55. Ekbom A. Indeterminate colitis: the magnitude of the problem. Inflamm Bowel Dis. 2000;6:S14–15.
56. Geboes K, Ectors N, D'Haens G, Rutgeerts P. Is ileoscopy with biopsy worthwhile in patients presenting with symptoms of IBD? Am J Gastroenterol. 1998;93:201–6.
57. Panaccione R, Tremaine WJ, Batts KW, Sandborn WJ. Diagnosis of lymphocytic or collagenous colitis in patients with ulcerative colitis or Crohn's disease. Gastroenterology. 1999;116:A833.
58. Geboes K, Desreumaux P, Jouret A, Ectors N, Rutgeerts P, Colombel JF. Diagnostic histopathologique de l'activité des maladies inflammatoires chroniques de l'intestin: evaluation de l'effet des traitements médicamenteux, application des scores histologiques. Gastroentérol Clin Biol. 1999;23:1062–73.
59. Cottone M, Pietrosi G, Martorana G *et al.* Prevalence of cytomegalovirus infection in severe refractory ulcerative colitis and Crohn's colitis. Am J Gastroenterol. 2001;96:773–5.
60. Moonka D, Furth EE, MacDermott RP, Lichtenstein GR. Pouchitis associated with primary cytomegalovirus infection. Am J Gastroenterol. 1998;93:264–6.
61. Ruther U, Nunnensiek C, Muller HA, Bader H, May U, Jipp P. Interferon alpha (IFN alpha 2a) therapy for herpes virus-associated inflammatory bowel disease (ulcerative colitis and Crohn's disease). Hepatogastroenterology. 1998;45:691–9.
62. Warren BF, Shepherd NA, Bartolo DCC. Pathology of the defunctioned rectum in ulcerative colitis. Gut. 1993;34:514–16.
63. Joossens S, Cassagnon M, Vermeire S *et al.* Are anti-Saccharomyces cerevisiae antibodies (ASCA) and perinuclear antineutrophil cytoplasmic antibodies (PANCA) useful in indeterminate colitis? A prospective follow-up study. Gastroenterology. 2000;118:A886.
64. Kirschner BS. Implications for management: Medical approach. Inflamm Bowel Dis. 2000; 6:S16–17.

37
The neuromodulation of intestinal inflammation

S. M. COLLINS, S. GANGULI, F. GALEAZZI and A. RUHL

INTRODUCTION

The ability of nerves to modulate intestinal inflammation has been recognized for some time. In 1939, Lium showed that persistent stimulation of the canine colon with parasympathomimetic drugs induced colitis which resembled human ulcerative colitis, and which could not be mimicked by the administration of vasopressin, excluding an ischaemic mechanism[1]. In clinical studies, vagotomy and close denervation of the colon was used to treat refractory colitis, with apparent success[2]. These early studies were performed at a time when the role of the psyche in the development of IBD was a viable hypothesis. As our understanding of the role of the immune system in IBD has increased, enthusiasm for a role for the nervous system in IBD has waned[2].

PSYCHO-NEURO-IMMUNOLOGY

In the last 25 years, there has been a substantial increase in our understanding of the inter-relationships between the psyche, the nervous system and the immune system. Initially, it was established that nerves are in close anatomical proximity to immunocytes, and that organs such as the spleen are innervated[3–6].

A broad functional context for neuro-immune interactions was provided by MacQueen *et al.* who showed that mast cell degranulation could be induced by Pavlovian conditioning[7]. Thus, tangible functional linkages could be envisaged between neurons in the CNS, and immune effector cells in the gut.

OBSERVATIONS IN PATIENTS WITH INFLAMMATORY BOWEL DISEASE

There are both indirect and direct lines of evidence supporting the neuromodulation of intestinal inflammation in patients with inflammatory bowel disease.

The beneficial effect of cigarette smoke and nicotine in ulcerative colitis may be construed as evidence of a neurally mediated effect, although this cannot be confirmed in man by the use of ganglion blocking drugs such as hexamethonium. The deleterious effect of smoking in Crohn's disease suggests that the modulation of inflammation of cholinergic nerves is complex. The variables here are the type of immunological drive to the inflammation (i.e. Th-1 or Th-2) as well as the background autonomic balance which appears to differ in Crohn's disease and ulcerative colitis. Other evidence in favour of neuro involvement in IBD may be derived from the apparent benefit obtained from the use of clonidine in patients with ulcerative colitis. Although this demonstration is limited to one placebo-controlled study, the observation is not surprising in light of recent animal work.

The apparent therapeutic benefit of lidocaine in left-sided ulcerative colitis is limited to one study group[8]. It is debatable whether this constitutes evidence of an effect on sensory nerves. Studies in animals provide a clear demonstration, in several models, that sensory nerves are protective[9] and blockade of such nerves would be expected to have deleterious effects on the inflammatory process. Some studies in animals have suggested that the effect of lidocaine is a non-selective membrane-stabilizing infection that includes all cells including inflammatory cells[10].

Certainly, the most direct demonstration of neuromodulation of intestinal inflammation comes from a recently published case report in which spinal cord stimulation by an electrode placed on the dorsal aspect of the spinal cord induced two successive relapses in a 48-year-old gentleman with stable left-sided ulcerative colitis[11]. Following these two stimulation-induced relapses, the device was removed and the patient remained stable thereafter. The results were interpreted as a possible demonstration of direct neurostimulation of the inflammatory process in the gut. The authors speculated that the observed relapse was due to the stimulation of neurons in the spinal cord, resulting in changes along the gut–brain axis. Although this interpretation has been challenged, the results remain provocative and highly suggestive of a direct neurogenic stimulation of a relapse of IBD in man.

RESULTS FROM ANIMAL STUDIES

Stress and inflammation in animal models of IBD

Although the literature is controversial, the balance of existing evidence is in favour of a role for stress in triggering relapses of human inflammatory bowel disease. While there are no data supporting a role for stress or behavioural factors in the aetiology of IBD, although ulcerative colitis was once considered a psychosomatic disorder, it is not uncommon for patients to present with the onset of illness during or following a time of emotional stress. Animal work has shown that prior exposure to stress enhances the response to an inflammatory stimulus; mild stress applied to rats augmented the response to intrarectal administration of the hapten dinitrobenzene sulphonic acid, DNB[12]. The mechanism underlying this stress-induced enhancement of the inflammatory response is not known, and involvement of hypothalamic pituitary pathways by corticotrophin-releasing factor (CRF) and vasopressin has been excluded[12]. However, it has been shown that this stress-induced enhancement of DNB-induced colitis is more prominent in Lewis rats with defective hypothalamic CRF release on exposure to stress[13,14].

A recent study in mice demonstrated the ability of stress to reactivate quiescent colitis[15]. In that study, mice were allowed to recover for 8 weeks after colitis induced by intracolonic administration of the hapten dinitrobenzene sulphonic acid. At that time, the colon had returned to normal. Mice were then exposed to a combined restraint and acoustic stress, and a subthreshold dose of DNB. While neither the stress nor this dose of DNB induced colitis when applied alone, in combination, they caused a relapse of the colitis accompanied by mucosal ulceration and a marked inflammatory cell infiltrate in the colon. The mechanism by which stress reactivated colitis was via an increase in permeability, allowing entry of luminal antigen and activating presensitized T lymphocytes. The phenomenon could be adoptively transferred by grafting CD4+ T cells from mice with colitis into naive recipient mice. While transfer of T cells alone did not cause colitis in recipient mice, these mice developed colitis following subsequent exposure to stress and a subthreshold dose of hapten. These results provide a tangible demonstration of a psycho-neuro-immune interaction in a clinically relevant context.

The autonomic nervous system and colitis

To date, the existing literature suggests sympathetic nerves are proinflammatory while, under normal circumstances, parasympathetic nerves provide no significant modulation of colonic inflammation in rats. Chemical sympathectomy with 6-hydroxy-dopamine (6-HD) resulted in a less severe colitis induced by TNB than was observed in vehicle-treated rats[9]. In contrast, hexamethonium did not significantly alter TNB colitis in the rat[16]. However, large doses of nicotine were proinflammatory and the deleterious effects of cigarette smoke in rats with TNB-induced colitis could be attenuated by hexamethonium, indicating the involvement of parasympathetic nerves[16]. Taken together, these findings indicate that pharmacological stimulation of nicotinic nerves has proinflammatory consequences, at least in this model of colitis. As DNB colitis is generally considered to be a Th-1 model of colitis[17], the deleterious effect of smoking in this model coincides with the same effect seen in Crohn's disease, which is also Th-1 mediated, and contrasts with the beneficial effect of smoking in ulcerative colitis[18]. Results of a pilot study in man have shown that patients with distal colitis have evidence of sympathetic dominance, as reflected by changes in heart rate variability. In contrast, parasympathetic dominance was evident in patients with more extensive colitis. These observations, taken in conjunction with the data from animal studies, prompt speculation that patients with distal rather than extensive colitis may be those who benefit more from cigarette smoking or nicotine.

Substance P and sensory nerves

Substance P is a major neurotransmitter of sensory nerves. It has long been implicated in the phenomenon of neurogenic inflammation. In this process, sensory nerves are stimulated and release substance P in an antidromic direction at the nerve terminus in the periphery. At this site, substance P exerts its effects on precapillary venules, causing vasodilatation, and initiates the expression of adhesion molecules and the extravasation of neutrophils into the tissue. This has been demonstrated in several tissues including the skin and lung, and more recently in the gut[19–21]. Studies have indicated that this proinflammatory action of substance P is mediated largely via NK1 receptors[20–24]. This mechanism is, however, tightly regulated at several loci, the most important of which are the internalization and recycling of the NK receptors[25] and the degradation of ligand by neutral endopeptidase[26]. Studies have shown that this membrane bound endopeptidase causes down-regulation during intestinal inflammation, thereby substantially increasing the bioavailability of substance P[27].

These studies have prompted consideration of NK1 receptor antagonists as potential therapeutic agents in intestinal inflammation. Unfortunately, results to date have not been encouraging[28].

Substance P is not the only neurotransmitter of sensory nerves. Calcitonin gene-related peptide (CGRP) is an important sensory neurotransmitter and it possesses anti-inflammatory properties; immunoneutralization of CGRP aggravates experimental colitis[29]. Thus, the net impact of sensory neurotransmitters is the algebraic sum of the pro- and anti-inflammatory effects of substance P and CGRP, respectively.

Sensory nerves are a component of local reflexes and such reflexes initiate changes in gut physiology that involve secretory and motor functions. Ablation of primary afferent nerves, and the accompanying disruption of these reflexes, invariably results in worsening of intestinal inflammation[30–32]. Thus, sensory nerves are considered protective against inflammation, most likely by virtue of the local reflex changes in physiology. This seems at odds with the notion that local anaesthetics may be beneficial in conditions such as ulcerative colitis[8]. However, local anaesthetics such as lidocaine have membrane-stabilizing properties and studies in rats have shown that topical administration of lidocaine has a systemic anti-inflammatory effect[33] which may well confer its apparent protective effect.

The role of enteroglia in the neuromodulation of inflammation

Enteroglia are support cells of enteric neurones. These cells possess receptors of neurotransmitters and are able to secrete proinflammatory cytokines. Enteroglia may also express Major Histocompatibility Complex II, as has been shown in Crohn's disease, and may activate lymphocytes via antigen presentation. Thus, enteroglia may serve as a strategic link between the nervous and immune systems in the gut. A recent study showed that enteroglia from rat intestine also possess receptors for interleukin-1β (IL-1β) and interleukin-6 (IL-6). Activation of these receptors modulated the release of IL-6; IL-1 stimulated the synthesis and release of IL-6 which in turn inhibited its own secretion[34]. There is also a preliminary report that the neurotransmitter noradrenaline stimulates the release of IL-6 from enteroglia[35]. In addition to promoting inflammation, IL-6 acts synergistically to suppress the release of acetylcholine from myenteric nerves[36], causing further disruption of enteric physiology during intestinal inflammation[37]. Thus, enteroglia may be an integral part of the inflammatory process, generating cytokines that serve to amplify the inflammatory cascade in the myenteric plexus, and directly affecting the release of neurotransmitters. In addition, enteroglia may serve as an essential link between the nervous and immune systems in the gut, enabling neurotransmitters to modulate inflammation via the release of proinflammatory cytokines.

References

1. Lium R. Etiology of ulcerative colitis. II. Effects of induced muscular spasm on colonic explants in dogs with comment on relation of muscular spasm to ulcerative colitis. Arch Intern Med. 1939;63:210–17.
2. Thorek P. Vagotomy for idiopathic ulcerative colitis and regional enteritis. J Am Med Assoc. 1951;145:140–6.
3. Felten DL, Felten SY, Carlson SL, Olschowka JA, Livnat S. Noradrenergic and peptidergic innervation of lymphoid tissues. J Immunol. 1985;135:755s–65s.
4. Stead RH, Kosecka-Janiszewska U, Oestreicher AB, Dixon MF, Bienenstock J. Remodeling of B-50 (GAP-43)- and NSE-immunoreactive mucosal nerves in the intestines of rats infected with Nippostrongylus brasiliensis. J Neurosci. 1991;11:3809–21.
5. O'Dorisio MS, Hermina NS, O'Dorisio TM, Balcerzak SP. Vasoactive intestinal polypeptide modulation of lymphocyte adenylate cyclase. J Immunol. 1981;127:2551–4.
6. Ottaway CA, Greenberg GR. Interaction of VIP with mouse lymphocytes: Specific binding and the modulation of mitogen responses. J Immunol. 1984;132:417–23.
7. MacQueen G, Marshall J, Perdue M, Siegel G, Bienenstock J. Pavlovian conditioning of rat mucosal mast cells to secrete rat mast cell protease II. Science. 1989;243:83–5.
8. Bjorck S, Dahlstrom A, Johansson L, Ahlman H. Treatment of the mucosa with local anaesthetics in ulcerative colitis. Agents Actions. 1992;10:C61–72.
9. McCafferty DM, Wallace JL, Sharkey KA. Effects of chemical sympathectomy and sensory nerve ablation on experimental colitis in the rat. Am J Physiol. 1997;272(2 Pt 1):G272–80.
10. McCafferty DM, Sharkey KA, Wallace JL. Beneficial effects of local or systemic lidocaine in experimental colitis. Am J Physiol. 1994;266(4 Pt 1):G560–77.
11. Kemler MA, Barendse GA, Van Kleef M. Relapsing ulcerative colitis associated with spinal cord stimulation [In Process Citation]. Gastroenterology. 1999;117(1):215–17.
12. Gue M, Bonbonne C, Fioramonti J *et al.* Stress-induced enhancement of colitis in rats: CRF and arginine vasopressin are not involved. Am J Physiol. 1997;272:G84–91.
13. Million M, Tache Y, Anton P. Susceptibility of Lewis and Fischer rats to stress-induced worsening of TNB-colitis: protective role of brain CRF. Am J Physiol. 1999;276(4 Pt 1):G1027–336.
14. Kiliaan AJ, Saunders PR, Bijlsma PB *et al.* Stress stimulates transepithelial macromolecular uptake in rat jejunum. Am J Physiol. 1998;275(5 Pt 1):G1037–444.
15. Qiu BS, Vallance BA, Blennerhassett PA, Collins SM. The role of CD4+ lymphocytes in the susceptibility of mice to stress-induced reactivation of experimental colitis. Nat Med. 1999;5(10): 1178–822.
16. Galeazzi F, Blennerhassett PA, Qiu B, O'Byrne PM, Collins SM. Cigarette smoke aggravates experimental colitis in rats [see comments]. Gastroenterology. 1999;117(4):877–83.
17. Neurath MF, Fuss I, Kelsall BL, Stuber E, Strober W. Antibodies to interleukin 12 abrogate established experimental colitis in mice. J Exp Med. 1995;182(5):1281–90.
18. Tobin MV, Logan RF, Langman MJS. Cigarette smoking and inflammatory bowel disease. Gastroenterlogy. 1987;93:316–21.
19. Appleyard CB, Wallace JL. Reactivation of hapten-induced colitis and its prevention by anti-inflammatory drugs. Am J Physiol. 1998;269:G119–25.
20. Belvisi MG, Barnes PJ, Rogers DF. Neurogenic inflammation in the airways: characterisation of electrical parameters for vagus nerve stimulation in the guinea pig. J Neurosci Meth. 1990;32:159–67.
21. Figini M, Emanueli C, Grady EF *et al.* Substance P and bradykinin stimulate plasma extravasation in the mouse gastrointestinal tract and pancreas. Am J Physiol. 1998;272:G785–93.
22. Baluk P, Bertrand C, Geppetti P, McDonald DM, Nadel JM. NK-1 receptors mediate leucocyte adhesion in neurogenic inflammation in the rat trachea. Am J Physiol. 1995;268:L263–9.
23. Piedimonte G, Hoffman IE, Husseini WK, Snider RM, Desai MC, Nadel JA. NK-1 receptors mediate neurogenic inflammatory increases in blood flow in rat airways. J Appl Physiol. 1993;74:2462–8.

24. Sternini C, Su D, Gamp PD, Bunnett NW. Cellular sites of expression of the neurokinin-1 receptor in the rat gastrointestinal tract. J Comp Neurol. 1998;358:531–40.
25. Bohm SK, Khitin LM, Grady EF, Aponte G, Payan DG, Bunnett NW. Mechanisms of desensitization and resensitization of proteinase-activated receptor-2. J Biol Chem. 1996;271:22003–16.
26. Sturiale S, Barbara G, Qiu B *et al.* Neutral endopeptidase (EC 3.4.24.11) terminates colitis by degrading substance P. Proc Natl Acad Sci USA. 1999;96(20):11653–8.
27. Hwang L, Leichter R, Okamoto A, Payan D, Collins SM, Bunnett NW. Downregulation of neutral endopeptidase (EC 3.4.24.11) in the inflamed rat intestine. Am J Physiol. 1993;264: G735–43.
28. Wallace JL, McCafferty DM, Sharkey KA. Lack of beneficial effect of a tachykinin receptor antagonist in experimental colitis. Regul Pept. 1998;73(2):95–101.
29. Eysselein VE, Reinshagen M, Patel A, Davis W, Nast C, Sternini C. Calcitonin gene-related peptide in inflammatory bowel disease and experimentally induced colitis. Ann N Y Acad Sci. 1992;657:319–27.
30. Swain MG, Agro A, Blennerhassett P, Stanisz A, Collins SM. Increased levels of substance P in the myenteric plexus of Trichinella-infected rats. Gastroenterology. 1992;102:1913–19.
31. Evangelista S, Meli A. Influence of capsaicin-sensitive fibres on experimentally-induced colitis in rats. J Pharm Pharmacol. 1989;41:574–5.
32. McCafferty DM, Wallace JL, Sharkey KA. Effects of chemical sympathectomy and sensory nerve ablation on experimental colitis in the rat. Am J Physiol. 1997;272:G272–80.
33. McCaffert D-M, Sharkey KA, Wallace JL. Beneficial effects of local or systemic lidocaine in experimental colitis. Am J Physiol. (Gastrointest Liver Physiol). 2001;266:G560–7.
34. Ruhl A, Collins SM, Stremmel W. Interleukin-6 expression and regulation in rat enteric glial cells. Am J Physiol. (Gastrointest Liver Physiol). 2001; 280[6], G1163–71.
35. Ruhl A, Collins SM. Enteroglial cells are an integral part of the neuroimmune axis in the gut. Gastroenterology. 1994;107:1226A.
36. Ruhl A, Hurst S, Collins SM. Synergism between interleukins 1 beta and 6 on noradrenergic nerves in rat myenteric plexus. Gastroenterology. 1994;107(4):993–1001.
37. Collins SM, Blennerhassett PA, Blennerhassett MG, Vermillion DL. Impaired acetylcholine release from the myenteric plexus of Trichinella-infected rats. Am J Physiol. 1989; 257:G898–903.

38
Relationship between stress, neuroimmune function and gut inflammation

A. L. HART and M. A. KAMM

INTRODUCTION

Ulcerative colitis and Crohn's disease appear to be associated with an interaction between genetic susceptibility and immune dysregulation. The immune dysregulation may be triggered by an environmental factor; in particular it appears to be directed towards the gut flora. The role of psychological factors in the initiation and perpetuation of inflammatory bowel disease remains a subject of debate. As knowledge increases in the immunological and microbiological aspects of pathogenesis of inflammatory bowel disease, and as the mechanisms by which psychological factors affect gut physiology become clearer, it is timely to consider how these factors may interact and contribute to the inflammatory process.

THE ROLE OF STRESS IN INFLAMMATORY BOWEL DISEASE

Both doctors[1] and patients[2] have long believed that stress may be involved in the initiation, perpetuation or relapse of inflammatory bowel disease. Ulcerative colitis was initially thought to be a purely psychosomatic disorder[3]. Although this view soon became obsolete, early observations suggested a link between psychological stress and disease exacerbation. The movement of nomadic Bedouin Arabs into government housing was associated with an increased prevalence of ulcerative colitis[4] and this has been attributed to the attendant social stress, although other environmental factors, such as diet or altered gut flora, cannot be excluded. Subsequent studies reported a positive association between inflammatory bowel disease and certain personality traits, such as neuroticism, introversion, obsessive–compulsive behaviours, dependency and perfectionism[5] and positive associations with psychiatric diagnoses have been found[6].

There are many reports in the literature of clinical studies assessing the link between psychological factors and inflammatory bowel disease activity. The retrospective literature is mixed. Some[7], but not all, controlled studies[8] find that ulcerative colitis patients recall increased life stress before an exacerbation. However, recall bias limits the interpretation of these studies.

Seven studies have prospectively assessed the relationship between psychological factors and inflammatory bowel disease. Most have reported a positive relationship between stress and exacerbations of disease[9–12], which includes not only subjective measures, but also objective endoscopic measures[13]. Recently, it has been shown that short-term stress does not appear to trigger exacerbations in ulcerative colitis but that long-term perceived stress increases the risk of exacerbations over a period of months to years[14].

However, not all the prospective studies concur with the association between stressful events and disease relapse[15]. There are methodological difficulties with these studies and their results should be interpreted with caution. Major life events and chronic daily stressors give rise to different responses and, importantly, the individual's perception of stressful events plays a role.

Psychological treatments have been used as a management modality in inflammatory bowel disease and have yielded some[16], but not exclusively[17] positive results. Again, these studies are challenging to perform and interpret.

Further evidence for an association between stress and inflammatory bowel disease comes from animal studies. Animal studies have provided evidence that stress can not only reactivate inflammation in colitis models[18], but also cause primary inflammation in a naïve host[19–21]. It has been shown that inflammation can develop spontaneously in animals subjected to stressful situations. For example, Gibbon monkeys subjected to social upheaval develop a fatal colitis[22]. In addition, it is speculated that the colitis found in cotton-top tamarins (*Saguinus oedipus*), a primate regarded as the animal model most closely resembling idiopathic colitis in humans, may be a reflection of captivity and the associated stress, although other environmental factors may play a role[23]. A direct demonstration of chronic stress inducing primary inflammation in a naïve host has recently been described[19–21]. It has also been demonstrated that longer-term life stresses, at least those that pertain to early maternal deprivation used in animal models, may predispose the mucosal barrier to permeability abnormalities when there is an additional acute stressor[24].

In addition to the development of spontaneous colitis in stressed animals, animal models of colitis display a relapse of their disease at times of stress. For example, in the study by Collins *et al.*[18], acute colitis, induced in rats by intrarectal administration of trinitrobenzene sulphonic acid (TNBS), can reactivate when the animals are subjected to restraint stress[25]. Not only acute stress, but also chronic stress, appears to exacerbate inflammation[26].

THE GUT–BRAIN–IMMUNE AXIS

The association between psychological factors and inflammatory bowel disease has stimulated interest in the mechanism of action of stress on bowel function and particularly on the inflammatory process. The brain clearly influences gut motor, sensory and secretory function via autonomic pathways. In addition, there is compelling evidence for an axis between the brain, the gut and the immune system, which provides the scientific plausibility for an association between stress and inflammatory bowel disease.

There is universal awareness of the impact of emotion on gut function, as highlighted by everyday expressions, such as 'a gut feeling'. In the expanding field of psycho-neuro-immunology, stress has been shown to modulate immune function through changes in immune cells[27], cytokine profiles[28], or susceptibility to infection[29] or vaccination[30]. Caution is needed in interpreting this field. In particular, there does appear to be a difference between the effects of acute and chronic stress on immune function, the latter having a more demonstrable immunosuppressive effect.

Some of the most compelling evidence for a brain–gut–immune link is the marked placebo effect seen in Crohn's disease and ulcerative colitis[31]. The placebo effect in ulcerative colitis is not limited to improvement in patients' symptoms or their perception of their illness, but also includes objective improvement in mucosal inflammation. It is difficult to explain the mechanism of this placebo response without invoking a classic conditioning paradigm. There is anatomical and functional evidence for bidirectional and reciprocal neuroimmune interactions within the intestinal mucosa. The mucosal system is innervated. Regulatory peptides, which include cytokines, growth factors, local hormones and neuropeptides, share functional ligands and receptors[32]. Neuroendocrine contact with cells of the mucosal immune system includes paracrine, neurocrine and endocrine routes.

MECHANISMS OF ACTION OF STRESS ON MUCOSAL BARRIER FUNCTION

The integrity of the intestinal epithelial barrier to antigens comprises mechanical barriers, secreted mucus/fluid barriers, microbiological and immunological barriers. Each of these barriers is a potential target to be modified by acute or chronic stress, resulting in changes in intestinal barrier function, which may subsequently permit the penetration of luminal bacteria into the epithelium and give the potential for an infiltration of inflammatory cells into the lamina propria. The mechanisms by which psychological factors can affect intestinal physiology and mucosal barrier function hold the key to a greater understanding of the effects of stress on mucosal inflammation.

In particular, stress can alter epithelial permeability, ion and water secretion and mucin release. It can also affect immune cells and their cytokine production. Lastly, it can influence the enteric microflora. There appears to be a stress-activated pathway from the central nervous system to mucosal immune cells, in particular mast cells, involving neuroendocrine factors such as corticotrophin releasing factor (CRF), and cholinergic and adrenergic mediators. Resulting changes in intestinal permeability, mucus and ion secretion, enteric microflora, immune cells and their cytokine production may result in invasion of luminal antigens that may initiate or perpetuate inflammation.

An increase in intestinal permeability in response to stress has been shown, in both animals and humans and with acute[33–36] and chronic[20,21,37] stress. The permeability defect influences all parts of the gastrointestinal tract[38], both transcellular and paracellular pathways and both small inert probes and biologically important macromolecules[35]. A change in secretion, a primary defence mechanism of the epithelial barrier, also occurs with acute and chronic stress in animals and humans[33,34,37,39,40]. It has been shown in animals that acute stress causes increased colonic mucin release. In addition, goblet cell depletion occurs[41,42]. Rapid mucin release during acute stress is thought to increase barrier properties and provides a degree of protection for the epithelial barrier. However, goblet cell depletion may be deleterious due to a reduced capacity to respond to ongoing threats.

Microbiological changes occur with stress in animal models. A decrease in *Lactobacillus* species has been shown[43] and an increase in bacterial adherence to the mucosa[44], which may occur secondary to a decrease in mucosal secretory IgA[45]. Bacteria have been shown to adhere to and penetrate the epithelial barrier in rats subjected to chronic stress[20].

MEDIATORS OF STRESS-INDUCED CHANGES

The changes in epithelial barrier function appear to be mediated via factors such as corticotrophin releasing factor (CRF), neurotensin and substance P. For example, the permeability and secretory changes noted when rats are subjected to acute stress are mediated by peripheral CRF[36]. In addition, the sequence of events leading to changes in mucin release is mediated by CRF[41]. Neurotensin, a peptide released from intestinal and non-intestinal sources that stimulates the release of ACTH and corticosterone levels, has also been shown to stimulate mucin secretion[42]. Cholinergic and adrenergic nerves and steroids play a role and there is complex integrative central processing in the brain. For example, cholinergic antagonists inhibit the effects of stress on the increased permeability[33] and Meddings and Swain have shown that the permeability increase disappears after adrenalectomy or pharmacological blockade of glucocorticoid receptors and that dexamethasone treatment of control animals mimics the changes seen with stress[38]. The cell types that appear to be involved include mast cells and CD4+ T cells.

Mast cells play an important role in the regulation of gut epithelial transport function and are activated by stress in humans[40]. They appear to mediate the effects of CRF on intestinal permeability and ion and mucin secretion[36,37,46]. A clear role for CD4+ T cells has been demonstrated in animal models of colitis. The stress-induced reactivation process observed in TNBS-treated rats was immune-dependent in that it was not induced in severe combined immune-deficient (SCID) or athymic mice. Moreover, CD4+ T cells taken from mice with experimental colitis could adoptively transfer the susceptibility to reactivation by stress to SCID mice[25].

SUMMARY

The concept of the gut–brain axis, the immune–brain axis and the extrapolation to the gut–brain–immune axis serves as a logical foundation for a role for psychological factors contributing to the initiation and reactivation of inflammatory bowel disease. The relationship between stress and inflammatory bowel disease comes from observational, clinical and animal studies. Furthermore, an insight has been gained into the mechanism of action of stress on mucosal function. It would seem that the effect of stress is to alter the threshold or balance of the response to neuroendocrine factors (for example CRF or neurotensin) in the gut wall by one of several mechanisms. CRF or other neuroendocrine factors may act directly or indirectly on the epithelium via mast cells or other immune cells. Resulting changes in intestinal permeability, mucin and ion secretion, microbial balance and bacterial adherence may result in invasion of luminal antigens that may perpetuate inflammation. The result of this inflammation may feed back centrally to further aggravate stress and stimulate further CRF-responsive events. Cholinergic and adrenergic nerves appear to play a role in this pathway.

References

1. Mitchell CM, Drossman DA. Survey of the AGA membership relating to patients with functional gastrointestinal disorders. Gastroenterology. 1987;92(5 Pt 1):1282–4.
2. Theis MK, Boyko EJ. Patient perceptions of causes of inflammatory bowel disease [letter]. Am J Gastroenterol. 1994;89(10):1920.
3. Alexander T. An objective study of psychological factors in ulcerative colitis in children. Appl Ther. 1965;7(10):837–9.
4. Salem SN, Shubair KS. Non-specific ulcerative colitis in Bedouin Arabs. Lancet. 1967;1(7488):473–5.
5. Robertson DA, Ray J, Diamond I, Edwards JG. Personality profile and affective state of patients with inflammatory bowel disease. Gut. 1989;30(5):623–6.
6. Helzer JE, Chammas S, Norland CC, Stillings WA, Alpers DH. A study of the association between Crohn's disease and psychiatric illness. Gastroenterology. 1984;86(2):324–30.
7. Hislop IG. Onset setting in inflammatory bowel disease. Med J Aust. 1974;1(25):981–4.
8. Riley SA, Mani V, Goodman MJ, Lucas S. Why do patients with ulcerative colitis relapse? Gut. 1990;31(2):179–83.
9. Duffy LC, Zielezny MA, Marshall JR *et al.* Lag time between stress events and risk of recurrent episodes of inflammatory bowel disease. Epidemiology. 1991;2(2):141–5.
10. Duffy LC, Zielezny MA, Marshall JR *et al.* Relevance of major stress events as an indicator of disease activity prevalence in inflammatory bowel disease. Behav Med. 1991;17(3):101–10.
11. Porcelli P, Zaka S, Centonze S, Sisto G. Psychological distress and levels of disease activity in inflammatory bowel disease. Ital J Gastroenterol. 1994;26(3):111–15.
12. Greene BR, Blanchard EB, Wan CK. Long-term monitoring of psychosocial stress and symptomatology in inflammatory bowel disease. Behav Res Ther. 1994;32(2):217–26.
13. Levenstein S, Prantera C, Varvo V *et al.* Psychological stress and disease activity in ulcerative colitis: a multidimensional cross-sectional study [see comments]. Am J Gastroenterol. 1994;89(8):1219–25.
14. Levenstein S, Prantera C, Varvo V *et al.* Stress and exacerbation in ulcerative colitis: a prospective study of patients enrolled in remission. Am J Gastroenterol. 2000;95(5):1213–20.
15. North CS, Alpers DH, Helzer JE, Spitznagel EL, Clouse RE. Do life events or depression exacerbate inflammatory bowel disease? A prospective study. Ann Intern Med. 1991;114(5):381–6.
16. Milne B, Joachim G, Niedhardt J. A stress management programme for inflammatory bowel disease patients. J Adv Nurs. 1986;11(5):561–7.
17. Schwarz SP, Blanchard EB. Evaluation of a psychological treatment for inflammatory bowel disease. Behav Res Ther. 1991;29(2):167–77.
18. Collins SM, McHugh K, Jacobson K *et al.* Previous inflammation alters the response of the rat colon to stress. Gastroenterology. 1996;111(6):1509–15.
19. Santos J, Antolin M, Malagelada JR. Social stress induces reversible inflammation and persistent barrier dysfunction in the rat intestine. Gastroenterology. 2001;120:A56 (abstr.).
20. Soderholm JD, Yang PC, Vohra A *et al.* Chronic psychological stress induces epithelial barrier disruption, bacterial penetration and mucosal inflammation in ileum and colon of naive rats. Gastroenterology. 2001;120:A70 (abstr.).
21. Soderholm JD, Yang PC, Vohra A, Riddell R, Perdue MH. Chronic psychological stress induces mucosal inflammation in the ileum and colon of naive rats: Role of mast cells. Gastroenterology. 2001;120:A694 (abstr.).

22. Stout C, Snyder RL. Ulcerative colitis-like lesion in Siamang gibbons. Gastroenterology. 1969;57(3):256–61.
23. Wood JD, Peck OC, Tefend KS *et al.* Evidence that colitis is initiated by environmental stress and sustained by fecal factors in the cotton-top tamarin (Saguinus oedipus). Dig Dis Sci. 2000;45(2):385–93.
24. Soderholm JD, Yates D, MacQueen G, Perdue MH. Early maternal deprivation predisposes adult rats to colonic mucosal barrier dysfunction in response to mild stress. Gastroenterology. 2001;120:A23 (abstr.).
25. Qiu BS, Vallance BA, Blennerhassett PA, Collins SM. The role of CD4+ lymphocytes in the susceptibility of mice to stress-induced reactivation of experimental colitis. Nat Med. 1999;5(10):1178–82.
26. Million M, Tache Y, Anton P. Susceptibility of Lewis and Fischer rats to stress-induced worsening of TNB-colitis: protective role of brain CRF. Am J Physiol. 1999;276(4 Pt 1):G1027–36.
27. Kiecolt-Glaser JK, Garner W, Speicher C, Penn GM, Holliday J, Glaser R. Psychosocial modifiers of immunocompetence in medical students. Psychosom Med. 1984;46(1):7–14.
28. Kiecolt-Glaser JK, Marucha PT, Malarkey WB, Mercado AM, Glaser R. Slowing of wound healing by psychological stress [see comments]. Lancet. 1995;346(8984):1194–6.
29. Cohen S, Tyrrell DA, Smith AP. Psychological stress and susceptibility to the common cold [see comments]. N Engl J Med. 1991;325(9):606–12.
30. Glaser R, Kiecolt-Glaser JK, Bonneau RH, Malarkey W, Kennedy S, Hughes J. Stress-induced modulation of the immune response to recombinant hepatitis B vaccine. Psychosom Med. 1992;54(1):22–9.
31. Ilnyckyj A, Shanahan F, Anton PA, Cheang M, Bernstein CN. Quantification of the placebo response in ulcerative colitis. Gastroenterology. 1997;112(6):1854–8.
32. Shanahan F. A gut reaction: lymphoepithelial communication in the intestine. Science. 1997; 275(5308):1897–8.
33. Saunders PR, Kosecka U, McKay DM, Perdue MH. Acute stressors stimulate ion secretion and increase epithelial permeability in rat intestine. Am J Physiol. 1994;267(5 Pt 1):G794–9.
34. Saunders PR, Hanssen NP, Perdue MH. Cholinergic nerves mediate stress-induced intestinal transport abnormalities in Wistar-Kyoto rats. Am J Physiol. 1997;273(2 Pt 1):G486–90.
35. Kiliaan AJ, Saunders PR, Bijlsma PB *et al.* Stress stimulates transepithelial macromolecular uptake in rat jejunum. Am J Physiol. 1998;275(5 Pt 1):G1037–44.
36. Santos J, Saunders PR, Hanssen NP *et al.* Corticotropin-releasing hormone mimics stress-induced colonic epithelial pathophysiology in the rat. Am J Physiol. 1999;277(2 Pt 1):G391–9.
37. Santos J, Benjamin M, Yang PC, Prior T, Perdue MH. Chronic stress impairs rat growth and jejunal epithelial barrier function: role of mast cells. Am J Physiol Gastrointest Liver Physiol. 2000;278(6):G847–54.
38. Meddings JB, Swain MG. Environmental stress-induced gastrointestinal permeability is mediated by endogenous glucocorticoids in the rat. Gastroenterology. 2000;119(4):1019–28.
39. Barclay GR, Turnberg LA. Effect of psychological stress on salt and water transport in the human jejunum. Gastroenterology. 1987;93(1):91–7.
40. Santos J, Saperas E, Nogueiras C *et al.* Release of mast cell mediators into the jejunum by cold pain stress in humans. Gastroenterology. 1998;114(4):640–8.
41. Castagliuolo I, LaMont JT, Qiu B *et al.* Acute stress causes mucin release from rat colon: role of corticotropin releasing factor and mast cells. Am J Physiol. 1996;271(5 Pt 1):G884–92.
42. Castagliuolo I, Leeman SE, Bartolak-Suki E *et al.* A neurotensin antagonist, SR 48692, inhibits colonic responses to immobilization stress in rats. Proc Natl Acad Sci USA. 1996;93(22): 12611–15.
43. Bailey MT, Coe CL. Maternal separation disrupts the integrity of the intestinal microflora in infant rhesus monkeys. Dev Psychobiol. 1999;35(2):146–55.
44. Spitz J, Hecht G, Taveras M, Aoys E, Alverdy J. The effect of dexamethasone administration on rat intestinal permeability: the role of bacterial adherence. Gastroenterology. 1994;106(1):35–41.
45. Wira CR, Sandoe CP, Steele MG. Glucocorticoid regulation of the humoral immune system. I. In vivo effects of dexamethasone on IgA and IgG in serum and at mucosal surfaces. J Immunol. 1990;144(1):142–6.
46. Castagliuolo I, Wershil BK, Karalis K, Pasha A, Nikulasson ST, Pothoulakis C. Colonic mucin release in response to immobilization stress is mast cell dependent. Am J Physiol. 1998;274 (6 Pt 1):G1094–100.

39
Medical therapy of ulcerative colitis

S. B. HANAUER

Medical therapy for ulcerative colitis continues to evolve, awaiting a better understanding of the aetiopathogenesis of the underlying disease process. To date, therapy has been applied to patients according to the paradigm of a therapeutic pyramid (Figure 1) based upon the extent and severity of disease. Nevertheless, despite a series of controlled clinical trials to justify therapeutic algorithms, there remain substantial gaps in our evidence base pertaining to both short- (induction of remission) and long-term management of individual disease scenarios.

Aminosalicylates remain the foundation of treatment for mild–moderate ulcerative colitis[1,2]. Sulphasalazine is the prototype agent and, to date, no other aminosalicylate has been proven more efficacious when administered in doses providing equal amounts of mesalazine[3]. There is a dose-response for both sulphasalazine and the various mesalazine formulations which, in the case of sulphasalazine, is compromised by dose-related intolerance[3]. In contrast, the dose-response for mesalazine formulations is disassociated from significant toxicity at least up to 4.8 g/day (equivalent to 12 g of sulphasalazine)[2].

In the setting of left-sided or distal colitis, there were no differences in response to oral aminosalicylates compared with treatment of extensive colitis; however, topical (rectal) mesalazine is superior to oral formulations at equal doses[2]. There does not appear to be a dose-response above 1 g for topically administered mesalazine to patients with active distal UC[4].

Aminosalicylates also form the foundation for maintenance therapy to prevent relapse of UC[5]. In this setting the dose-response has been less well defined. Traditionally, the maintenance dose for sulphasalazine has been reduced from the induction dose (primarily related to tolerance rather than efficacy)[1,2]. However, in the absence of dose-related adverse events with mesalazine and sufficiently powered dose-ranging maintenance trials[3], it is most rational to continue the same dose required to induce remissions to maintain remissions. In addition, controversy continues regarding the optimal means of maintaining remissions for patients with distal UC who have required rectal mesalazine to induce remission. Again, clinical trials suggest that rectal formulations of

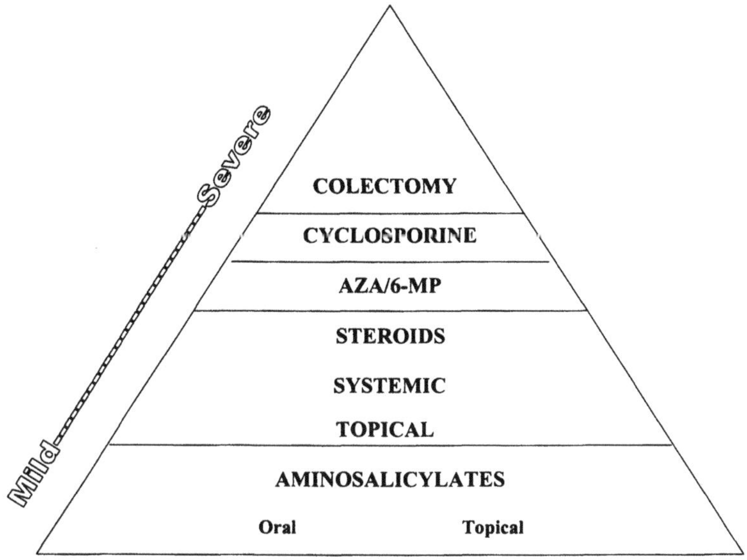

Figure 1 Therapeutic pyramid for ulcerative colitis

mesalazine are more effective than equal (weekly) doses of oral agents[2]. With regard to comparability amongst the oral aminosalicylates for treatment of distal UC, there are limited data that the conjugated formulations (sulphasalazine, olsalazine, balsalazide) may be more effective than the pH-release formulations of mesalazine[5,6].

One area where the utility of aminosalicylates as maintenance agents needs to be reassessed is their effectiveness after steroids have been required to induce remission. In a recent trial comparing mesalazine (1.2 g/day) with a probiotic (*E. coli* Nissle strain) after steroid-induced remission, both agents were associated with relapse rates between 65% and 75%[7]. Many from North America argue that the dose of mesalazine was too small, despite the aforementioned debate regarding maintenance dosing with mesalazine for UC. Nevertheless, it may be necessary to re-examine the efficacy of aminosalicylates as concomitant therapy with, or compared to, purine antimetabolites for prevention of relapse after steroid-induced remission.

Moving up the therapeutic pyramid, corticosteroids have been the primary therapy for moderate–severe acute ulcerative colitis but remain ineffective as maintenance agents[4]. Topical corticosteroids are efficacious for treating distally active UC[8] although these have not been as effective as topical mesalazine, nor has a dose-response been adequately assessed for individual corticosteroid formulations. Corticosteroid enemas are also considered a component of the intensive therapy for patients with severe colitis in combination with parenteral steroids[9].

Systemically active steroids have been used for nearly 40 years to quell acute attacks of UC. Still, dose-ranging data are quite limited for oral prednisone[10] for out-patient therapy of moderate–severe disease as well as for parenteral glucocorticoids in severe attacks[11]. There is no advantage of doses up to 1 g/day of methylprednisolone compared with conventional dosing of up to 60 mg/day[4,12], yet better dosing studies and comparisons of delivery systems (bolus infusions, intermittent infusions or continuous infusions) would be helpful in clinical practice. In addition, attempts to develop an oral delivery system for rapidly metabolized ('less-systemic') steroids, such as budesonide, have not been successful to date. It remains to be determined whether variability in colonic transit times, pH and metabolism by microflora will preclude clinically effective oral formulations for pan-colonic or left-sided UC.

Despite 'acceptance' of the clinical utility of the purine antimetabolites for refractory or steroid-dependent UC[1], the evidence base is extremely thin. A few older trials demonstrated steroid-sparing benefits, but the majority of the 'data' derive from the Mt. Sinai and Lennox Hill experience in New York published as case series rather than controlled trials[13,14]. A single controlled trial has been published that supports a role for azathioprine as a maintenance agent to prevent relapse in patients who required the immunomodulators to achieve remission[15] and we, as well as others, have found that azathioprine or mercaptopurine is useful to maintain remissions for patients who have required cyclosporine to treat acute severe UC[16–18]. With recognition of the genetic polymorphism in the thiopurine methyltransferase enzyme and potential for therapeutic drug monitoring of 6-thioguanine metabolite levels, prospective trials that examine dosing, utility of therapeutic drug monitoring and value of leukopenia are warranted to clarify the ultimate utility of these agents in UC.

In recent years, the utility of cyclosporine has been verified in controlled trials for severe UC[19] as well as in subsequent clinical experience[16,20]. In most series, cyclosporine has been administered in conjunction with corticosteroids; however, in a recent trial from the Leuven group, cyclosporine alone was as efficacious as intravenous corticosteroids[21]. Future trials may attempt to clarify optimal dosing and therapeutic drug monitoring of levels[22]. Likewise, trials of similar immunosuppressants with improved oral absorption, such as microemulsion cyclosporine or tacrolimus, may improve the ability to treat moderate–severe patients without hospitalization for intravenous cyclosporine[23–25]. In addition, it would be of benefit to define the optimal duration of treatment of cyclosporine before transitioning to the purine antimetabolites and whether there is any benefit for co-administration of immunomodulators with aminosalicylates.

A number of novel developments have been described for the treatment of UC that are generating enthusiasm and the need for additional clinical trials. A potential role for heparin was first described in a series of cases from Ireland[26] but remains to be confirmed in clinical trials. Similarly, the Japanese have advocated leukocyte apheresis to treat UC[27] but additional controlled trials comparing more conventional Western approaches, and determination of the specific cell types for removal, are needed to assess the short- and long-term value of this expensive and time-consuming technique. One could also envision the evolution of a series of novel anti-inflammatory compounds and additional immunomodulators to treat UC as well as targeted therapy for virtually all the known cascades of pro-inflammatory cytokines and chemokines now recognized to participate in the inflammatory cascades of active UC. These would also include inhibition of the adhesion molecules on inflammatory cell and endothelial cell surfaces.

Finally, recent studies on the impact of probiotic therapy have been most promising in UC. Evidence in favour of the Nissle 1917 strain of *E. coli* as a maintenance agent for UC has been reported[7,28], as have trials of combination probiotics to prevent the development of pouchitis after ileoanal anastomoses[29]. It remains to be determined whether pharmaceutical development will proceed along the lines of conventional dose-ranging, safety and efficacy studies or whether probiotics will be introduced to the general public as 'nutriceuticals' without the formal clinical scientific rigour of additional controlled clinical trials. Hopefully, clinicians (and patients) will have the opportunity to evaluate controlled trials that are required to identify the ultimate positioning of probiotics within our therapeutic armamentarium.

In the meantime, medical therapy for ulcerative colitis remains sequential, aimed at inducing, then maintaining, remissions. The current therapeutic algorithm begins with aminosalicylates for mild–moderate disease and continues these for patients who respond to this first-line therapy. Moderate–severely ill patients, or those not responding to aminosalicylates, require a course of steroids to induce remission. While aminosalicylates have been the standard approach to maintenance after corticosteroid induction of remission, there remains some doubt as to their ultimate efficacy in this setting, and whether the immunomodulators (or probiotics) offer a more-effective long-term approach and whether adherence to these more simplified dosing schedules will improve long-term outcomes. It does seem that the purine antimetabolites are required, at least as an adjunct to aminosalicylates, after cyclosporine inductive therapy. In this setting, the requirement for aminosalicylates has not been evaluated. Ultimately, we might consider 'reversing' the therapeutic pyramid for (at least severe) ulcerative colitis. The evidence for efficacy of cyclosporine without steroids calls into question whether we will ever need corticosteroids to treat ulcerative colitis, thereby offering the potential to avoid the considerable toxicity associated with these agents. In the meantime, numerous segments of our evidence base remain insufficiently answered by controlled trials, offering both the need and opportunity to continue clinical research to optimize treatment of this medically controllable but incurable disease.

References

1. Kornbluth A, Sachar DB. American College of Gastroenterology, Practice Parameters Committee. Ulcerative colitis practice guidelines in adults. Am J Gastroenterol. 1997;92(2): 204–11.
2. Hanauer SB. Aminosalicylate therapy for ulcerative colitis. In: Bayless TM, Hanauer SB, editors, Advanced Therapy of Inflammatory Bowel Disease. Hamilton, Ontario, Canada: B.C. Decker Inc, 2001:123–6.
3. Sutherland L, Roth D, Beck P, May G, Makiyama K. Oral 5-aminosalicylic acid for inducing remission in ulcerative colitis. Cochrane Database Syst Rev. 2000. 2.
4. Hanauer S. Medical therapy for ulcerative colitis. In: Kirsner J, editor, Inflammatory Bowel Disease. Philadelphia, PA: WB Saunders, 2000:529–77.
5. Courtney MG, Nunes DP, Bergin CF *et al.* Randomised comparison of olsalazine and mesalazine in prevention of relapses in ulcerative colitis [see comments]. Lancet. 1992; 339(8804):1279–81.
6. Green JR, Gibson JA, Kerr GD *et al.* Maintenance of remission of ulcerative colitis: a comparison between balsalazide 3 g daily and mesalazine 1.2 g daily over 12 months. ABACUS Investigator group [In Process Citation]. Aliment Pharmacol Ther. 1998;12(12):1207–16.

7. Rembacken BJ, Snelling AM, Hawkey PM, Chalmers DM, Axon AT. Non-pathogenic *Escherichia coli* versus mesalazine for the treatment of ulcerative colitis: a randomised trial [see comments]. Lancet. 1999;354(9179):635–9.
8. Marshall JK, Irvine EJ. Rectal corticosteroids versus alternative treatments in ulcerative colitis: a meta-analysis. Gut. 1997;40(6):775–81.
9. Blomberg B, Jarnerot G. Clinical evaluation and management of acute severe colitis. Inflamm Bowel Dis. 2000;6(3):214–27.
10. Baron JH. Outpatient treatment of ulcerative colitis. Br Med J. 1962;2:441–4.
11. Lennard-Jones JE. Toward optimal use of corticosteroids in ulcerative colitis and Crohn's disease. Gut. 1983;24(3):177–81.
12. Hodgson H. Systemic corticosteroids in inflammatory bowel disease. In: Bayless T, Hanauer S, editors, Advanced Therapy of Inflammatory Bowel Disease. Hamilton, Ontario, Canada: BC Decker Inc, 2001:127–31.
13. Adler DJ, Korelitz BI. The therapeutic efficacy of 6-mercaptopurine in refractory ulcerative colitis. Am J Gastroenterol. 1990;85(6):717–22.
14. George J, Present DH, Pou R, Bodian C, Rubin PH. The long-term outcome of ulcerative colitis treated with 6-mercaptopurine. Am J Gastroenterol. 1996;91:1711–14.
15. Hawthorne AB, Logan RF, Hawkey CJ *et al.* Randomised controlled trial of azathioprine withdrawal in ulcerative colitis. Br Med J. 1992;305(6844):20–2.
16. Cohen RD, Stein R, Hanauer SB. Intravenous cyclosporin in ulcerative colitis: a five-year experience. Am J Gastroenterol. 1999;94(6):1587–92.
17. Fernandez-Banares F, Bertran X, Esteve-Comas M *et al.* Azathioprine is useful in maintaining long-term remission induced by intravenous cyclosporine in steroid-refractory severe ulcerative colitis. Am J Gastroenterol. 1996;91(12):2498–9.
18. Ramakrishna J, Langhans N, Calenda K, Grand RJ, Verhave M. Combined use of cyclosporine and azathioprine or 6-mercaptopurine in pediatric inflammatory bowel disease. J Pediatr Gastroenterol Nutr. 1996;22(3):296–302.
19. Lichtiger S, Present DH, Kornbluth A *et al.* Cyclosporine in severe ulcerative colitis refractory to steroid therapy [see comments]. N Engl J Med. 1994;330(26):1841–5.
20. Van Gossum A, Schmit A, Adler M *et al.* (Belgian IBD Group). Short- and long-term efficacy of cyclosporin administration in patients with acute severe ulcerative colitis. Acta Gastroenterol Belg. 1997;60(3):197–200.
21. D'Haens G, Lemmens L, Geboes K *et al.* Intravenous cyclosporine versus intravenous corticosteroids as single therapy for severe attacks of ulcerative colitis. Gastroenterology. 2001;120(6):1323–9.
22. Cohen RD. Intravenous cyclosporine in severe ulcerative colitis: ready to stand alone? Gastroenterology. 2001;120(6):1541–3.
23. Actis GC, Aimo G, Priolo G, Moscato D, Rizzetto M, Pagni R. Efficacy and efficiency of oral microemulsion cyclosporin versus intravenous and soft gelatin capsule cyclosporin in the treatment of severe steroid-refractory ulcerative colitis: an open-label retrospective trial. Inflamm Bowel Dis. 1998;4(4):276–9.
24. Oppong K, Record CO. Neoral may be as effective as intravenous cyclosporine in the treatment of steroid-resistant ulcerative colitis [letter]. Am J Gastroenterol. 1998;93(7):1188–9.
25. Matsuhashi N, Nakajima A, Watanabe K *et al.* Tacrolimus in corticosteroid-resistant ulcerative colitis. J Gastroenterol. 2000;35(8):635–40.
26. Gaffney PR, Doyle CT, Gaffney A, Hogan J, Hayes DP, Annis P. Paradoxical response to heparin in 10 patients with ulcerative colitis. Am J Gastroenterol. 1995;90(2):220–3.
27. Ayabe T, Ashida T, Kohgo Y. Centrifugal leukocyte apheresis for ulcerative colitis. Ther Apher. 1998;2(2):125–8.
28. Kruis W, Schutz E, Fric P, Fixa B, Judmaier G, Stolte M. Double-blind comparison of an oral *Escherichia coli* preparation and mesalazine in maintaining remission of ulcerative colitis. Aliment Pharmacol Ther. 1997;11(5):853–8.
29. Shanahan F. Inflammatory bowel disease: immunodiagnostics, immunotherapeutics, and ecotherapeutics. Gastroenterology. 2001;120(3):622–35.

Section VIII
Complications of ileal-pouch anastomosis

40 Postoperative complications after ileal pouch–anal anastomosis

G. POGGIOLI, S. LAURETI, F. PIERANGELI, M. RAVAIOLI, F. UGOLINI, P. GIONCHETTI and M. CAMPIERI

INTRODUCTION

Restorative proctocolectomy with ileal pouch–anal anastomosis (IPAA) has been progressively accepted as the first choice procedure for the treatment of ulcerative colitis (UC) refractory to medical therapy and familial adenomatous polyposis (FAP). Since its introduction, the original technique has been progressively modified, mostly by the use of the stapled technique, which has shortened the duration of the procedure and reduced the complication rates. Indeed, currently, many major centres report good outcomes for the vast majority of the patients. In addition, pouch excision or permanent rediversion rates are low, ranging between 3.5% and 10%[1–3]. However, while this retrospective review of the results confirms the safeness of the procedure, long-term results remain variable in the series published. In particular, the long-term complication rate is controversial and the treatment is under discussion.

MATERIALS AND METHODS

From 1 November 1984 to 1 June 2001, 391 patients underwent restorative proctocolectomy with IPAA.

Almost all the operations were carried out by one of the investigators (G.P.) and the late G. Gozzetti*. Among the 391 patients, 347 were affected by idiopathic colitis, 43 by FAP and one by multiple synchronous large bowel cancer involving the rectum (MSLBC). Two hundred and thirty (58.8%) were male and 161 (41.2%) female; the mean age was 35 years.

All the patients subjected to IPAA for idiopathic colitis had been diagnosed preoperatively as UC. Among the 347 patients with idiopathic colitis, 321 were finally found to be affected by UC and 26 (7.5%) by indeterminate colitis (IC). Of

*Former Chief of the Department from 1981 to 1995.

the patients who underwent an ileal pouch procedure for UC, 266 (76.6%) had the ileoanal anastomosis stapled (St) and 81 handsewn (Hs), while 40 out of 43 of those operated on for FAP had an Hs anastomosis. In 3 patients with FAP a stapled anastomosis without loop ileostomy was carried out: all these patients presented with multiple advanced colorectal cancer and needed early adjuvant therapy.

All the patients were followed for a mean period of 7.2 years (range 0.1–17 years). Data collected prospectively in an IPAA computerized database included: preoperative data, surgical technique, early (within 30 days of surgery; divided into general, abdominal, pelvic and ileostomy closure-related) and late complications with their treatment: perianal fistulas (pouch–anal and pouch–vaginal), intestinal obstruction and anastomotic stricture occurring later than 30 days p.o. were considered as late complications.

The follow-up consisted of clinical examination and interview gathered by the investigators at 1, 3, 6 and 12 months postoperatively and yearly thereafter.

Pouch failure was defined as removal of the reservoir, whether converted to a permanent stoma or not, or removal of a failed reservoir with a loop ileostomy functioning as terminal. To investigate the risk factors for surgical complications, patients were divided into different groups, according to:

(1) Sequence of construction,
(2) Fashioning or not of protective ileostomy during IPAA procedure,
(3) Type of ileoanal anastomosis,
(4) Period of construction,
(5) Perioperative blood transfusions.

Functional results

Analysis of the influence of complications on functional outcome was then performed, comparing results at 1, 3 and 5 or more years (mean follow-up 6.1 years). Factors included in the analysis were: mean number of bowel movements during 24 h, mean number of nocturnal bowel movements, pad usage, presence of any grade of leakage and modifications of sexual activity.

Late complications

The number and type of late complications did not allow any statistical analysis of the risk factors.

We divided late complications into two groups:

(1) Procedure-related, more serious, represented by pouch–anal and pouch–vaginal fistulas;
(2) Others, not procedure-related, which are a consequence of any major abdominal operations (e.g. intestinal obstruction).

Statistical analysis

Results are expressed as mean ($\pm$ standard deviation): proportions of events were compared by means of the χ^2 test and a value of $p < 0.05$ was considered as statistically significant. Ordinal variables were compared in two groups using the Wilcoxon rank sum test.

RESULTS

Data on patient distribution and technical characteristics of procedures are shown in Table 1.

Among the 391 patients submitted to IPAA, 370 (94.6%) are now functioning. There was no perioperative mortality. Five patients died (1.3%) subsequently; all of them had a coexisting colorectal neoplasm at the time of surgery. Four are now waiting for the closure of the diverting ileostomy. Twelve patients (3.1%)

Table 1 Patient distribution and technical characteristics of procedures

Characteristic	*Number*	*Percentage*
Gender		
Male	230	58.8
Female	161	41.2
Period of construction		
1984–1990	104	26.6
1991–1995	142	36.3
1996–2001	145	37.1
Preoperative diagnosis		
UC	347	88.7
FAP	43	11
MSLBC	1	0.3
Sequence of construction		
IRA	25	6.4
Completion proctectomy with stoma	116	29.7
Completion proctectomy no stoma	98	25.1
Single stage with stoma	125	32
Single stage no stoma	27	6.9
Ileostomy		
Yes	259	66.2
No	132	33.8
Anastomosic fashion		
Handsewn	119	30.4
Stapled	272	69.6
Shape of pouch		
J	383	98
S	4	1
W	2	0.5
H	2	0.5
Blood transfusions		
No transfusion	209	54.7
1–2 U	103	27
3–5 U	55	14.4
>5 U	15	3.9
Final diagnosis		
UC	321	82.1
FAP	43	11
MSLBC	1	0.3
Indeterminate colitis	19	4.8
Crohn's disease	7	1.8

were converted to permanent ileostomy. Respectively, eight patients presented with chronic post-surgical sepsis and had the reservoir excised with conversion to permanent ileostomy; in two of them, final diagnosis of the disease is still uncertain. Two patients refused excision of the reservoir but their loop ileostomy must be considered as definitive. One patient was converted to permanent ileostomy two years after IPAA at another centre for intra-abdominal desmoid tumour. One patient had his pouch excised recently for cancer which developed in the anal transitional zone below the HS ileoanal anastomosis. Finally, two patients had their pouch removed for multiple fistulization due to Crohn's disease (CD) misdiagnosed at the time of surgery. In conclusion, 10 patients (2.5%) have a non-functioning pouch due to post-surgical complications.

Early complications

General complications

General complications occurred in 18 patients (4.6%; Table 2). The incidence of general complications was significantly higher in patients submitted to the single-stage procedure with ileostomy compared with the others (Table 3).

Abdominal complications

Abdominal abscesses occurred in 12 patients (3.1%). In five (1.3%), the abscess was related to a proximal pouch fistula and was treated surgically. In the remaining seven patients (1.8%), it was not related to a proximal pouch fistula and was treated

Table 2 Incidence and type of general complications

Complication	*Number*	*Percentage*
Dehydration	6	1.5
Lung infection	2	0.5
Cardiac failure	1	0.3
Renal failure	4	1.0
Deep venous thrombosis	5	1.3
Total	18	4.6

Table 3 General complications and sequence of construction

Sequence of construction	*General complications*	*No general complications*
Previous IRA	1 (4.0)	24 (96.0)
CP + stoma	2 (1.7)	114 (98.3)
CP no stoma	2 (2.0)	96 (98.0)*
Single-stage + stoma	13 (10.4)	112 (89.6)
Single-stage, no stoma	0 (0)	27 (100)
Total	18 (4.6)	373 (95.4)

*$p < 0.05$; figures in parentheses are percentages.

Table 4 Types of abdominal complications

Abdominal complication	*Number*	*Percentage*
Minor		
Wound infection	43	11.0
Major		
Abscess	12	3.1
Proximal fistula	5	1.3
Obstruction	19	4.9
Bleeding	8	2.0

Table 5 Risk factors for abdominal abscess

	Abdominal abscess	*No abdominal abscess*	*p-value*
Period of construction			
1984–1990	10 (9.6)	94 (90.4)	
1991–1995	1 (0.7)	141 (99.3)	< 0.05
1996–2001	1 (0.7)	144 (99.3)	
Sequence of construction			
Previous IRA	1 (4.0)	24 (96)	
CP + stoma	4 (3.4)	112 (96.6)	
CP, no stoma	1 (4.0)	97 (99)	NS
Single-stage + stoma	6 (4.8)	119 (95.2)	
Single-stage, no stoma	0	27 (100)	
Blood transfusions			
No transfusion	1 (0.5)	208 (99.5)	
1–2 U	6 (5.8)	97 (94.2)	0.004
3–5 U	3 (5.5)	43 (94.5)	
>5 U	2 (13.3)	11 (86.7)	
Anastomotic fashion			
Handsewn	9 (7.6)	110 (92.4)	0.001
Stapled	3 (1.1)	269 (98.9)	
Gender			
Male	6 (2.6)	224 (97.4)	
Female	6 (3.7)	155 (96.3)	NS
Ileostomy			
Yes	11 (4.2)	248 (95.8)	
No	1 (0.8)	131 (99.2)	< 0.05
Final diagnosis			
UC	9 (2.8)	313 (97.8)	
FAP	1 (2.3)	42 (97.7)	NS
IC	2 (10.5)	17 (89.5)	
CD	0	7 (100)	
Total	12 (3.1)	379 (96.9)	

Figures in parentheses are percentages.

conservatively with i.v. antibiotics or locally through drainage (Table 4). The incidences of abdominal abscess and proximal pouch fistula were significantly higher in patients submitted to blood transfusions, in those with handsewn anastomosis and in those operated early in the surgical experience (Table 5).

Table 6 Incidence and type of pelvic complications

Complication	*Number*	*Percentage*
Disruption	4	1.0
Pelvic abscess	1	0.3
Dehiscence	5	1.3
Ischaemia	1	0.3
Anastomotic fistula	13	3.3
Pouch–vaginal fistula	4	1.0
Pouch–urethral fistula	1	0.3
Torsion	2	0.5
Stenosis	4	1.0
Bleeding	3	0.8
Total	38*	9.6

*More than one complication in some patients.

Pelvic complications

Early pelvic complications occurred in 36 patients (9.2%), the vast majority being of septic type (Table 6).

Specifically, septic complication with anastomotic involvement occurred in 22 patients (5.6%). Patients with anastomotic dehiscence were all treated surgically, while, among those with anastomotic fistula, protective ileostomy was constructed if not done at the time of IPAA; the remaining patients were treated conservatively. Finally, minor anastomotic disruption (1%) in handsewn anastomoses was treated with transanal resuture. All of them had complete *restitutio ad integrum*.

Pelvic complications were not significantly related to the anastomotic fashion; on the other hand, they were significantly more frequent in patients operated early in the surgical experience and in those submitted to a single-stage procedure, without protective ileostomy and in patients submitted to blood or plasma transfusion (Table 7).

Loop ileostomy closure-related

Ileostomy closure-related complications occurred in 19 patients (4.9%); treatment of these patients is shown in Figure 1.

Pouch failure

A significantly higher incidence of failure was found in patients previously submitted to IRA, in those submitted to one or more units of RBC in the perioperative period and in those with pelvic complications (Table 8).

Re-do pouch

The re-do pouch procedure was carried out in 13 patients. Six of them had been submitted to IPPA in other centres. Indications for this treatment are shown in Table 9. The rate of salvage was 84.6%.

Table 7 Risk factors for pelvic complications

	Pelvic complications	*No pelvic complications*	*p-value*
Period of construction			
1984–1990	15 (14.4)	89 (85.6)	
1991–1995	9 (6.3)	133 (93.7)	0.03
1996–2001	12 (8.3)	133 (91.7)	
Sequence of construction			
Previous IRA	6 (24.0)	19 (76.0)	
CP + stoma	10 (8.6)	106 (91.4)	
CP no stoma	8 (8.2)	90 (91.8)	0.05
Single-stage + stoma	6 (4.8)	119 (95.2)	
Single-stage, no stoma	6 (22.8)	21 (77.8)	
Blood transfusions			
No transfusions	13 (6.2)	196 (93.8)	
1–2 U	6 (5.8)	97 (94.2)	< 0.05
3–5 U	12 (21.8)	43 (78.2)	
>5 U	5 (27)	11 (73)	
Anastomotic fashion			
Handsewn	15 (12.6)	104 (87.4)	NS
Stapled	21 (7.7)	251 (92.3)	
Gender			
Male	21 (9.1)	209 (90.9)	
Female	15 (9.3)	146 (90.7)	NS
Ileostomy			
Yes	22 (8.5)	237 (91.5)	
No	14 (10.6)	118 (89.4)	NS
Final diagnosis			
UC	34 (10.4)	288 (89.6)	
FAP	2 (4.7)	41 (95.3)	NS
IC	0	19 (100)	
CD	0	7 (100)	
Total	36 (9.2)	355 (90.8)	

Figures in parentheses are percentages.

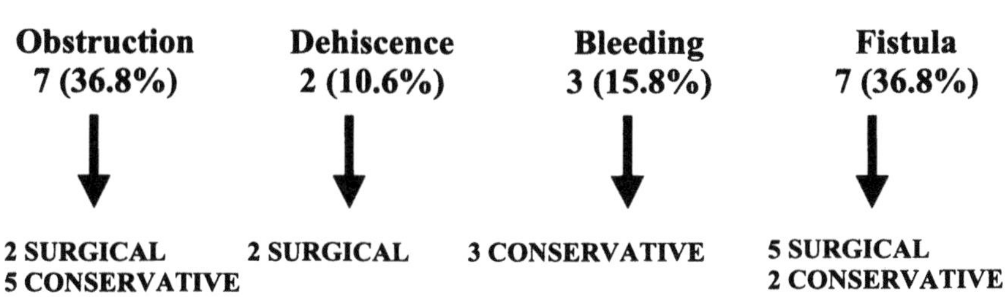

Figure 1 Incidence and treatment of ileostomy closure-related complications

Table 8 Risk factors for pouch failure

	Pouch failure	*No failure*	*p-value*
Period of construction			
1984–1990	6 (5.8)	98 (94.2)	
1991–1995	5 (3.5)	137 (96.5)	0.06
1996–2001	1 (0.7)	144 (99.3)	
Sequence of construction			
Previous IRA	2 (8.0)	23 (92.0)	
CP + stoma	7 (6.0)	109 (94.0)	
CP, no stoma	0	98 (100)	0.04
Single-stage + stoma	3 (2.4)	122 (97.6)	
Single-stage, no stoma	0	27 (100)	
Blood transfusions			
No transfusions	3 (1.4)	206 (98.6)	
1–2 U	2 (2.0)	101 (98.0)	<0.05
3–5 U	4 (7.3)	51 (92.7)	
>5 U	3 (20.0)	12 (80.0)	
Anastomotic fashion			
Handsewn	9 (7.6)	110 (92.4)	0.001
Stapled	3 (1.1)	269 (98.9)	
Gender			
Male	7 (3.0)	223 (97.0)	
Female	5 (3.1)	156 (96.9)	NS
Ileostomy			
Yes	12 (4.6)	247 (95.4)	
No	0	132 (100)	<0.05
Pelvic sepsis			
Yes	6 (21.4)	22 (78.6)	
No	6 (1.7)	357 (98.3)	NS
Final diagnosis			
UC	8 (2.4)	314 (97.6)	
FAP	2 (4.7)	41 (95.3)	<0.05
IC	0	19 (100)	
CD	2 (28.5)	5 (71.5)	
Total	12 (3.1)	379 (96.9)	

Figures in parentheses are percentages.

Table 9 Indications for re-do pouch

Indication	*Number*	*Percentage*
Pelvic fibrosis	1	7.7
Pouch fistula	8	61.5
Pouch–urethral fistula	1	7.7
Rotation	1	7.7
Mega-pouch	1	7.7
Ischaemia	1	7.7

Late complications

Intestinal obstruction

Eleven patients experienced intestinal obstruction (2.8%).

Other abdominal complications

One patient presented with a late proximal J-pouch fistula, and was treated conservatively with antibiotics. It developed between the apex of the pouch and the perineum in the presacral space behind the reservoir. This was probably due to a granuloma in the blind loop of the J pouch without relevant abscess demonstrated at CT scan.

Strictures of the pouch–anal anastomosis

Patients with minor anastomotic strictures, easily treated with outpatient digital dilatation, have not been included in this series. They are frequent in all series, mainly in handsewn anastomoses, but they do not present a serious medical problem.

The incidence of late stenosis was not significantly higher in patients with handsewn anastomosis.

All these patients have been treated conservatively by means of dilatation with anal dilators: none of them needed revisional surgery.

Pouch–anal and pouch–vaginal fistulas

This complication occurred in 17 cases (4.3%). Twelve patients presented with pouch–anal fistula, either *in ano* (90.9%) or anastomotic (9.1%). In 5, a pouch–vaginal fistula occurred.

The treatment for pouch–anal fistulas was conservative in all cases, through placement of drainage with a Prolene seton; in 1 of these patients, however, additionally to the placement of seton, a diverting stoma was constructed. Two of the 5 cases of pouch–vaginal fistula were treated conservatively (seton). In these patients the conservative treatment did not lead to a real *restitutio ad integrum* but was effective for the control of the sepsis, providing the patients with an acceptable quality of life. One patient was successfully treated with surgical aggressive therapy, by means of a gracile-muscle flap interposition and loop ileostomy, successively closed.

A fourth patient was firstly submitted, without success, to a perineal re-do anastomosis (neo-ileoanal anastomosis) as suggested by Fazio *et al.*[4], and subsequently to a successful muscular flap interposition.

In a fifth patient, who presented with a wide pouch–vaginal fistula, a diverting stoma has been constructed; this has to be considered as permanent since the patient refused surgical treatment with muscular flap interposition.

Indeterminate colitis and late complications

The role of diagnosis in late complications such as fistulas is crucial. We have classified the idiopathic colitis submitted to IPAA as UC, Crohn's colitis and IC.

Among this last group, we have classified three different subgroups, according to Wells *et al.*[5]. The first group includes all the cases in which the diagnosis was impossible: IC *tout court*. The second group includes colitis not clearly definable as UC but more easily assimilable to them: IC probable UC. The last group is represented by indeterminate probable Crohn's colitis, including those colitises not clearly identifiable as CD but presenting features that resemble it.

Among the 26 patients originally diagnosed as having IC, 12 had indeterminate colitits not subsequently specifed, which we called 'true IC'. Four cases were called 'IC probable UC' and 3 cases 'IC probable CD'.

In our experience, the clinical outcome of patients with IC varies. Patients with IC and the indeterminate forms 'probable UC' and 'probable CD' have an absolutely similar outcome to those with UC.

Out of the 7 patients with definite Crohn's colitis, 2 were submitted to removal of the reservoir for recurrence of the disease in our centre. The other 5 patients are in good health although 1 of them has reported recurrent episodes of pouchitis and another has a jejuno–ileal fistula ('by-pass fistula').

In our experience, IC does not lead to an increased risk of late perianal fistula. Indeed, among the 17 patients who presented with this complication, only 2 had IC (1 of these was subsequently diagnosed as having CD). In these 2 cases, however, the removal of the pouch with permanent ileostomy was necessary for intractable perianal disease.

Effect of postoperative complications on functional results

Functional results in all patients are shown in Table 10.

Table 10 Functional results

	1 year	*2–3 years*	*≥5 years*
Use of pads			
Yes	43 (14)	26 (11.5)	22 (13.8)
No	264 (86)	200 (88.5)	138 (86.3)
Leakage			
Yes	161 (52.4)	107 (47.3)	68 (42.5)
No	146 (47.6)	119 (52.7)	92 (57.5)
Return to work			
Yes	260 (84.7)	196 (87.1)	138 (86.3)
No	47 (15.3)	29 (12.9)	22 (13.8)
Sexual activity			
Improved	24 (7.8)	21 (9.3)	17 (10.6)
Worsened	17 (5.5)	13 (5.7)	10 (6.3)
Unchanged	266 (86.7)	192 (85.0)	133 (83.1)
Bowel movements (mean)			
Minimal	4.5	4.4	4.3
Maximal	7.5	7.7	7.2
Nocturnal	0.9	0.8	0.7

Figures in parentheses are percentages.

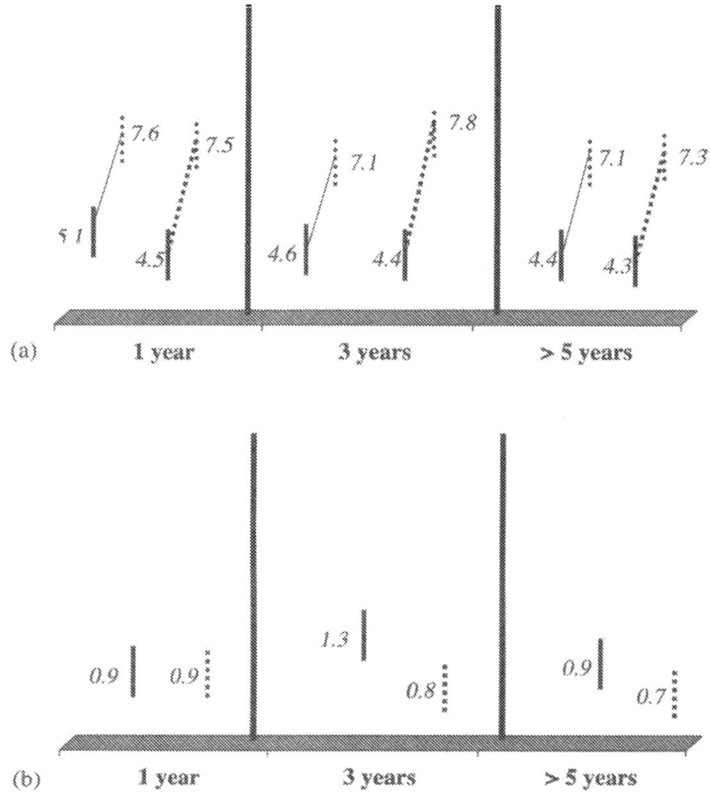

Figure 2 Effect of pelvic sepsis on bowel movements. (**a**) Number of bowel movements/24 h in patients with (...) or without (——) pelvic sepsis (p = NS). (**b**) Number of bowel movements during the night in patients with (...) or without (——) pelvic sepsis (p = NS)

The occurrence of postoperative pelvic complications did not significantly influence the functional outcome of patients. Specifically, the mean number of bowel movements/24 h and number of nocturnal bowel movements was similar in the two groups (Figure 2a, 2b).

Similarly, no differences were found in incidence of seepage, soiling, modifications of sexual activity or pad usage between the two groups (Table 11).

DISCUSSION

IPAA has reached 'legal age' by now: indeed, it is more than 20 years ago that Sir Alan Parks[6] first described this operation. Both the short- and the long-term outcomes, as well as a consistent reduction in complication rates, make this procedure the 'gold standard' in surgical treatment of UC and FAP.

Table 11 Functional results and pelvic sepsis

	Pelvic complications	*No pelvic complications*	*p-value*
Pad usage			
1 year	5 (20.8)	38 (13.4)	
3 years	3 (13.6)	23 (11.3)	NS
>5 years	1 (5.6)	21 (14.8)	
Leakage			
1 year	12 (50)	147 (51.9)	
3 years	13 (59.1)	94 (46.1)	NS
>5 years	9 (50)	58 (40.8)	
Sexual activity			
1 year			
Not modified	20 (83.3)	246 (86.9)	
Worsened	2 (8.3)	15 (5.3)	NS
Improved	2 (8.3)	22 (7.8)	
3 years			
Not modified	20 (90.9)	172 (84.3)	
Worsened	1 (4.5)	12 (5.9)	NS
Improved	1 (4.5)	20 (9.8)	
>5 years			
Not modified	17 (94.4)	116 (81.7)	
Worsened	0	10 (6.3)	NS
Improved	1 (5.6)	16 (10.6)	

Figures in parentheses are percentages.

The incidence of these complications is acceptable and most of them can be successfully managed, often with local therapy[7,8]. In addition, as shown in other major reports[1,9] and in our series, experience has reduced the incidence of pelvic sepsis, which represents the most devastating complication, since it can lead to pelvic fibrosis, ultimate failure of the operation and pouch excision.

Pelvic sepsis represents the most dangerous complication, since, overall, it is the most common cause of pouch failure. Recent series have shown sepsis rates to be between 5% and 14% after IPAA[2–3,10]. In a recent report from the Mayo Clinic[11], it represented the main reason for pouch removal, bearing in mind that 63% of patients with this complication required a permanent stoma. In our experience, pelvic sepsis occurred in 7.7% of patients. Treatment was never surgical if anastomosis was not involved; on the other hand, all the patients with dehiscence were treated surgically. The treatment is described above. However, we would like to stress here the possibility of treating even major complications with a re-do pouch.

Looking at the risk factors, in addition to amount of experience, we found an important risk factor was the sequence of construction. In fact, previous IRA and single-stage procedure without ileostomy represent a high-risk procedure. Similar results were found by Williamson *et al.*[12] who described a higher incidence of septic complications in patients with single-stage procedure without ileostomy (22% vs. 14%). Better nutritional status and less need for steroids or immunosuppressive therapy in patients previously submitted to subtotal colectomy may account for the lower risk of pelvic complications in those patients. Finally, our experience shows that postoperative complications do not affect functional results or quality of life.

The Lahey Clinic Group[13] found a significant difference in number of bowel movements, leakage and pad usage between patients with and without pelvic sepsis, with a mean follow-up of 56 months, the major deterioration in function occurring after treatment for multiple perineal complications. However, in the case of successful treatment of complications, functional outcome was equivalent to that in patients with no perineal complications.

Similarly, the Mayo Clinic Group[14] described higher rates of incontinence, protective pad usage and requirement for constipating or bulking medications in patients with pelvic abscess formation.

Moreover, the Heidelberg Group[15] not only described a worse outcome in patients with pelvic complications, but also found in these patients a significantly higher incidence of 'secondary pouchitis' compared with other patients, requiring surgical treatment in nearly all cases.

The reason for the differences in functional outcome between our and other experiences can be found in our aggressive approach to surgical complications. In fact, even though some authors consider sepsis a contraindication to radical pouch revision[16,17], in our experience, the presence of complicating pelvic sepsis does not mandate the removal of the reservoir and the construction of a permanent ileostomy, provided that re-do pouch procedures are attempted prior to the establishment of pelvic fibrosis[18–20].

Pouch failure rates range in the literature from 3.5% to 10%; poor functional results, pelvic sepsis and unsuspected CD represent the major causes of pouch failure[1,2].

The overall incidence of pouch failure in this series was 3.1%; the incidence has decreased in the last 5 years to 0.7% from the initial 5.8%. Similar data have been found by the Toronto Group[9], who excluded from the analysis the first 200 pouches performed, in order to minimize the effects of the learning curve.

More controversial is the treatment of late complications. In fact their appearance is not only a treatment problem but also introduces the issue of evolutionary change of diagnosis from ulcerative colitis to indeterminate colitis or even Crohn's disease. Often, the development of late perianal fistulas is not a septic phenomenon, so we must consider such a complication as the deepening of an ulcer. Indeed, the internal orifice of the fistula is usually placed below the anastomosis[21]. Our approach in the presence of late perianal fistula is conservative, since the goal, in these cases, is exclusively the control of the sepsis.

Indeed, the discovery of a pouch–anal or pouch–vaginal fistula could be a sign of misdiagnosed colitis other than the ulcerative one. Fazio *et al.*[22] reported that more than 50% of patients with late perianal fistulas after IPAA suffer from CD. In our opinion, this assumption is not always true. There is no doubt, however, that the issue of indeterminate colitis has grown increasingly important in the 'pouch era'. Indeed, this particular condition has become important since Crohn's disease has been widely considered a contraindication to the fashioning of an ileoanal pouch, even though Panis described a failure rate of 10% in patients with colorectal CD submitted to IPAA[23].

The problem of the differential diagnosis of the colitis has led to some considerations:

(1) Some authors[24–26] report significantly higher complication rates for IC compared with UC. Indeed, this risk is reported as ranging from 30% to 50% vs. 3–20%, respectively. However, our experience did not confirm this finding. Indeed, in our series, pelvic sepsis rates were 3.8% in the IC group vs. 8.7% in the UC group. In addition, only one proximal pouch fistula developed in the IC group (3.8%), compared with four (1.3%) in patients with UC.
(2) Similarly, as highlighted above, our series does not show an increased risk for late complication rates in IC compared with UC. Indeed, among the 17 patients with late pouch–anal or pouch–vaginal fistulas, only one had IC and another was ultimately diagnosed as having CD.
(3) Finally, the risk for pouch removal ranges from 0.4% to 8% for UC compared to 20–28% in the IC group[25–28].

This increased risk, however, seems to be attributable to the occurrence of early or late complications in patients who were ultimately diagnosed as having a misdiagnosed CD.

The conclusion that we draw from our experience is that patients with either 'true IC' or 'probable UC' should be treated in the same way as those with definite UC. Crohn's colitis, when the diagnosis is preoperatively certain, represents a contraindication to the execution of an IPAA. In the case of 'IC probable CD', if the diagnosis is made preoperatively, a subtotal colectomy should be done and, if the diagnosis is confirmed after histological examination of the specimen, it is worth waiting for about two years before proceeding, when necessary, to IPAA and then only if, during this period, no signs of recurrence have occurred in the ileum.

Going back to the other surgical-related late complications, intestinal obstruction is the most important. There are not many thing to discuss regarding this issue. It is interesting to note that, while intestinal obstruction early after surgery is rarely the result of a mechanical obstruction and usually has a functional origin, mostly due to postoperative dehydration, late intestinal obstruction, which in our series occurred in 2.5%, usually requires reoperation because of the presence of postoperative adhesions. This is similar to all other major abdominal procedures.

CONCLUSIONS

In conclusion, the evolution of the techniques and technologies has given IPAA a wide popularity and the procedure is now performed successfully in an increasing number of centres. However, even though increased experience has led to simplification of the procedure, it is still a technically demanding operation that should be performed only in referral centres.

Our results confirm that complication rates have decreased to the same rates as those of other major abdominal procedures, but those involving the J-pouch are an unavoidable part of this sphincter-saving technique. Pelvic sepsis remains the most frequent and dangerous complication but, if reservoir-salvaging surgery is timely and appropriate, pouch failure rates are acceptable.

In addition, long-term complication rates and their treatment are still controversial especially concerning the major late complications represented by pouch–anal and pouch–vaginal fistulas. Correct preoperative diagnosis of inflammatory colitis is important. It is not clear whether the incidence of long-term complications increases with time, whether they are due to retained rectal mucosa or whether they are dependent on the type of anastomosis.

Repeated studies with longer follow-up are thus necessary.

References

1. Gemlo BT, Wong DW, Rothemberger DA *et al.* Ileal pouch–anal anastomosis: patterns of failure. Arch Surg. 1992;127:784–7.
2. Marcello PW, Roberts PL, Schoetz DJ Jr *et al.* Long term results of the ileoanal pouch procedure. Arch Surg. 1993;128:500–4.
3. Fazio VW, Ziv Y, Church JM *et al.* Ileal pouch–anal anastomoses complications and function in 1005 patients. Ann Surg. 1995;222:120–7.
4. Fazio VW, Wu SJ, Lavery IC. Repeat ileal pouch–anal anastomosis to salvage septic complications of pelvic pouches. Clinical outcome and quality of life assessment. Ann Surg. 1998;228;4:588–97.
5. Wells AD, McMillan I, Price AB *et al.* Natural history of indeterminate colitis. Br J Surg. 1991;78:179–81.
6. Parks AG, Nicholls RJ. Proctocolectomy without ileostomy for UC. Br Med J. 1978;2:85–8.
7. Cohen Z, McLeod RS, Stern HE *et al.* The pelvic pouch and ileoanal anastomosis procedure: surgical technique and initial results. Am J Surg. 1985;160:601–7.
8. Zmora O, Efron JE, Nogueras JJ *et al.* Reoperative abdominal and perineal surgery in ileoanal pouch patients. Dis Colon Rectum. 2001;1310–14.
9. MacRae HM, McLeod RS, Cohen Z *et al.* Risk factors for pelvic pouch failure. Dis Col Rectum. 1997;40n3:257–62.
10. Johnson E, Carlsen E, Nazir M, Nygard K. Morbidity and functional outcome after restorative proctocolectomy for ulcerative colitis. Eur J Surg. 2001;167:40–5.
11. Meagher AP, Farouk R, Dozois RR *et al.* J ileal pouch anal anastomosis for chronic ulcerative colitis: complications and long-term outcome in 1310 patients. Br J Surg. 1998;85:800–3.
12. Williamson ME, Lewis WG, Sagar PM *et al.* One-stage restorative proctocolectomy without temporary ileostomy for ulcerative colitis: a note of caution. Dis Colon Rectum. 1997;40: 1019–22.
13. Breen E, Schoetz DJ, Marcello PW *et al.* Functional results after perineal complications of ileal pouch–anal anastomosis. Dis Colon Rectum. 1998;41:691–5.
14. Farouk R, Dozois RR, Pemberton JH. Incidence and subsequent impact of pelvic abscess after ileal pouch–anal anastomosis for chronic ulcerative colitis. Dis Colon Rectum. 1997; 41:1239–43.
15. Heuschen UA, Autschbach F, Allemeyer EH *et al.* Long-term follow-up after ileoanal pouch procedure. Dis Colon Rectum. 2001;44(4):487–99.
16. Sagar PM, Dozois RR, Wolff BG *et al.* Disconnection, pouch revision and reconnection of the ileal pouch–anal anastomosis. Br J Surg. 1996;83:1041–5.
17. Ogunbiya OA, Korsgen S, Keighley MRB. Pouch salvage. Long term outcome. Dis Colon Rectum. 1997;40:548–52.
18. Poggioli G, Marchetti F, Selleri S *et al.* Redo pouches: salvaging of failed ileal pouch–anal anastomoses. Dis Rectum. 1993;36:492–6.
19. Korsgen S, Nikiteas N, Ogunbiya OA *et al.* Results from pouch salvage. Br J Surg. 1996;83:372–4.
20. Lindquist K, Nilsell K, Liljeqvist L. Cuff abscess and ileoanal anastomotic separations in pelvic pouch surgery. Dis Colon Rectum. 1987;30:355–9.
21. Groom JS, Nicholls RJ, Hawley PR *et al.* Pouch–vaginal fistula. Br J Surg. 1993;80:936–40.
22. Lee P, Fazio VW, Church JM *et al.* Vaginal fistula following restorative proctocolectomy. Dis Colon Rectum. 1997;40(7):752–9.
23. Regimbeau JM, Panis Y, Pocard M *et al.* Long-term results of ileal pouch–anal anastomosis for colorectal Crohn's disease. Dis Colon Rectum. 2001;44:769–78.

24. Atkinson KG, Owen DA, Wankling G. Restorative proctocolectomy and indeterminate colitis. Am J Surg. 1994;167:516–18.
25. Marcello PW, Schoetz DJ, Roberts PL *et al.* Evolutionary changes in the pathologic diagnosis after the ileoanal pouch procedure. Dis Colon Rectum. 1997;40:263–9.
26. Koltun WA, Schoetz DJ, Roberts PL *et al.* Indeterminate colitis predisposes to perineal complications after ileal pouch–anal anastomosis. Dis Colon Rectum. 1991;34(10):857–60.
27. McIntyre PB, Pemberton JH, Wolff BG *et al.* Indeterminate colitis. Dis Colon Rectum. 1995;38(1):51–4.
28. Sagar PM, Dozois RR, Wolff BG. Long term results of ileal pouch–anal anastomosis in patients with Crohn's disease. Dis Colon Rectum. 1996;39(8):893–8.

41
Complications of the ileoanal pouch: medical complications

W. J. SANDBORN

INTRODUCTION

The causes of pouch dysfunction following abdominal colectomy with ileal pouch–anal anastomosis include anastomotic stricture, pouchitis, cuffitis, and Crohn's disease of the ileoanal pouch[1]. This chapter reviews the diagnostic approach to ileoanal pouch dysfunction, and the medical therapy of ileoanal pouch disorders in patients with a history of ulcerative colitis who have undergone colectomy with ileoanal pouch.

DIAGNOSTIC APPROACH TO POUCH DYSFUNCTION

Patients with ileoanal pouch dysfunction can be broadly categorized by their presenting complaints into: patients with difficulty evacuating, patients with excess stool frequency, and patients experiencing symptoms of bloating and colic[1]. Patients with difficulty evacuating must be evaluated for anastomotic stricture. When an anastomotic stricture is identified, these patients should undergo dilation of the anastomosis under anaesthesia by a colorectal surgeon. Patients with symptoms of difficult evacuation in whom an anastomotic stricture is not identified by digital examination should undergo a pouchogram X-ray. This study may identify patients with a significant pouch septum (which can be divided with a GIA stapler), or a long efferent limb (this is particularly common in S pouches and lateral pouches) that can be surgically revised by shortening the 'spout' of the pouch.

Patients who present with complaints of excess stool frequency should undergo a stool culture to exclude parasites and bacterial pathogens. Pouchoscopy is indicated to evaluate for evidence of cuffitis, pouchitis or Crohn's disease. The endoscope must be advanced through the pouch and into the prepouch ileum. The finding of prepouch ileitis is highly suggestive of Crohn's disease. Findings of patchy ulceration or friability within the pouch would suggest pouchitis. This endoscopic diagnosis should be confirmed by biopsy that demonstrates villous atrophy, chronic inflammatory cell (lymphocyte) infiltration, and acute inflammation (neutrophil infiltration)[2]. For patients with a stapled anastomosis, the residual 1–2 cm rectal cuff distal to the anastomosis must be examined for evidence of inflammation in the residual rectum which is termed 'cuffitis' or 'strip pouchitis'. Patients with excess stool frequency who have a normal endoscopy should be evaluated for compliance and capacity of the pouch with pouchogram X-ray, nuclear scintigraphic emptying study, and examination under anaesthesia by a colorectal surgeon. Patients with normal pouch compliance and capacity may be treated symptomatically with antidiarrhoeal medication and dietary advice. Patients with evidence of low pouch capacity should be carefully assessed with pelvic CT/MRI or ultrasound to evaluate for a peripouch abscess, which may require treatment with antibiotics, radiologic drainage, and sometimes defunctionalization of the pouch.

Patients who have presenting symptoms of bloating and colic should undergo small bowel follow-through X-ray to exclude partial small bowel obstruction caused by Crohn's disease or adhesions. Patients with a normal small bowel X-ray should be treated for irritable bowel syndrome.

POUCHITIS

Treatments which are reported to possibly be effective for pouchitis include antibiotics, probiotic bacteria, oral or rectal mesalamine, oral or rectal corticosteroids, immune modifier drugs such as azathioprine or 6-mercaptopurine, short chain fatty acids enemas, glutamine suppositories, and bismuth carbomer enemas[3]. These therapies will be discussed further below.

Madden and colleagues performed a randomized double-blind placebo-controlled trial of metronidazole for chronic pouchitis[4]. Thirteen patients with an ileoanal pouch and chronic pouchitis in the setting of a history of ulcerative colitis were enrolled in a crossover trial. Patients were treated with oral metronidazole 400 mg three times daily or placebo for 14 days. They underwent a 7-day washout prior to crossover from the first to the second therapy. Eleven of thirteen patients completed the crossover trial. The mean stool frequency in patients treated with metronidazole decreased from 10 to 9. Conversely, the mean stool frequency for patients treated with placebo increased from 8.9 up to 10.7. This difference was statistically significant. Side effects occurred in 55% of metronidazole-treated patients, including nausea, vomiting, abdominal discomfort, headache, and skin rash. Hurst and colleagues reported a case series of antibiotic treatment of pouchitis in 104 consecutive patients with ileoanal pouch for ulcerative colitis[5]. Fifty-two patients (50%) had at least one episode of pouchitis. Metronidazole was reported to be effective in 41 of those 52 patients (79%). Metronidazole was not tolerated in 5/52 (10%), and was not effective in 6/52 (12%). Ciprofloxacin, which was used for metronidazole-intolerant or -refractory patients, was effective in 8/11 (73%). Pouch excision with ileostomy was ultimately required in 2 of 3 patients who were refractory to both metronidazole and ciprofloxacin. The overall response rate to antibiotic therapy was 96%.

Gionchetti and colleagues reported on the use of probiotic bacteria for maintenance therapy in patients with chronic pouchitis[6]. Forty patients with a history of chronic pouchitis in remission after induction therapy with antibiotics were enrolled in a randomized double-blind placebo-controlled study. Patients were randomized to oral VSL#3 which consists of a probiotic bacterial cocktail containing four strains of lactobacilli, three strains of bifidobacteria, and one strain of strep-salivarius subspecies Thermophillus or placebo for 9 months. At the end of 9 months, relapse had occurred in 3 of 20 patients (15%) in the VSL#3 group as compared to 20 of 20 (100%) in the placebo group. This difference was statistically significant. This same group also utilized probiotic bacteria as prophylaxis against the onset of pouchitis in patients undergoing ileoanal pouch surgery for ulcerative colitis[7]. Forty consecutive patients who underwent colectomy with ileoanal pouch for ulcerative colitis were randomized to oral VSL#3 or placebo for 12 months. Over the 12 months, acute pouchitis occurred in 2 of 20 (10%) patients in the VSL#3 compared with 8 of 20 (40%) patients in the placebo group; $p < 0.01$.

The efficacy of drugs that are commonly used to treat ulcerative colitis (mesalamine, corticosteroids, immunosuppressives) for pouchitis is unclear[3]. Patients who fail with antibiotic therapy are frequently treated with mesalamine suppositories or enemas, and, in some cases, with oral mesalamine or sulphasalazine. Anecdotal experience suggests that these therapies are not very beneficial in antibiotic-refractory patients. Similarly, corticosteroid enemas are commonly used in patients with refractory pouchitis, again with anecdotal experience suggesting little benefit. Oral corticosteroids are typically reserved for patients who are more seriously ill, and for patients for whom the underlying diagnosis is changed from pouchitis to Crohn's disease. There is very little published information about the role of azathioprine or 6-mercaptopurine for refractory chronic pouchitis but anecdotal experience suggests that these therapies may not be beneficial.

There is very little data available regarding the efficacy of short chain fatty acid enemas for pouchitis. One case report suggested that 2 of 2 patients improved with enemas containing sodium acetate, sodium propionate, and sodium butyrate[8]. In contrast, a subsequent report from Tremaine and colleagues suggested that only 3 of 8 patients improved using short chain fatty acid enemas of exactly the same composition[9]. In patients with distal ulcerative colitis, short chain fatty acid enemas were ultimately proven to be ineffective in placebo-controlled trials.

There was a small study from the Mayo Clinic by Wischmeyer and colleagues in which 19 patients with chronic pouchitis were randomized to sodium butyrate suppositories or glutamine suppositories[10]. Three of nine patients (33%) treated with sodium butyrate suppositories improved compared with 6 of 10 patients (60%) treated with glutamine suppositories. It is unclear whether these therapies are equally effective, or equally ineffective.

Bismuth has both antimicrobial and antidiarrhoeal properties. Tremaine *et al.* conducted a randomized, double-blind, placebo-controlled trial of bismuth carbomer (an acrylic acid polymer) foam enemas in 40 patients with active chronic pouchitis refractory to standard therapy[11]. After 3 weeks, 9 of 20 patients (45%) treated with bismuth improved compared with 9 of 20 patients (45%) treated with placebo. The placebo was xanthem gum, and subsequent studies have suggested that xanthem gum and other gums or resins may be therapeutic for distal ulcerative colitis. Thus, the possibility exists that this study had a therapeutic placebo control. A subsequent open-label study from the same authors suggested that bismuth subsalicylate may be beneficial for patients with chronic pouchitis[12].

The overall treatment algorithm for patients with symptoms of pouchitis begins with endoscopy and biopsy as discussed above[2]. For patients with endoscopic evidence of pouchitis, the initial treatment should be metronidazole. Most patients will respond to 1–2 weeks of metronidazole, without relapse when therapy is discontinued. For patients who relapse, repeat treatment with metronidazole is recommended, and some patients may require maintenance therapy with metronidazole at the lowest effective dose. Patients who do not respond to metronidazole or who are intolerant of metronidazole should be treated with ciprofloxacin. In patients who fail to respond to both metronidazole and ciprofloxacin, other therapy such as oral or rectal mesalamine, or rectal corticosteroids can be attempted, but there is little evidence that these medications are of clinical benefit in this setting. Likewise, there is little evidence that nutritional therapy such as short chain fatty acid enemas or glutamine suppositories is effective. In countries where VSL#3 is available, this therapy can be recommended for maintenance of remission in patients with chronic pouchitis. There is not yet sufficient data to recommend that all patients undergoing ileoanal pouch surgery receive empiric prophylactic therapy with VSL#3. For patients with chronic pouchitis who cannot be managed with medical therapy, surgical consultation to consider pouch excision or diversion with loop ileostomy is recommended.

CUFFITIS

Patients who undergo abdominal colectomy with a stapled ileoanal pouch will have 1–2 cm of residual rectal mucosa distal to the anastomosis. These patients are at risk for ongoing inflammation of the remaining rectum which is a form of proctitis commonly termed ‘cuffitis’ or ‘strip pouchitis’[13]. Open-label clinical experience has suggested that mesalamine or corticosteroid suppositories are an effective therapy for this condition in most situations[14]. About half of patients with active inflammation of the residual rectal cuff will also have evidence of active pouchitis, and will require simultaneous therapy with antibiotics[14]. In patients with refractory cuffitis, a transanal mucosectomy of the remaining rectal mucosa can be undertaken by an experienced colorectal surgeon.

CROHN'S DISEASE OF THE ILEOANAL POUCH

About 5% of patients who undergo colectomy with ileoanal pouch for ulcerative colitis will later have their diagnosis changed to Crohn's disease. Findings that can lead to a change in diagnosis include inflammation of the prepouch ileum or more proximal gastrointestinal tract, complex perianal fistulizing disease, and rereview of the original colectomy specimen by an experienced pathologist with a change in pathological diagnosis to Crohn's disease. Anecdotally, these patients with Crohn's disease of the ileoanal pouch appear to gain clinical benefit from antibiotic therapy. In addition, these patients often require medical therapy for moderate to severe Crohn's disease including oral or intravenous corticosteroids, azathioprine or 6-mercaptopurine, methotrexate, and in some cases infliximab, cyclosporine, or tacrolimus[3]. A typical approach would be to treat patients with a combination of antibiotics, a tapering course of oral cortico-steroids, and azathioprine or 6-mercaptopurine (reserving methotrexate for azathioprine/ 6-mercaptopurine-intolerant patients). Patients who fail to respond to this combination therapy may benefit from infliximab[15]. In rare cases, calcineurin inhibitor therapy with cyclosporine or tacrolimus may be beneficial in patients with complex perianal fistulas in the setting of Crohn's disease of the ileoanal pouch[16].

CONCLUSIONS

One placebo-controlled trial suggested efficacy of metronidazole for chronic pouchitis. Up to 96% of patients will respond to treatment with either metronidazole or ciprofloxacin. Two placebo-controlled trials have demonstrated efficacy of probiotic bacteria to prevent pouchitis and maintain remission. Uncontrolled trials have suggested possible benefit for mesalamine, corticosteroids, azathioprine, or 6-mercaptopurine. Short chain fatty acid enemas and butyrate or glutamine suppositories appear to be of little value. Bismuth carbomer enemas are not effective for pouchitis. Most patients will respond to antibiotics, some require suppressive therapy, and a minority require pouch excision or exclusion with ileostomy.

References

1. Sagar PM, Pemberton JH. Ileo-anal pouch function and dysfunction. Dig Dis. 1997;15:172–88.
2. Sandborn WJ, Tremaine WJ, Batts KP, Pemberton JH, Phillips SF. Pouchitis after ileal pouch–anal anastomosis: a Pouchitis Disease Activity Index. Mayo Clin Proc. 1994;69:409–15.
3. Sandborn WJ. Pouchitis following ileal pouch–anal anastomosis: definition, pathogenesis, and treatment. Gastroenterology. 1994;107:1856–60.
4. Madden MV, McIntyre AS, Nicholls RJ. Double-blind crossover trial of metronidazole versus placebo in chronic unremitting pouchitis. Dig Dis Sci. 1994;39:1193–6.
5. Hurst RD, Molinari M, Chung TP, Rubin M, Michelassi F. Prospective study of the incidence, timing and treatment of pouchitis in 104 consecutive patients after restorative proctocolectomy. Arch Surg. 1996;131:497–500.
6. Gionchetti P, Rizzello F, Venturi A *et al.* Oral bacteriotherapy as maintenance treatment in patients with chronic pouchitis: a double-blind, placebo-controlled trial. Gastroenterology. 2000;119:305–9.
7. Gionchetti P, Rizzello F, Venturi A *et al.* Prophylaxis of pouchitis onset with probiotic therapy: a double-blind, placebo controlled trial. Gastroenterology. 2000;118:A190.
8. de Silva HJ, Ireland A, Kettlewell M, Mortensen N, Jewell DP. Short-chain fatty acid irrigation in severe pouchitis. N Engl J Med. 1989;321:1416–17.
9. Tremaine WJ, Sandborn WJ, Phillips SF, Pemberton JH, Carpenter HA. Short chain fatty acid (SCFA) enema therapy for treatment-resistant pouchitis following ileal pouch–anal anastomosis (IPAA) for ulcerative colitis (UC). Gastroenterology. 1994;106:A784.
10. Wischmeyer P, Pemberton JH, Phillips SF. Chronic pouchitis after ileal pouch–anal anastomosis: responses to butyrate and glutamine suppositories in a pilot study. Mayo Clin Proc. 1993;68:978–81.
11. Tremaine WJ, Sandborn WJ, Wolff BG, Carpenter HA, Zinsmeister AR, Metzger PP. Bismuth carbomer foam enemas for active chronic pouchitis: a randomized, double-blind, placebo-controlled trial. Aliment Pharmacol Ther. 1997;11:1041–6.
12. Tremaine WJ, Sandborn WJ, Kenan ML. Bismuth subsalicylate tablets for chronic antibiotic-resistant pouchitis. Gastroenterology. 1998;114:A1101.
13. Rauh SM, Schoetz DJ Jr, Roberts PL, Murray JJ, Coller JA, Veidenheimer MC. Pouchitis – is it a wastebasket diagnosis? Dis Colon Rectum. 1991;34:685–9.

14. Lavery IC, Sirimarco MT, Ziv Y, Fazio VW. Anal canal inflammation after ileal pouch–anal anastomosis. The need for treatment. Dis Colon Rectum. 1995;38:803–6.
15. Ricart E, Panaccione R, Loftus EV, Tremaine WJ, Sandborn WJ. Successful management of Crohn's disease of the ileoanal pouch with infliximab. Gastroenterology. 1999;117:429–32.
16. Sandborn WJ. Preliminary report on the use of oral tacrolimus (FK506) in the treatment of complicated proximal small bowel and fistulizing Crohn's disease. Am J Gastroenterol. 1997;92:876–9.

42
Inflammatory bowel disease: how does basic science help clinical management?

D. K. PODOLSKY

It is axiomatic that basic science will only achieve its full potential for improving clinical care with the complete identification of the cause(s) and the pathogenesis of inflammatory bowel diseases. However, it is already clear that interval progress can still result in significant advances in clinical management. These benefits are both direct and indirect.

Progress in efforts to identify the genetic basis of inflammatory bowel disease should soon enable more precise and direct approaches to diagnosis, stratification and prognostication. Much of this promise remains to be fulfilled with identification of the specific genes responsible for the linkages established by initial genomic screening efforts. More importantly basic science is already resulting in new and more effective therapeutics for patient management. The available and evolving cytokine and anticytokine therapies provide demonstration of the benefit of progress in the knowledge of the actions of the pro- and anti-inflammatory cytokines. Other examples that only hint at the overall long-term potential opportunities include definition of the role of luminal bacteria in driving inflammatory responses.

Recent progress has given us a glimpse of the power of basic science to transform the clinical management of patients with inflammatory bowel disease. The future will hopefully enable the realization of that potential.

The past several years have seen an accelerating expansion in the scope of basic research efforts focused on definition of the causes and mechanisms underlying inflammatory bowel disease. With this investment of time, effort and research funding, one may plausibly ask: what impact have the results of research had on the care of patients with major forms of inflammatory bowel disease?

Defined narrowly, the direct impact of basic research on patient care has so far been relatively modest. Nevertheless, there are some advances in clinical diagnosis and management which clearly have been the outgrowth of basic laboratory investigation. First among these is the characterization of the mechanisms of actions and toxicity of commonly used therapeutic agents. Definition of the pharmacology and metabolism of the active moiety within sulphasalazine, 5-ASA, has served as the foundation for the development of alternative forms of 5-ASA which have significantly expanded its clinical utility. Availability of formulations which benefit patients with small bowel disease and variations which are tolerated by the minority of patients who are vulnerable to hypersensitivity reactions to the prototypic sulphasalazine have clearly enabled improved care for many patients with both ulcerative colitis and Crohn's disease. Definition of the variations among patients in metabolism of 6-mercaptopurine due to genotype TPMT enables better prediction of toxicity to this important agent and may enhance its utility in overall care of patients with chronic inflammatory bowel disease. Similarly, basic pharmacological characterization of the variant corticosteroid budesonide, and most particularly its highly efficient first-pass clearance, offer an increased therapeutic index for those patients requiring corticosteroids. Still another advance which can clearly be seen as an outgrowth of basic laboratory studies is promised refined diagnostic accuracy. Thus, demonstration of the relatively specific association of the presence of pANCA and ASCA with ulcerative colitis and Crohn's disease is facilitating more accurate diagnosis, at least among a small subset of patients in whom diagnosis may not be clear on the basis of the traditional clinical and physical laboratory findings. In summary, a number of discrete improvements in the diagnosis and care of patients with Crohn's disease can be reasonably well attributed to findings that originated through basic laboratory research.

While sceptics might view these advances as modest in proportion to the effort, it is important to recognize that many of the most profound advances in the basic investigation of IBD have only been relatively recently achieved. As a result of the inevitable need for further work before basic discovery may be translated into clinical practice, the more proper question to pose at this time is: how will basic laboratory advances alter clinical practice? Considerably more optimism can be offered in response to that question. To properly outline the improvements in clinical care that may be anticipated, a brief overview of key advances provides a useful perspective. It should also be noted that the pace of discovery can be expected to accelerate further because of more general advances in science that can be applied to unanswered questions relevant to inflammatory bowel disease. Some of these large-scale trends include completion of the human genome project, development of proteomics, improving bioinformatics and computational biology techniques as well as high throughput screening to rapidly identify therapeutic agents that can achieve a pharmacological role once a suitable target has been identified.

Given these trends, what have been the most important basic science advances relevant to prognostication for future improvements in clinical care? These include definition of the basic mechanisms underlying mucosal immune response and determinants that lead to either active immunity (both adaptive and innate) or tolerance. It is increasingly evident that mucosal homeostasis depends on exquisite balance determined by the interface between this mucosal immune system and luminal constituents. The central features of the mucosal immune system include distinct lymphocyte subsets as well as mucosal macrophages, the former comprising both Th-1 and Th-2 lymphocytes, which in general are counterbalanced by regulatory T-cells variably identified as Tr-1 or Th-3 lymphocytes. Each of these are now recognized to be distinguished by production of stereotypical combinations of cytokines and other mediators. Indeed, more complete definition of the complexity of the network of regulatory peptides coordinating interactions among the full variety of cell types present in the mucosa is another highly important achievement of basic research over the past several years.

Definition of the functional importance of these cell subsets and the various cytokines and other regulatory peptides has been enabled by the development of powerful approaches allowing either transgenic expression or targeted gene deletion to create robust murine models for characterization of relevant mechanisms. Indeed, general development of these mutant murine cell lines is another very important threshold accomplishment of the past several years and they have shed light on many observations made using reductionist models *in vitro* as well as direct study of patient populations. Insights made possible by these murine models include demonstration of the contributory roles that altered immune response or epithelial barrier function may play in rendering animals susceptible to chronic inflammation. In addition, these models have allowed direct proof of the concept of genetic susceptibility and of the ability of multiple genetic loci to interact and determine distinct phenotypes in the various mutant murine lines. Finally, these models have also provided opportunity for direct proof of the role of environmental factors and more specifically components of the 'normal' flora as essential co-factors for the actual development of the disease in the susceptible host. All of these findings in mice augment direct studies in man.

Studies of patients and murine models have also led to important advances in the characterization of the intermediate mechanisms involved in the recruitment of inflammatory cells and their activation at sites of inflammatory disease activities. These intermediate mechanisms include expression of adhesion molecules that mediate leukocyte recruitment, signalling pathways involved following recruitment of these leukocytes and the variety of 'non-specific' mediators of inflammation, ranging from arachidonic acid metabolites to neuropeptides.

An especially important very recent advance which sets the stage for evolution in diagnosis and management in the very near term has been the identification of the first gene with proven causal involvement in susceptibility to a major form of inflammatory bowel disease. Thus the IBD-1 locus on chromosome 16, encoding a protein designated nod-2, can confer susceptibility to Crohn's disease when mutated. Just as importantly, this gene product appears to serve as an intracellular receptor for the bacterial product lipopolysaccharide and promises to shed further light on the overall mechanisms that result in chronic intestinal inflammation, consistent with other lines of recent research and progress described below. Importantly, several other putative genetic loci have been implicated in initial microsatellite genomic screens and follow-up additional linkage studies suggest that, in the near future, a more complete definition of the range of genes which confer and define the overall risk of given individual to develop inflammatory bowel disease will be achieved. As noted above, the studies using mutant murine lines underscore the potential importance of interactions among loci to define the eventual clinical features of the resulting inflammatory bowel disease.

As these genetic loci are being defined, current progress in identifying environmental factors which seem to be necessary for the actual development of the disease are especially important. While undoubtedly a number of external factors (e.g. smoking behaviour, NSAID use) may have a significant impact on these processes, at least as implied by results of epidemiological studies, it is increasingly clear that microflora may be a central factor. Of interest, the role of the microbial population within the lumen as a disease cofactor is quite distinct from classical paradigms of transmissible disease, i.e. they appear to contribute to disease without actual invasion, tissue destruction or toxin formation. Definition of the molecular basis of the microbial–mucosal interaction is a very important area that is undergoing rapid progress; these seem to be mediated in substantial part by an evolutionarily ancient set of receptors that comprise a key part of the innate immune system. These receptors include members of at least two families, the Toll-like receptors and the Nod family (especially including the protein encoded by the IBD-1 gene) and collectively known as pathogen associated with molecular pattern (PAMP) receptors.

A final area of important recent progress which sets the stage for improvements in clinical care is an understanding of the molecular basis of tissue response to injury and repair, and the factors which may determine whether this can be accelerated or whether these will be a non-homeostatic end result, including fibrosis and stricture formation which serves as the key feature of Crohn's disease in many patients.

Given these recent advances, what are the improvements in clinical management that patients and clinicians can expect? What is the impact of the definition of IBD susceptibility genes? The impact will be quite profound and may indeed become practically available over the next few years. The potential improvements include the ability for more precise diagnosis in a way which will certainly supersede the current limitations of serologic markers as well as the more historically useful criteria of clinical history, physical examination, histology, radiology and endoscopy. With more objective and reproducible criteria for patient diagnosis, substratification should be possible with the ability to make a more accurate assessment of the prognosis and natural history itself. These capabilities will be of great benefit to patients and allow more rational thinking with respect to the use of prophylactic or maintenance therapies. Similarly, patient substratification may allow definition of response to specific therapeutic agents, which will also streamline the treatment of patients to more rapidly achieve the therapeutic endpoint that is currently possible only through empiric trials of a range of different medications. Certainly, identification of gene variants which confer susceptibility will be able to identify the risk for a patient prior to the development of the disease. As with the diagnosis of any other genetic disorder, this will involve complicated ethical issues, which will need to be carefully considered before they can be applied to general clinical practice. It is likely that this will have the most immediate impact on family members of patients identified with inflammatory bowel disease. What remains to be determined is whether the ability to identify risk will permit interventions that can actually prevent disease, the ultimate goal for understanding the underlying basis of any disorder.

How will definition of the mechanisms of mucosal immunity and tolerance affect clinical care? Regulation of the mucosal immune system to assure a normal response to the environment will be a focal point of future treatments. Empiric evidence suggests that immune regulation can be quite effective in achieving disease control. However, currently, this regulation is achieved only in a highly non-specific way through broadly active agents which have concurrent severe potential side effects, in part because of the breadth of their suppression. Targeted selective immune suppression, perhaps immune deletion of the relevant aberrant clonal cells, should permit the desired endpoint of effective therapy without concurrent side effects. Just as importantly, these interventions should provide the ability to maintain remission, another of the important unmet needs in patient care.

How will determination of the composition of the microflora and its role in driving mucosal inflammation impact on clinical care? The implications of the definition of the microflora that contribute to inflammation and the mechanisms through which these effects are achieved are quite immediate. Already empiric evidence suggests the promise for improved management as reflected in the benefit achieved by some patient subsets, e.g. patients with perineal disease or Crohn's colitis through the use of antibiotics (e.g. metronidazole) and through the recent provocative findings of the therapeutic benefit of administration of probiotics to provide a more compatible commensal flora to patient subsets. The promise that these approaches hold lies not only in their potential effectiveness, but also in their promise to be free of serious side effects. It is quite possible that therapeutic manipulation of the flora will turn out to be the most powerful tool available for the long-term treatment of patients with inflammatory bowel disease. Notwithstanding the importance of identifying the genetic basis that confers susceptibility for IBD, once identified, there will be few practical options to actually alter that genotypic profile. In contrast, environmental factors and, most particularly, the microflora will be directly accessible for therapeutic intervention and, insofar as the actions are discrete from the host and therefore are one step removed, may be especially free of side effects compared with manipulation of the underlying mucosal immune system or host mucosal integrity.

How will definition of the molecular basis of intestinal barrier and repair translate into improved patient care? As noted briefly above, it is possible that alterations in the integrity of the mucosal barrier *per se* are sufficient to confer susceptibility, even in the presence of normal immune responses as suggested by studies in mutant murine lines. Until there is full identification of IBD-associated genes, it remains to be seen whether there are parallels in man but indirect evidence supports this inference. Thus agents (e.g. NSAIDs) which alter the barrier function can lead to chronic intestinal inflammation. Definition of the molecular basis may therefore allow new strategies to enhance the integrity of the barrier function as an entirely novel therapeutic approach. Just as importantly, characterization of the repair mechanisms may not only allow new insights into approaches to accelerate repair, but may ensure that tissue recovery after the inflammatory process has been down-regulated is achieved in a way which restores normal structure and function, rather than lead to the complication which frequently dominates the clinical picture, i.e. fibrosis and stricture formation.

In addition to the ability to identify genetic loci conferring susceptibility to IBD, other genomic studies will have an impact on the clinical management in the future. Most promising is the possibility of pharmacogenomic profiling, i.e. defining the specific forms of genes relevant to absorption, mechanisms of action, metabolism and toxicity of given therapeutic agents. Already there is an obvious example of this potential in the relatively crude precedent of TPMT profiling to predict risk of toxicity to 6MP. The accelerating pace by which genotyping can be done (through broad advances in technology as mentioned above), in particular the ability to identify single nucleotide polymorphisms (SNPs) will soon make possible actual profiling of pharmacologically relevant genes, at least those responsible for metabolism and toxicity, for broad clinical usage in the near future.

In summary, what will basic science do for clinical practice? In most general terms it is reasonable to expect the possibility of more accurate diagnosis and more precise prognosis. In addition, these advances should facilitate the development of progressively more effective therapies with reduced toxicity. It remains unclear whether the ultimate definition of the mechanistic basis of disease will provide opportunities for actual disease prevention, though that should continue to serve as the ultimate goal of further research. The time frame in which these possibilities will be realized remains unclear, but it is worth noting that many are already on the horizon, at least with respect to more effective therapies based on more well-founded experimental rationales. Definition of the cytokine networks is a significant underpinning of the development of the recently available anti-TNF agents, as well as other cytokines moving through clinical developments of pathways as exemplified by interleukin-11 and others. Definition of the mechanism of leukocyte recruitment has also resulted in a number of agents that block key adhesion in molecules as exemplified by antibodies targeting the integrins α-4 or α-4 β7 that are under advanced clinical development at this time. The definition of signalling pathways, most notably the activation NF-κB, has also already served as the foundation of the development of agents which can modulate their activity. All these represent very specific examples of new therapeutic agents that have been specifically enabled by progress in basic laboratory research. Others have been developed in the context of this progress in general, as exemplified by the variety of immunomodulatory agents which have now been evaluated for potential use and, to a varying degree, are now integrated into therapeutic options as exemplified by methotrexate and thalidomide. The timeframe in which there will be general clinical availability of the promised advances for some of the other areas remains unclear, but it is likely that many of these too will materialize over the next three to five years, including a general introduction of the ability to use genetic markers for diagnosis and prognosis as well as pharmacogenomic profiling.

Four other factors will influence success in achieving the full potential suggested by recent basic promising research. Certainly, material resources, especially research funding, will be a key determinant. Equally important will be the ability to attract, train and engage an even larger number of both basic and clinical investigators necessary to pursue all the currently promising avenues for further basic investigation and application. All this, however, can only be realized by dynamic bidirectional interaction between basic research and clinical practice, which has, in many ways, served as the basis for much of the recent progress highlighted in this brief overview. Thus, clinical observation of epidemiology first pointed to the important role of genetic susceptibility in inflammatory bowel disease, and served as the springboard for the identification of IBD-susceptibility genes.

Similarly, epidemiological studies which have shown a direct or inverse relationship between environmental factors, such as smoking, early appendectomy or manipulation of the microflora, have served as the basis for the formulation of hypotheses that have framed studies in each of these important directions. Similarly, clinical characterization of response to empiric therapies in defining those which seem to be effective, as well as those that are ineffectual, helps to focus the research community on important areas for further study. Conversely, intense study on the basic level of mechanisms has already prompted the development of new emphasis on immunomodulatory and cytokine therapies as suggested above, and the still-incomplete understanding of the full role of luminal flora in driving chronic inflammation, as also already mentioned, has led to active application in the clinical arena through the study of probiotics and antibiotics. The bidirectional nature of progress through the interaction of basic research and clinical practice in communities is perhaps best highlighted by the development of anti-TNF as a therapeutic agent. Clinical development of anti-TNF agents was an outgrowth of more basic studies characterizing production of pro-inflammatory cytokines and associating them with inflammatory bowel disease. In turn, the demonstration of efficacy of anti-TNF has helped to focus further studies of the role of TNF as a mediator involved in mechanisms central to disease pathogenesis.

While progress in basic research holds great promise, it is certainly important to note the many unmet needs of IBD patients. Among these are the need for better approaches for predicting relapse and response to therapy. Especially pressing is the need for more-effective and less-toxic therapies as an alternative to corticosteroids, and well-tolerated agents which are effective in maintaining 'remission'. The latter includes, in specific instances, the ability to offer effective prophylaxis after remission in patients with Crohn's disease. Unfortunately, many patients with the most severe disease still need better forms of highly active primary therapy.

How will these unmet needs be addressed? Predicting relapse and response may be possible on the basis of characterization of markers of immune and inflammatory activation. Better understanding of immune response should allow more specific targeting of particular lymphocyte subsets that will offer a much more-effective and less-toxic alternative to steroids. Similarly, effective maintenance will be possible once we have a more complete understanding of the factors that sustain, in the normal individual, mucosal immune cell equilibrium and the integrity of the mucosa, while prophylaxis and maintenance in general should be enabled by understanding the mechanisms through which the luminal flora interacts with the mucosa. Understanding the basic mechanisms of the disease should offer more potent antagonism of non-specific mediators for patients with the most severe refractory disease a primary effective therapy.

All these opportunities, made possible through the evolution of large-scale technology and progress on many fronts, also present some ironic challenges for both basic and clinical research. Basic science has provided a rapidly expanding number of drug targets. The number of new investigational agents will challenge clinicians and clinical investigators to prioritize those for development. The need for prioritization will therefore place a premium on efficiency of their clinical evaluation, and thus conversely raises a challenge for basic science to provide intermediate markers for rapid determination of response and potentially more efficient allocation of study patients based on the better understanding of genotype and phenotype. Although there are many challenges, progress has already been made and that progress should lead to optimism for future advances that will indeed yield significant benefits to patients in the years ahead.

Acknowledgements

The perspective described in this chapter summarizes the work of a large number of committed investigators and clinicians who are actively endeavouring to understand IBD and improve care for patients with these disorders all over the world.

Index

99. Goebell H, Holtmann G, Talley NJ, eds. *Functional Dyspepsia and Irritable Bowel Syndrome: Concepts and Controversies.* Falk Symposium 99. 1998 ISBN 0-7923-8735-X

100. Blum HE, Bode Ch, Bode JCh, Sartor RB, eds. *Gut and the Liver.* Falk Symposium 100. 1998 ISBN 0-7923-8736-8

101. Rachmilewitz D, ed. *V International Symposium on Inflammatory Bowel Diseases.* Falk Symposium 101. 1998 ISBN 0-7923-8743-0

102. Manns MP, Boyer JL, Jansen PLM, Reichen J, eds. *Cholestatic Liver Diseases.* Falk Symposium 102. 1998 ISBN 0-7923-8746-5

102B. Manns MP, Chapman RW, Stiehl A, Wiesner R, eds. *Primary Sclerosing Cholangitis.* International Falk Workshop. 1998. ISBN 0-7923-8745-7

103. Häussinger D, Jungermann K, eds. *Liver and Nervous System.* Falk Symposium 102. 1998 ISBN 0-7924-8742-2

103B. Häussinger D, Heinrich PC, eds. *Signalling in the Liver.* International Falk Workshop. 1998 ISBN 0-7923-8744-9

103C. Fleig W, ed. *Normal and Malignant Liver Cell Growth.* International Falk Workshop. 1998 ISBN 0-7923-8748-1

104. Stallmach A, Zeitz M, Strober W, MacDonald TT, Lochs H, eds. *Induction and Modulation of Gastrointestinal Inflammation.* Falk Symposium 104. 1998 ISBN 0-7923-8747-3

105. Emmrich J, Liebe S, Stange EF, eds. *Innovative Concepts in Inflammatory Bowel Diseases.* Falk Symposium 105. 1999 ISBN 0-7923-8749-X

106. Rutgeerts P, Colombel J-F, Hanauer SB, Schölmerich J, Tytgat GNJ, van Gossum A, eds. *Advances in Inflammatory Bowel Diseases.* Falk Symposium 106. 1999 ISBN 0-7923-8750-3

107. Špičák J, Boyer J, Gilat T, Kotrlik K, Mareček Z, Paumgartner G, eds. *Diseases of the Liver and the Bile Ducts – New Aspects and Clinical Implications.* Falk Symposium 107. 1999 ISBN 0-7923-8751-1

108. Paumgartner G, Stiehl A, Gerok W, Keppler D, Leuschner U, eds. *Bile Acids and Cholestasis.* Falk Symposium 108. 1999 ISBN 0-7923-8752-X

109. Schmiegel W, Schölmerich J, eds. *Colorectal Cancer – Molecular Mechanisms, Premalignant State and its Prevention.* Falk Symposium 109. 1999 ISBN 0-7923-8753-8

110. Domschke W, Stoll R, Brasitus TA, Kagnoff MF, eds. *Intestinal Mucosa and its Diseases – Pathophysiology and Clinics.* Falk Symposium 110. 1999 ISBN 0-7923-8754-6

110B. Northfield TC, Ahmed HA, Jazwari RP, Zentler-Munro PL, eds. *Bile Acids in Hepatobiliary Disease.* Falk Workshop. 2000 ISBN 0-7923-8755-4

111. Rogler G, Kullmann F, Rutgeerts P, Sartor RB, Schölmerich J, eds. *IBD at the End of its First Century.* Falk Symposium 111. 2000 ISBN 0-7923-8756-2

112. Krammer HJ, Singer MV, eds. *Neurogastroenterology: From the Basics to the Clinics.* Falk Symposium 112. 2000 ISBN 0-7923-8757-0

113. Andus T, Rogler G, Schlottmann K, Frick E, Adler G, Schmiegel W, Zeitz M, Schölmerich J, eds. *Cytokines and Cell Homeostasis in the Gastrointestinal Tract.* Falk Symposium 113. 2000 ISBN 0-7923-8758-9

114. Manns MP, Paumgartner G, Leuschner U, eds. *Immunology and Liver.* Falk Symposium 114. 2000 ISBN 0-7923-8759-7

Falk Symposium Series

115. Boyer JL, Blum HE, Maier K-P, Sauerbruch T, Stalder GA, eds. *Liver Cirrhosis and its Development.* Falk Symposium 115. 2000 ISBN 0-7923-8760-0
116. Riemann JF, Neuhaus H, eds. *Interventional Endoscopy in Hepatology.* Falk Symposium 116. 2000 ISBN 0-7923-8761-9

116A. Dienes HP, Schirmacher P, Brechot C, Okuda K, eds. *Chronic Hepatitis: New Concepts of Pathogenesis, Diagnosis and Treatment.* Falk Workshop. 2000 ISBN 0-7923-8763-5

117. Gerbes AL, Beuers U, Jüngst D, Pape GR, Sackmann M, Sauerbruch T, eds. *Hepatology 2000 – Symposium in Honour of Gustav Paumgartner.* Falk Symposium 117. 2000 ISBN 0-7923-8765-1

117A. Acalovschi M, Paumgartner G, eds. *Hepatobiliary Diseases: Cholestasis and Gallstones.* Falk Workshop. 2000 ISBN 0-7923-8770-8

118. Frühmorgen P, Bruch H-P, eds. *Non-Neoplastic Diseases of the Anorectum.* Falk Symposium 118. 2001 ISBN 0-7923-8766-X
119. Fellermann K, Jewell DP, Sandborn WJ, Schölmerich J, Stange EF, eds. *Immunosuppression in Inflammatory Bowel Diseases – Standards, New Developments, Future Trends.* Falk Symposium 119. 2001 ISBN 0-7923-8767-8
120. van Berge Henegouwen GP, Keppler D, Leuschner U, Paumgartner G, Stiehl A, eds. *Biology of Bile Acids in Health and Disease.* Falk Symposium 120. 2001 ISBN 0-7923-8768-6
121. Leuschner U, James OFW, Dancygier H, eds. *Steatohepatitis (NASH and ASH).* Falk Symposium 121. 2001 ISBN 0-7923-8769-4

121A. Matern S, Boyer JL, Keppler D, Meier-Abt PJ, eds. *Hepatobiliary Transport: From Bench to Bedside.* Falk Workshop. 2001 ISBN 0-7923-8771-6

122. Campieri M, Fiocchi C, Hanauer SB, Jewell DP, Rachmilewitz R, Schölmerich J, eds. *Inflammatory Bowel Disease – A Clinical Case Approach to Pathophysiology, Diagnosis, and Treatment.* Falk Symposium 122. 2002 ISBN 0-7923-8772-4

www.ingramcontent.com/pod-product-compliance
Ingram Content Group UK Ltd.
Pitfield, Milton Keynes, MK11 3LW, UK
UKHW021828170926
475607UK00007B/42

9780792387725